Melasma and Vitiligo in Brown Skin

$119.20

Evangeline B. Handog
Maria Juliet Enriquez-Macarayo
Editors

Melasma and Vitiligo in Brown Skin

Springer

Editors
Evangeline B. Handog
Asian Hospital and Medical Center
Muntinlupa
Philippines

Maria Juliet Enriquez-Macarayo
Angeles University Foundation
Medical Center
Pampanga
Philippines

ISBN 978-81-322-3662-7 ISBN 978-81-322-3664-1 (eBook)
DOI 10.1007/978-81-322-3664-1

Library of Congress Control Number: 2017930224

Printed on acid-free paper

This Springer imprint is published by Springer Nature
The registered company is Springer (India) Pvt. Ltd.
The registered company address is: 7th Floor, Vijaya Building, 17 Barakhamba Road, New Delhi 110 001, India

Foreword

It is indeed my pleasure to welcome the reader to *Melasma and Vitiligo in Brown Skin*. The editors, Evangeline B. Handog and Maria Juliet Enriquez-Macarayo, have gathered an impressive group of experts to share their knowledge and experience gained from caring for thousands of patients with these two common disorders. Improving the lives of all individuals with vitiligo and melasma is essential, but especially so for those with brown skin in whom the diseases are either more obvious or more persistent. This book's global perspective for a global audience is noteworthy and unique. Its contents will certainly have an enormous impact on the quality of life of patients from around the world with these two disorders of pigmentation.

New Haven, CT, USA　　Jean Bolognia

Preface

Melasma and vitiligo are disfiguring dermatological concerns, from its discovery many centuries ago up to present time. Both entities remain to be a challenge for the skin expert and the patient. The qualities of life of these individuals are affected invariably. Because of a wide range of therapeutic options, expectations of resolution are high. However, there is no simple regimen to claim success in handling both skin disorders.

In this book, we have opted to focus on melasma and vitiligo, particularly in the brown skin. There is much discussion among the white and black skin, but we discovered a paucity among people of brown race. We are fortunate to have gathered a great selection of contributors whose involvement in treating people of brown skin has become a passion. To our knowledge, this is the first book to devote a comprehensive dissertation of melasma and vitiligo in brown skin, from how it came about to how it can be assessed, diagnosed, and treated.

The management of melasma and vitiligo is difficult, sometimes even frustrating. Many articles, reviews, lectures, and clinical trials have been done and are being carried out, as this book is published. With the clarity being shed as to their pathogenesis, there is now a trend of evidence-based management from topical and oral preparations, procedural techniques, and even laser therapy. Clinicians are aided in utilizing these knowledge and skills to give hope to patients suffering from these disorders. More so, armed with cosmeceuticals, cosmetics, and camouflage, the quality of life of our patients may well be further alleviated.

This initial undertaking, gathering experiences of the skin experts dealing with melasma and vitiligo in brown-skinned people, hopes to provide a plethora of information and measures to help our patients. To the patients suffering from melasma and vitiligo, we dedicate this endeavor.

Muntinlupa, Philippines — Evangeline B. Handog
Pampanga, Philippines — Maria Juliet Enriquez-Macarayo

About the Editors

Dr. Evangeline B. Handog, the first woman president of the International Society of Dermatology, is currently the chair of the Department of Dermatology, Asian Hospital and Medical Center, Philippines, and head of the Cosmetic Unit of the Department of Dermatology, Research Institution for Tropical Medicine, Philippines.

As chair of the Pigmentary Disorders Advisory Board of the Philippines, her research interest is primarily on melasma and other pigmentary disorders. She has published more than 30 papers and written 14 chapters for international books, mostly on lightening agents.

She is a member of the editorial board of the *International Journal of Dermatology*, faculty of F1000 and contributor to UpToDate.

Maria Juliet Enriquez-Macarayo, an active dermatologist consultant at Angeles University Foundation Medical Center, Pampanga, Philippines, is currently the editor in chief of the *International Society of Dermatology's Connection Newsletter*, an associate faculty of F1000, and a contributor to UpToDate.

She has coauthored local and international book chapters on pigmentary disorders, acne, and diseases in Asian skin. With her valuable insights, she is a well-appreciated lecturer and a key opinion leader.

Contents

Part I
The Brown Skin

Chapter 1
The Concept of Brown Skin

Maria Juliet Enriquez-Macarayo and Evangeline B. Handog

The Color of One's Skin Speaks of So Many Facets in One's Life

It reflects one's physical traits, genetic components, history, nationality, and geographic roots. And by these, we mean one's race. Scientifically, skin color depends on many factors, genetics aside: inflammation, blood hemoglobin level, carotenoids in the dermis and increased melanin deposition. Melanin in itself is a polymer that comes as pheomelanin (red-yellow) and eumelanin (black-brown).

Brown, as a color, is a hue that runs between a mileage of the colors red and yellow, wooden, earthen or orange. Lightness is from medium to low, and saturation is from low to moderate [1, 2]. Figure 1.1 shows the different shades of brown among the Filipinos.

Brown skin people, as a category, may be considered a racial or ethnic classification, based on human skin color. As discussed by many learned authors as early as the eighteenth century, included in this category are populations from Africa (North), America (Latin and South) and Asia (Western, South, and Southeast).

Several classification schemes exist designating how a particular skin color reacts to several stimuli. For long, researches have followed the Fitzpatrick Phototyping Scale developed in 1975 by Dr. Thomas B. Fitzpatrick, based on the typical response of the different skin types to ultraviolet light. The majority of

M.J. Enriquez-Macarayo, MD (✉)
Dermatology Department, Angeles University Foundation Medical Center, Angeles City, Pampanga, Philippines
e-mail: majulietmacarayomd@gmail.com

E.B. Handog
Department of Dermatology, Asian Hospital and Medical Center, 2205 Civic Drive, Muntinlupa, Philippines, 1780
e-mail: vangee@handog.net

E.B. Handog, M.J. Enriquez-Macarayo (eds.), *Melasma and Vitiligo in Brown Skin*, DOI 10.1007/978-81-322-3664-1_1

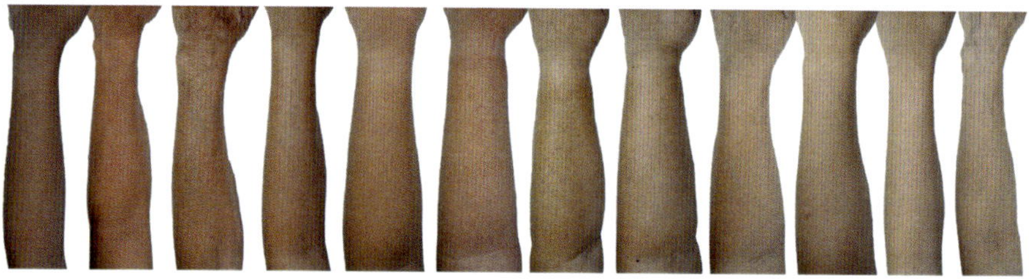

Fig. 1.1 Different shades of brown among Filipinos

brown skin people are categorically placed in the skin phototypes IV–V. The skin burns minimally to rarely but tans uniformly or more easily [3–5].

The Lancer Ethnicity Scale (LES), introduced in 1998 by Dr. Harold A. Lancer, added ancestry to the existing Fitzpatrick skin type. With ethnicity background included, it aids in defining potential risks for patients undergoing cosmetic procedures. Higher risks abound a higher rate/score on this ethnicity scale. Moderate, significant, and considerable risks are seen in the LES types 3, 4, and 5, respectively. Asians (Chinese, Koreans, Japanese, Thai, Vietnamese, Filipinos), Polynesians, Americans (Latin, Central, South) and American Indians (Central and South) have skin type IV and LES type 4. Africans (Central, North, East, and West), Eritreans and Ethiopians, Middle East Arabic and Indians have skin type V and LES type 4 [6].

The Roberts Skin Type Classification System, proposed by Dr. Wendy Roberts in 2006, deals with identifying a patient's skin type characteristics. It further went on to predict the response of the skin to insult, injury and inflammation, detecting the susceptibility of sequelae for individuals of global skin types. Using four indices (phototype, hyperpigmentation, photoaging and scarring), optimal outcomes may then be identified for each patient [5, 7].

In today's society, differences in skin color have evolved due to environmental, dietary, and adaptive factors. Migration patterns and intermarriage practices have contributed to a montage in the races and ethnicities we were all familiar with. Geneticists have reported a very high percentage of variations within races rather than between races [8].

An individual's skin color still speaks of one's race or ethnic roots. But in a world of skin afflictions, one's color speaks strongly of the ability of that individual to respond to specific treatments and procedures.

We took the courage to embark on this book, particularly giving opportune time to specifically deal with melasma and vitiligo in brown skin, believing there is a special need for this category of human skin.

References

1. American Heritage® Dictionary of the English Language, 5th ed. Boston: Houghton Mifflin Harcourt Publishing Co; 2011.
2. Butterfield J. Collins English dictionary: complete and unabridged. Glasgow: Harper Collins Publishers; 2003.

3. Fitzpatrick TB. Soleil et peau [Sun and skin]. Journal de Médecine Esthétique. 1975;2:33–4.
4. Fitzpatrick TB. Ultraviolet-induced pigmentary changes: benefits and hazards. Curr Probl Dermatol. 1986;15:25–38.
5. Roberts WE. Skin types classification old and new. Dermatol Clin. 2009;27(4):529–33.
6. Lancer HA. Lancer ethnicity scale (LES). Lasers Surg Med. 1998;22:9.
7. Roberts WE. The Roberts skin type classification system. J Drugs Dermatol. 2008;7(5):452–6.
8. Taylor SC, Cook-Bolden F. Defining skin of color. Cutis. 2002;69:435–7.

Chapter 2
Prevalent Skin Disorders in Brown Skin

Maria Juliet Enriquez-Macarayo and Evangeline B. Handog

2.1 Introduction

How does one compare white, black, brown, and all the colors in between? The differences in color hue may be easily identifiable. But what constitutes the individuals bearing the different skin colors may be not that easy to fathom. Though we are all unique, grouping the colors in a cluster helps in understanding how one's skin may react to the different cutaneous diseases. Continents around the world are beset with people of different colors. Intermarriages and travel have been a major factor in the distribution of races and ethnic groupings around the globe.

There is much data abounding white skin and this is on a continuum. Lately, there is an accumulation of data for black skin with the interest in the skin of color. But for brown skin, as a group, there is paucity of data. For us to come up with correct database, we have to correlate data from different countries.

M.J. Enriquez-Macarayo (✉)
Dermatology Department, Angeles University Foundation Medical Center, Angeles City, Pampanga, Philippines
e-mail: majulietmacarayomd@gmail.com

E.B. Handog
Department of Dermatology, Asian Hospital and Medical Center, 2205 Civic Drive, Muntinlupa, Philippines, 1780
e-mail: vangee@handog.net

E.B. Handog, M.J. Enriquez-Macarayo (eds.), *Melasma and Vitiligo in Brown Skin*,
DOI 10.1007/978-81-322-3664-1_2

2.2 Factors to Consider

Variations in the enlisted prevalent skin disorders are dependent on multiple factors, which we have to keep in mind when dissecting data in different sources:

- Environmental condition – humidity and seasonal variation [1, 2]
- Lifestyle – overcrowding, water availability, occupation, customs, religion and beliefs, and hygiene [2–6]
- Socioeconomic status and education [3, 4]
- Different methodologies for studies carried out; no definite uniform method

2.3 Prevalent Skin Disorders Among Brown Skin

India is a vast country comprised mostly of brown skin people. Patterns of skin diseases, influenced by various factors, differ from region to region. The consequent morbidities have a profound effect on the individual and the community [3]. The most prevalent cutaneous conditions noted in the past years were eczema and dermatitis, urticaria, fungal skin infections, acne, and alopecia [4, 7, 8]. In the past decade, eczemas, fungal infections, pyodermas, and scabies were the major patterns of skin morbidities [9, 10]. Infectious dermatoses were led by scabies followed by tinea infections; acne, eczema, and dermatitis were the most common noninfectious dermatoses [3]. A more recent prospective study revealed similar common skin conditions, but acne with or without post-inflammatory hyperpigmentation (PIH) topped the list [2].

In an early study conducted in Nepal, a Himalayan country in the Indian subcontinent, cutaneous infections were the most common dermatologic condition followed by eczemas [11]. Fungal infections, acne, and melasma were recorded topping the list in another study done much later [1]. More recently, Shrestha et al. documented the topmost common diseases as eczemas, pigment disorders (melasma, PIH, ephelides, and vitiligo), infections, acne, and urticaria [5].

The Nepalese, with skin type falling mostly into Fitzpatrick type III and IV, tan more easily with resultant pigmentary disorders induced or aggravated by ultraviolet radiation (UVR) exposure. Melasma was the most common pigment disorder, attributed to repeated exposure to UVR in addition to racial factors and genetic predisposition [5].

Asia is a diverse continent with its multiracial population bearing mostly Fitzpatrick skin type III–V. A study conducted in Singapore, where patients were mostly Chinese, listed atopic dermatitis, acne vulgaris, and viral infections as the most common diagnoses among its populace. Urticaria predominated among the Chinese, psoriasis and alopecia in Indians, and PIH in Malays and Indians who tend to have darker skin compared with the Chinese [12]. Asian pediatric population in Singapore presenting with skin diseases showed a prevalence of eczemas, infections (viral, bacterial, fungal, parasitic), and pigmentation disorders [13].

In a population-based survey in Indonesia, the prevalence of fungal infections was twice as high as dermatitis [14].

In the Philippines, the most common skin disorders recorded from 2011 to 2015 were acne vulgaris, contact dermatitis (allergic and irritant), scabies, seborrheic dermatitis, atopic dermatitis, lichen simplex chronicus, verruca (vulgaris and plana), tinea corporis, and psoriasis. PIH and melasma were the most frequently encountered pigmentary disorders [15].

High melanin content may confer better photoprotection against UVR damage, but it is also a reason for several pigmentary disorders among darker skin-colored people, including Asians [16, 17]. Epidermal disorders commonly encountered by physicians are melasma, freckles, lentigines, and PIH. Nevus of Ota and acquired bilateral nevus of Ota-like macules are common dermal pigmentary disorders [16].

Less common skin conditions that may be seen among Asians include Mongolian spot, nevus of Ota, nevus of Ito, Kawasaki disease, primary cutaneous amyloidosis (lichen or macular), Kikuchi-Fujimoto disease, and lipodystrophia centrifugalis abdominalis infantilis (LCAI) [18–22].

Cutaneous diseases commonly affecting Hispanics/Latinos are acne vulgaris, eczema, verruca vulgaris, and pigmentary disorders (PIH, melasma). The incidence of melasma in this group is as high as 80%, especially in pregnant Mexican women [23, 24]. Uncommon in the general population but with a predilection for Hispanics/Latinos are Hermansky-Pudlak syndrome and erythema dyschromicum perstans [24].

References

1. Jha AK, Gurung D. Seasonal variation of skin diseases in Nepal: a hospital based annual study of out-patient visits. Nepal Med Coll J. 2006;8(4):266–8.
2. Sajith M, Lokhande KD, Padma S, Pawar AP. Prevalence of various skin disorders and prescribing pattern of antihistamines in tertiary care hospital, Pune. Int J Pharma Sci Res (IJPSR). 2014;5(3):73–7.
3. Baur B, Sarkar J, Manna N, Bandyopadhyay L. The pattern of dermatological disorders among patients attending the skin O.P.D of a tertiary care hospital in Kolkata, India. IOSR J Dent Med Sci (JDMS). 2013;3(4):4–9.
4. Joel JJ, Jose N, Shastry CS. Patterns of skin disease and prescribing trends in rural India. Sch Acad J Pharm. 2013;2(4):304–9.
5. Shrestha R, Lama L, Gurung D, Shresta DP, Rosdahl I. Pattern of skin diseases in a rural village development community of Nepal. Nepal J Dermatol Venereol Leprol (NJDVL). 2014; 12(1):41–4.
6. Lilly E, Kundu RV. Dermatoses secondary to Asian cultural practices. Int J Dermatol. 2012;51: 372–82.
7. Patel NG, Patel NJ. Epidemiological study of skin (dermatological) diseases and its treatment in North Gujarat. Asian J Pharma Clin Res. 2010;3(4):40–2.
8. Saravanakumar RT, Prasad GS, Ragul G, Mohanta GP, Manna PK, Moorthi C. Study of prescribing pattern of topical corticosteroids in the department of dermatology in a multispecialty tertiary care teaching hospital in South India. Int J Res Pharm Sci. 2012;3(4):685–7.
9. Devi TB, Zamzachin G. Pattern of skin diseases in Imphal. Ind J Dermatol. 2006;51(2): 149–50.

10. Asokan N, Prathap P, Ajithkumar K, Ambooken B, Binesh VG, George S. Pattern of skin diseases among patients attending a tertiary care teaching hospital in Kerala. Ind J Dermatol Venereol Leprol. 2009;75(5):517–8.
11. Sarkar C, Das B, Sripathi H. Drug prescribing pattern in dermatology in a teaching hospital in Western Nepal. J Nepal Med Assoc (JNMA). 2001;41:241–6.
12. Chua-Ty G, Goh CL, Koh SL. Pattern of skin diseases at the National Skin Centre (Singapore) from 1989–1990. Int J Dermatol. 1992;31:555–9.
13. Goh CL, Akarapanth R. Epidemiology of skin disease among children in a referral skin clinic in Singapore. Pediatr Dermatol. 1994;11:125–8.
14. Saw SM, Koh D, Adjani MR, Wong ML, Hong CY, Lee J, et al. A population-based prevalence survey of skin diseases in adolescents and adults in rural Sumatra, Indonesia, 1999. Trans R Soc Trop Med Hyg. 2001;95:344–8.
15. Philippine Dermatological Society Health Information Systems. Philippine Dermatological Society. c2011 [updated (2016 Feb); cited (26 Mar 2016)]. Available by request from: pdshis@outlook.com.
16. Ho SGY, Chan HHL. The Asian dermatologic patient: review of common pigmentary disorders and cutaneous diseases. Am J Clin Dermatol. 2009;10(3):153–68.
17. Talakoub L, Wesley NO. Differences in perceptions of beauty and cosmetic procedures performed in ethnic patients. Semin Cutan Med Surg. 2009;28:115–29.
18. Lee CS, Lim HW. Cutaneous diseases in Asians. Dermatol Clin. 2003;21(4):669–77.
19. Wong C. Cutaneous amyloidosis. Int J Dermatol. 1987;26:273–7.
20. Wang WJ, Chang YT, Huang CY, Lee DD. Clinical and histopathological characteristics of primary cutaneous amyloidosis in 794 Chinese patients. Zhonghua Yi Xue Za Zhi (Taipei). 2001;64(2):101–7.
21. Rasi A, Khatami A, Javaheri SM. Macular amyloidosis: an assessment of prevalence, sex, and age. Int J Dermatol. 2004;43:898–9.
22. Juan CC, Hwang B, Lee PC, Lin YJ, Chien JC, Lee HY, Meng CCL. The clinical manifestations and risk factors of a delayed diagnosis of Kawasaki disease. J Chin Med Assoc. 2007;70(9):374–9.
23. Taylor SC. Epidemiology of skin diseases in people of color. Highlight Skin Color. 2003;71:271–5.
24. Sanchez MR. Cutaneous diseases in Latinos. Dermatol Clin. 2003;21(4):689–97.

Part II
Melasma in Brown Skin

Chapter 3
Definition, Incidence, and Etiology of Melasma in Brown Skin

Tania Cestari, Juliano Peruzzo, and Natalia Giongo

3.1 Definition

Melasma is an acquired disorder of melanogenesis leading to hyperpigmentation and manifested by almost always symmetrical brown to gray-black macules and patches with serrated irregular edges. It occurs especially in sun-exposed areas and typically affects young to middle-aged women [1]. It is most commonly seen on the face and, less commonly, on extrafacial locations such as the neck, arms, and chest [2]. In spite of being asymptomatic, melasma lesions cause aesthetic impairment and significantly affect the quality of life.

The word melasma comes from the Greek "melas" which means black and refers to its brownish clinical presentation [3]. Disease descriptions are recognized since the reports of Hippocrates (470–360 BC), when its worsening was referred to occur after sun exposure, fire heat, cold, and skin inflammations [3].

Three clinical patterns are usually described: *centrofacial,* with patches on the frontal region, nasal dorsum, cheekbones, and chin areas (65 % of the cases); *malar*, which occurs in 20 % of the cases; and *mandibular*, seen in about 15 % of the patients [4, 5].

T. Cestari (✉) • J. Peruzzo • N. Giongo
University of Rio Grande do Sul, Hospital de Clínicas de Porto,
Santo Inacio 500 ap 1002, RS 90570-150 Porto Alegre, Brazil
e-mail: tcestari@terra.com.br

E.B. Handog, M.J. Enriquez-Macarayo (eds.), *Melasma and Vitiligo in Brown Skin*,
DOI 10.1007/978-81-322-3664-1_3

3.2 Incidence

Pigmentation disorders, including melasma, are the third most frequent complaint in dermatological appointments and predominate in the age between 30 and 40 years [5].

Although occurring in all ethnic groups, the incidence of melasma varies according to the studied population. It is known that there is a predominance among Asian, Hispanic, and African descendants [2, 6], as well as among those who live in intertropical areas where the exposure to ultraviolet radiation (UVR) is inevitable [2, 7]. Its prevalence is also higher in intermediate phototypes (III, IV, V) [3, 6]. In lighter skin phototypes (Fitzpatrick skin type II and III), it is usually influenced by the presence of family history, in contrast to a negative family history in Fitzpatrick's phototypes IV and V [8, 9].

In India, the demographic and clinical findings show regional variability, ranging from 4 to 10 % in urban areas and up to 41 % in rural settings. Taking into consideration the different regions and their ethnic compositions, the incidence of melasma is estimated to occur in 15–35 % of adult Brazilian women [10]. In Iran, melasma was identified in 39.5 % of women, 9.5 % of which were pregnant women [3]. In the United States, melasma affects five to six million people [6, 11].

Melasma is more prevalent in women, in an estimated 9:1 ratio compared to men [3, 7], although this ratio can vary depending on the populations. In Southeast Asia, for example, the prevalence reaches 40 % in adult women and 20 % in adult men [12]. In Puerto Rico, on the other hand, men formed only 10 % of the total melasma patients [13]. In India, 20–25 % of patients with melasma are men. This difference is probably related to the country's climate, a large number of outdoor workers, and a greater cosmetic awareness among male patients [14].

Most cases develop between 20 and 40 years of age [3], with a decreasing prevalence after menopause [8] suggesting a hormonal relationship in its pathogenesis. The extrafacial forms of melasma, on the other hand, are most common in postmenopausal women.

3.3 Etiology

Although the exact cause of melasma is unknown, several factors are associated with its development and worsening. The most commonly reported precipitating factors are pregnancy, oral contraceptives, and sun exposure [7].

The family history of melasma occurs in about 50 % of patients, particularly in those with darker skin types [15]. These rates suggest a hereditary etiological component which is being considered the most important risk factor for melasma development [4]. With a family history of melasma, patients tend to have the disorder earlier [16] and to present longer duration of symptoms [8]. A recent discovery found the role of the H19 gene in melasma. This gene transcribes a noncoding ribonucleic acid and is downregulated in melasma lesions, inducing melanogenesis and the transference of melanin from melanocytes to keratinocytes [1, 17]. In addition, several other genes associated with melanogenesis were analyzed, and studies showed that they are upregulated in melasma skin, when compared to unaffected areas [18].

The association between ultraviolet radiation (UVR) and melasma is well established, and it is seen as the main triggering factor for the disorder [3, 7, 19]. The UVR increases melanogenic activity, causing darker epidermal pigmentation in regions with melasma than in the adjacent skin [3]. Intense and long-term exposure to UVR activates an inflammatory cascade mainly through oxidative stress and the formation of reactive oxygen species. Inflammatory signals stimulated by UVR, which include cytokines and alpha-melanocyte-stimulating hormone, can also cause melanogenesis [16]. In most patients melasma onset happens predominantly in the summer [4], and reports of worsening and higher recurrence rates with sun exposure are common. There is also a high prevalence of the disease in places of greater solar irradiation. Moreover, centrofacial melasma is more prevalent in the regions corresponding to the areas where the UVR focuses more directly. Other radiation wavelengths such as visible light and infrared also have a melanogenic potential, although to a lesser degree [3].

Melasma is also sensitive to hormonal influence. The use of oral contraceptives (OCP), hormone replacement therapy (HRT), ovarian tumors, and endocrine disorders have been linked to the pigmentation onset or worsening [19, 20]. The relationship with hormonal activity is supported by the fact that women are more frequently affected, and the beginning of melasma usually occurs after adolescence, during pregnancy, or while using OCP. Moreover, its prevalence decreases after menopause and rarely manifests before puberty [20]. Estrogen and progesterone increase the activity of tyrosinase. It has been demonstrated by immunohistochemical analysis that the skin affected by melasma has increased expression of estrogen receptor beta as well as progesterone receptors around small vessels when compared to the adjacent normal skin [16, 21]. Thus, it is believed that the pigmentation is related to the effects of estrogen and progesterone in melanocytes.

In male patients, luteinizing hormone (LH) circulating levels are higher, while testosterone concentration is lower in melasmic men when compared to controls, suggesting a role of subtle testicular resistance in the pathogenesis of melasma [1, 14, 22].

The association of melasma occurrence and the use of OCP are well known and reported by around 25 % of patients [15]. This is seen especially in cases with a positive family history for the disorder. Its discontinuation or change for a lower estrogenic dose, however, did not seem to improve the pigmentation [7]. Thus, a systematic change in hormonal contraception in melasma patients seems unwarranted. Melasma occurs in up to 75 % of pregnancies [23], and 26–29 % of women have reported to have their onset during pregnancy [8, 15]. The stimulus for melanogenesis occurs especially in the third trimester and can be explained by the increase of placental, ovarian, and pituitary hormones [3].

There are some studies correlating the appearance of melasma to endocrine diseases, especially thyroid abnormalities. In a recent study, the frequency of thyroid disorders in patients with melasma was around 20 %, almost five times greater than in control subjects [24]. It was also observed that the association between thyroid autoimmunity and melasma was mainly seen in women whose melasma developed during pregnancy or after the ingestion of OCP [25].

The use of light and laser technologies may trigger or exacerbate preexisting clinical or subclinical melasma. In addition, they may predispose to a rebound effect after using intense pulsed light by the association to post-inflammatory hyperpigmentation [26]. Other cosmetic procedures, such as chemical peelings, which may cause skin inflammation, can also lead to exacerbation of melasma. These changes are seen most frequently in people of higher phototypes [27].

In addition to OCPs, other drugs also can cause melasma. Photosensitizing drugs may activate melasma or dark preexisting lesions, and the mechanism is probably similar to that of exacerbation after cosmetic procedures. Pigmentation resembling melasma develops in 10 % of patients receiving phenytoin. The drug exerts direct action on melanocytes causing dispersion of melanin granules and also induces increased pigmentation in the basal epidermis [1]. Finasteride's inhibition of 5α-reductase may lead to increased levels of progesterone in the skin, inducing hyperpigmentation, relating to the appearance of melasma [28]. Diethylstilbestrol for treatment of prostate cancer was also related to melasma onset [1].

The psychosocial stress and impairment in the quality of life caused by melasma cannot be overemphasized. Stressful events had already been reported as a disease trigger. One study showed that patients with melasma presented a higher level of anxiety as well as an increased use of antidepressants and anxiolytics compared with control. Stress and depression are associated with higher cortisol levels and melanocortin production, which exert melanogenic activity [7, 29, 30].

Cosmetics have been rarely implicated to cause melasma [31]. However, patients with melasma have demonstrated a high prevalence of contact sensitivity to cosmetics. Pigmented cosmetic dermatitis and cosmetic contact sensitivity should be considered in the etiologic factors when melasma is not associated with pregnancy, lactation, or hormone therapy [27]. In India, the common practice of using vegetable oils (mustard oil) on the face after bath may predispose to the appearance of pigmentation secondary to sun exposure [32], since it is a common photosensitizer [14].

3.4 New Concepts

A major angiogenic factor is suggested in the pathogenesis of melasma. There is an increased expression of vascular endothelial growth factor (VEGF) in keratinocytes and blood vessels of greater diameter and number in the affected skin when compared to the adjacent healthy skin [33]. Though it is unclear whether the increased vasculature is specific or just the result of chronic UV accumulation accompanying epidermal hyperpigmentation, there is a clear relationship between the number of blood vessels and the intensity of pigmentation in melasma [33].

Exposure to different light wavelengths seems to be related to the appearance of hyperchromic lesions on the face. There is no consensus for this role, but there is evidence showing that in addition to the wavelength in the UV range, visible light (VL) is also able to induce increased pigmentation of the skin, especially in patients with higher phototype [2, 19]. Visible light, as well as UVR exposure, appears to cause direct damage to melanocytes' DNA and to promote the synthesis, release, and activation of epidermal factor through cytokines aimed to control the proliferation and survival of melanocytes [34, 35]. VL-induced pigmentation is more intense and stable in these patients, when compared to the pigmentation induced by UVA exclusively. This would explain the partial protection of most sunscreens [19].

Pollution can be considered a possible synergistic factor to already established melasma and other facial pigmentary dyschromias [36]. Correlation between the exposure to air pollution and signs of aging, more specifically pigmentary spots, has been described. The suggested mechanism for that association is the triggering of oxidative stress [37].

Melasma is a very prevalent disease that causes great aesthetic and psychological damage, especially in people of higher phototype. Although several triggering factors are already known, new discoveries are emerging and may represent a breakthrough in the pigmentation's therapeutic management and prevention, especially in the toughest cases.

References

1. Sarkar R, Arora P, Garg VK, Sonthalia S, Gokhale N. Melasma update. Indian Dermatol Online J. 2014;5:426–35.
2. Cestari TF, Dantas LP, Boza JC. Acquired hyperpigmentations. An Bras Dermatol. 2014;89:11–25.
3. Handel AC, Miot LDB, Miot HA. Melasma: a clinical and epidemiological review. An Bras Dermatol. 2014;89:771–82.
4. Sanchez NP, Pathak MA, Sato S, Fitzpatrick TB, Sanchez JL, Mihm MC. Melasma: a clinical, light microscopic, ultrastructural, and immuno-fluorescence study. J Am Acad Dermatol. 1981;4:698–710.
5. Pandya AG, Guevara IL. Disorders of hyperpigmentation. Dermatol Clin. 2000;18:91–8.
6. Sheth VM, Pandya AG. Melasma: a comprehensive update: part I. J Am Acad Dermatol. 2011;65:689–97.
7. Tamegade A, Miot LDB, Bonfietti C, Gige TC, Marques MEA, Miot HA. Clinical patterns and epidemiological characteristics of facial melasma in Brazilian women. J Eur Acad Dermatol Venereol. 2013;27:151–6.
8. Hexsel D, Lacerda DA, Cavalcante AS, Machado Filho CAS, Kalil CL, Ayres EL, et al. Epidemiology of melasma in Brazilian patients: a multicenter study. Int J Dermatol. 2014;53:440–4.
9. Melasma: a monography. 1st ed. New Delhi /Philadelphia: Jaypee Brothers Medical Publishers (P) Ltd; 2015. p 86.
10. Ishiy PS, Silva LRE, Penha MÁ, Handel AC, Miot HA. Skin diseases reported by workers from UNESP campus at Rubião Jr, Botucatu-SP (Brazil). An Bras Dermatol. 2014;89: 529–31.

11. Costa A, Moisés TA, Cordero T, Alves CRT, Marmirori J. Association of emblica, licorice and belides as an alternative to hydroquinone in the clinical treatment of melasma. An Bras Dermatol. 2010;85:613–20.
12. El-Essawi D, Musial JL, Hammad A, Lim HW. A survey of skin disease and skin-related issues in Arab Americans. J Am Acad Dermatol. 2007;56:933–8.
13. Vázquez M, Maldonado H, Benmamán C, Sánchez JL. Melasma in men. A clinical and histologic study. Int J Dermatol. 1988;27:25–7.
14. Sarkar R, Puri P, Jain RK, Singh A, Desai A. Melasma in men: a clinical, aetiological and histological study. J Eur Acad Dermatol Venereol. 2010;24:768–72.
15. Ortonne JP, Arellano I, Berneburg M, Cestari T, Chan H, Grimes P, et al. A global survey of the role of ultraviolet radiation and hormonal influences in the development of melasma. J Eur Acad Dermatol Venereol. 2009;23:1254–62.
16. Lieberman R, Moy L. Estrogen receptor expression in melasma: results from facial skin of affected patients. J Drugs Dermatol. 2008;7:463–5.
17. Kim N-H, Lee C-H, Lee A-Y. H19 RNA downregulation stimulated melanogenesis in melasma. Pigment Cell Melanoma Res. 2010;23:84–92.
18. Kang HY, Suzuki I, Lee DJ, Ha J, Reiniche P, Aubert J, et al. Transcriptional profiling shows altered expression of wnt pathway- and lipid metabolism-related genes as well as melanogenesis-related genes in melasma. J Invest Dermatol. 2011;131:1692–700.
19. Passeron T. Melasma pathogenesis and influencing factors - an overview of the latest research. J Eur Acad Dermatol Venereol. 2013;27 Suppl 1:5–6.
20. Achar A, Rathi SK. Melasma: a clinico-epidemiological study of 312 cases. Indian J Dermatol. 2011;56:380–2.
21. Jang YH, Lee JY, Kang HY, Lee E-S, Kim YC. Oestrogen and progesterone receptor expression in melasma: an immunohistochemical analysis. J Eur Acad Dermatol Venereol. 2010;24:1312–6.
22. Sialy R, Hassan I, Kaur I, Dash RJ. Melasma in men: a hormonal profile. J Dermatol. 2000;27:64–5.
23. Jadotte YT, Schwartz RA. Melasma: insights and perspectives. Acta Dermatovenerol Croat. 2010;18:124–9.
24. Rostami Mogaddam M, Iranparvar Alamdari M, Maleki N, Safavi Ardabili N, Abedkouhi S. Evaluation of autoimmune thyroid disease in melasma. J Cosmet Dermatol. 2015;14:167–71.
25. Lutfi RJ, Fridmanis M, Misiunas AL, Pafume O, Gonzalez EA, Villemur JA, et al. Association of melasma with thyroid autoimmunity and other thyroidal abnormalities and their relationship to the origin of the melasma. J Clin Endocrinol Metab. 1985;61:28–31.
26. Li Y-H, Chen JZS, Wei H-C, Wu Y, Liu M, Xu Y-Y, et al. Efficacy and safety of intense pulsed light in treatment of melasma in Chinese patients. Dermatol Surg Off Publ Am Soc Dermatol Surg Al. 2008;34:693–701.
27. Prabha N, Mahajan VK, Mehta KS, Chauhan PS, Gupta M. Cosmetic contact sensitivity in patients with melasma: results of a pilot study. Dermatol Res Pract. 2014;2014:316219.
28. Famenini S, Gharavi NM, Beynet DP. Finasteride associated melasma in a Caucasian male. J Drugs Dermatol. 2014;13:484–6.
29. Handel AC, Lima PB, Tonolli VM, Miot LDB, Miot HA. Risk factors for facial melasma in women: a case–control study. Br J Dermatol. 2014;171:588–94.
30. Freitag FM, Cestari TF, Leopoldo LR, Paludo P, Boza JC. Effect of melasma on quality of life in a sample of women living in southern Brazil. J Eur Acad Dermatol Venereol. 2008;22:655–62.
31. Grimes PE. Melasma. Etiologic and therapeutic considerations. Arch Dermatol. 1995;131:1453–7.
32. Sarkar R, Jain RK, Puri P. Melasma in Indian males. Dermatol Surg Off Publ Am Soc Dermatol Surg Al. 2003;29:204.
33. Kim EH, Kim YC, Lee E-S, Kang HY. The vascular characteristics of melasma. J Dermatol Sci. 2007;46:111–6.

34. Kang HY, Ortonne J-P. What should be considered in treatment of melasma. Ann Dermatol. 2010;22:373–8.
35. Mahmoud BH, Ruvolo E, Hexsel CL, Liu Y, Owen MR, Kollias N, et al. Impact of long-wavelength UVA and visible light on melanocompetent skin. J Invest Dermatol. 2010;130: 2092–7.
36. Roberts WE. Pollution as a risk factor for the development of melasma and other skin disorders of facial hyperpigmentation - is there a case to be made? J Drugs Dermatol. 2015;14:337–41.
37. Vierkötter A, Schikowski T, Ranft U, Sugiri D, Matsui M, Krämer U, et al. Airborne particle exposure and extrinsic skin aging. J Invest Dermatol. 2010;130:2719–26.

Chapter 4
Pathogenesis of Melasma

Kyoung Chan Park and In Su Kim

4.1 Introduction

Although genetic predisposition, ultraviolet radiation, and female sex hormones are classical influencing factors [1–4], recent evidences suggest that there are additional factors that may play a key role in the development and relapse of melasma. Researchers have focused on the activation of lesional melanocytes via paracrine and autocrine mediators [5–7]. Several proteins and cellular components, growth factors, and signaling mechanisms have been suggested to be deeply involved in the pathogenesis of melasma.

Different ethnic groups have a diverse range of skin phototypes, pigmentation, and varying incidences of melasma [8]. Thus, melasma has a complex pathogenesis that has not yet been fully elucidated. However, distinctive histopathologic features of melasma might provide new clues toward further understanding its pathogenesis.

K.C. Park, MD, PhD (✉)
Department of Dermatology, Seoul National University College of Medicine, Seoul National University Bundang Hospital, 82, Gumi-ro 173beon-gil, Bundang-gu, Seongnam-si, Gyeonggi-do 463-707, South Korea
e-mail: gcpark@snu.ac.kr

I.S. Kim
Department of Dermatology, Seoul National University Bundang Hospital, 82, Gumi-ro 173beon-gil, Bundang-gu, Seongnam-si, Gyeonggi-do 463-707, South Korea
e-mail: anel803@naver.com

E.B. Handog, M.J. Enriquez-Macarayo (eds.), *Melasma and Vitiligo in Brown Skin*,
DOI 10.1007/978-81-322-3664-1_4

4.2 Major Influencing Factors

4.2.1 Genetic Factors

Genetic component is the most important risk factor for melasma. However, no Mendelian pattern of segregation has been identified [9]. A case of melasma occurring in both identical twins was reported in England in 1987. It was triggered by hormonal stimulation, which worsened after sun exposure. Nevertheless, it did not occur in their other sister (not twin), which strengthens the hypothesis of genetic susceptibility to the development of melasma [10].

Several studies have attempted to recognize the prevalence of melasma in the general population. The reported prevalence of melasma ranges from 8.8 % in Hispanic female population in the Southern United States to as high as 40 % in Southeast Asian populations [11, 12]. In a self-administered questionnaire study that included 324 women, 48 % of patients with melasma had a family history of melasma (97 % in a first-degree relative). There was a low family history of melasma in patients with skin type I or II (34 %) compared with those in patients with skin types III to VI (57 %). Individuals with family history of melasma tended to have darker skin (90 % types III–VI) compared with those without family history (77 % types III–VI) [3].

4.2.2 Hormonal Factors

Sex hormones, such as estrogen and progesterone, are factors involved in the regulation of skin pigmentation [13]. Melasma is more common in women, accounting for 90 % of all cases. It has been reported in 50–70 % of pregnant women as well as in 10–20 % of women using oral contraceptives [14, 15]. These clinical evidences suggest that estrogen may be more likely to trigger melasma.

In an *in vitro* cell culture model, estradiol has been shown to upregulate tyrosinase, tyrosinase-related protein (TRP)-1, and TRP-2 transcription [16]. Melanin synthesis is also increased by 17β-estradiol in human melanocytes in culture [17]. In addition, estrogen receptor (ER)β expression showed an increasing tendency in the lesions compared with the unaffected area (mean ± standard deviation: 0.39 ± 0.17 vs. 0.31 ± 0.17, $p > 0.05$). The nuclear staining of progesterone receptor (PR) was also significantly increased in the lesions compared with the unaffected epidermis (0.47 ± 0.15 vs. 0.36 ± 0.14, $p = 0.03$) [18]. Interestingly, an increased immunoreactivity of ERβ was also noted in the dermis, especially around the small blood vessels and fibroblast-like cells compared with the unaffected dermis (1.33 ± 0.82 vs. 0.97 ± 0.59, $p = 0.04$). However, there was no significant difference in the expression of PR between the lesions and the unaffected dermis (1.24 ± 0.90 vs. 0.96 ± 0.68, $p = 0.17$) [18]. These results suggest that there may be an association between hormonal receptors and melasma.

4.2.3 UV Irradiation

The higher level of solar elastosis in melasma skin implies that chronic sun exposure is a prerequisite for the development of melasma. After ultraviolet B (UVB) irradiation, keratinocytes induce melanocyte proliferation and melanogenesis by secreting stem cell factor (SCF), basic fibroblast growth factor (bFGF), interleukin-1, endothelin-1, inducible nitric oxide synthase, α-melanocyte-stimulating hormone, and adrenocorticotropic hormone [19–22]. The secretion of prostaglandin E2 after UVB exposure results in larger and more dendritic melanocytes [23]. Furthermore, the solar damage of the dermis could induce the secretion of melanogenic cytokines, including SCF and hepatocyte growth factor, from the dermal fibroblasts, thereby influencing the development of hyperpigmentation in the overlying epidermis [24, 25]. The dermal fibroblasts secrete a soluble form of SCF during rapid growth or inflammation. Thus, it is possible that the inflammation in the dermis from the accumulated UV irradiation may be associated with the activation of fibroblasts, which can result in the upregulation of SCF in the skin affected with melasma. The SCF mRNA expression is significantly increased in melasma lesions compared with nonlesional skin (0.83 ± 0.5 vs. 0.51 ± 0.4, $p < 0.01$). RT-PCR of c-kit mRNA also revealed a significant difference in the expression between the lesional and nonlesional skin (0.78 ± 0.7 vs. 0.57 ± 0.6, $p < 0.01$). Thus, the increased production of soluble SCF in melasma skin is involved via SCF/c-kit-induced signaling in the activation of melanocytes, leading to their increased proliferation and melanogenesis [5].

4.3 Additional Factors

4.3.1 Gene Expression Change

The protein levels of melanogenesis-associated factors (tyrosinase, TRP-1, dopachrome tautomerase, silver) were increased in the melasma lesions, indicating a higher melanogenic activity in the lesional skin. Interestingly, the lipid metabolism-associated genes (peroxisome proliferator-activated receptor α (PPAR α), arachidonate 15-lipoxygenase (ALOX15), type B (ALOX15B), diacylglycerol O-acyltransferase2-like 3, and PPAR-γ coactivator 1α) were downregulated in the lesional skin. This finding was supported by an impaired barrier function in the lesional skin of melasma.

Wnt signaling-associated factors (Wnt inhibitory factor (WIF)-1, secreted frizzled-related protein 2 (SFRP2), and Wnt5a) were also found to be upregulated in the lesional skin [26]. The Wnt pathway has a critical role in the development of epidermal melanocytes, and microphthalmia-associated transcription factor (MITF) is a nuclear mediator of this pathway [27, 28]. As a consequence of WIF-1 overexpression, the melanin content and tyrosinase activity in normal human epidermal melanocyte were significantly increased. Therefore, WIF-1 may have the physiologic functions in melanocytes as an auto- or paracrine modulator of Wnt signaling [29]. The increased SFRP2 observed around fibroblasts also suggested the possibility of a cross talk between the dermis and epidermis via the Wnt pathway in the development of melasma [26].

Another interesting study showed that H19 downregulation stimulates melanogenesis in melasma patients [30]. H19 gene transcribes a 2.3 kb noncoding RNA that is thought to have a possible role in certain malignancies [31, 32]. H19 knockdown in a mixed cell culture system (keratinocytes and melanocytes) did induce a tyrosinase overexpression as well as an increase of melanosome transfer. A combination of estrogen treatment and H19 RNA knockdown induce more than additive effects on tyrosinase expression in the mixed cell culture system, whereas UV irradiation does not. These suggest that downregulation of H19 and a sufficient dose of estrogen might be involved in the development of melasma [30].

4.3.2 *Histopathologic Considerations*

4.3.2.1 Epidermal Hyperpigmentation

The most characteristic histologic feature of melasma is the increased melanin in the epidermis, and in a clinical study involving 56 Korean melasma patients, epidermal pigmentation was shown to be increased in the lesional skin of melasma [33]. Similar findings were seen in 11 melasma cases involving Fitzpatrick skin type IV and VI [34].

The paracrine linkages among keratinocytes, fibroblasts, and melanocytes play important roles in regulating the epidermal melanization [5]. Fontana-Masson staining has shown that the melanin content of the melasma skin is higher in all layers of the epidermis, including the stratum corneum [33, 35, 36]. An image analysis of the skin from 22 patients with melasma showed a significant difference in the density of melanin between the melasma skin (0.37 ± 0.02) and perilesional normal skin (0.34 ± 0.02) ($p < 0.01$) [37]. Based on these findings, it is suggested that the development of melasma involves accelerated melanin synthesis, increased levels of melanin transfer to the keratinocytes, and reduced melanosome degradation [33].

Reports on melanocyte numbers in melasma are inconsistent. Kang et al. found a higher melanin content and increased numbers of melanocytes in the melasma skin. Their study involved a quantitative image analysis of 56 Fontana-Masson-stained sections. Compared with perilesional normal skin, the number of melanocytes per millimeter of epidermal length and the number of melanocytes per millimeter of rete ridge length are increased by 24 % and 27 %, respectively. In addition, ultrastructural observations showed an increase in the numbers of melanosomes and melanocytes [33].

In contrast, a study by Grimes et al. did not find a significant increase in melanocyte numbers in melasma skin compared with perilesional normal skin in their study composed of 22 skin specimens from subjects with Fitzpatrick skin types IV–VI immunostained using Mel-5 [34]. Moreover, in their study of 44 patients with melasma, Miot et al. did not find any differences in melanocyte numbers between the melasma skin and perilesional normal skin sections labeled using a Melan-A antibody [37]. Electron microscopy showed higher numbers of mature melanosomes in keratinocytes and melanocytes in the melasma skin [37] and a significantly higher number of dendrites per keratinocyte in the melasma skin (7.55 ± 2.53 dendrites per keratinocyte) than in the perilesional normal skin (5.28 ± 1.85 dendrites per keratinocyte) ($p < 0.05$) [34]. Furthermore, electron microscopy demonstrated increased levels of activity within melanocytes in the melasma skin, which was deduced from the presence of higher organelle numbers, including mitochondria, Golgi apparatuses, rough endoplasmic reticula, and ribosomes [33].

There are immunohistochemical evidences that suggest melanogenesis-related proteins are increased. Immunohistochemistry using NKI-beteb, which recognizes the melanocyte lineage-specific pmel-17 antigen, showed a higher staining intensity in the melasma skin than in the normal skin (Fig. 4.1) [38]. Mel-5 immunostaining, which detects TRP-1, also increased in intensity in the melasma skin than in the normal skin, suggesting that the levels of TRP-1 are higher in melasma melanocytes

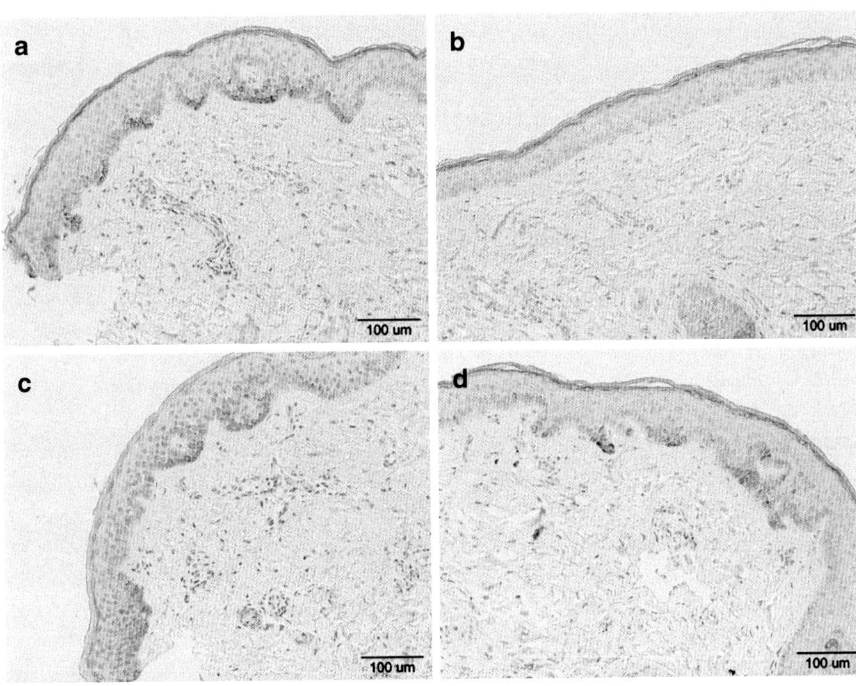

Fig. 4.1 Immunostaining for NKI-beteb and tyrosinase-related protein (TRP)-2 before and after treatment with a combination of soybean extract and niacinamide for 8 weeks. Immunostaining for (**a**) NKI-beteb before treatment (×100), (**b**) NKI-beteb after treatment (×100), (**c**) TRP-2 before treatment (×100), and (**d**) TRP-2 after treatment (×100) [38]

[33]. Moreover, we have observed the elevated expression of TRP-2 in the melasma skin (Fig. 4.1). These findings support the concept of an increased level of melanogenesis in the pathogenesis of melasma.

4.3.2.2 Basement Membrane Disruption

Some studies have investigated the status of the basement membrane in the melasma skin. Sanchez et al. demonstrated the presence of vacuolar degeneration of the basal cells and the focal vacuolar degeneration of the basement membrane in 3.9 % (3/76) of melasma skin specimens [39]. In contrast, Kang et al. did not observe any disruptions of the basement membrane in their evaluation of skin samples from 56 Korean patients with melasma using diastase-resistant periodic acid-Schiff (D-PAS) staining and electron microscopy [33]. However, the same authors reported that pendulous melanocytes associated with basement membrane abnormalities are a characteristic feature of melasma [6].

Another study of melasma patients with Fitzpatrick skin types IV and V revealed that PAS staining showed damage in the basal membrane in 95.8 % of the melasma lesions versus 58.3 % of the perilesional skin, and antibody to collagen type IV showed damage in 83 % of the melasma lesions versus 66 % of the perilesional skin [36].

Basement membrane disruption could be caused by elevated levels of matrix metalloproteinase (MMP)-2 and MMP-9, which degrade type IV and VI collagen during chronic UV exposure [40]. MMP-2 expression was found to be increased in the lesional skin compared with the perilesional normal skin (0.018 ± 0.014 vs. 0.004 ± 0.005, $p = 0.006$) [6]. Since free melanin and melanophages are present in the dermis of the melasma skin, disruption of the basement membrane could facilitate the descent or the movement of active melanocytes and melanin into the dermis, which is reflected in the constant hyperpigmentation of melasma [33, 36].

4.3.2.3 Solar Elastosis

Many observations strongly suggest that sun exposure is the primary trigger of melasma. Melasma affects particularly the face, a sun-exposed area, and the condition worsens in the summer. Solar elastosis is more marked in areas of melasma, compared with the unaffected facial skin [35]. Kang et al. reported a moderate-to-severe degree of solar elastosis in 93 % of melasma patients included in their study [33]. The melasma skin showed a significantly higher degree of solar elastosis than the perilesional normal skin (83 % vs. 29 %, $p < 0.05$) [36]. Furthermore, the amount of elastotic material was significantly higher in the melasma skin than that in the perilesional normal skin (13.3 ± 2.8 % vs. 10.2 ± 2.9 %, $p < 0.001$). Moreover, thick, highly curled, and more fragmented elastic fibers were observed in Verhoeff-van Gieson-stained sections of the melasma skin [33].

4.3.2.4 Increased Vascularization

Accumulating evidence has shown that the number of blood vessels is higher in the melasma lesions than in the perilesional normal skin [41–43]. The increase in the number of vessels was more prominent than the increase in vessel size. This finding represents that the erythema noticed in melasma patients could be due to angiogenesis and telangiectasia [41]. An immunohistochemical study of factor VIIIa-related antigen showed a considerable increase in the number of enlarged blood vessels, vessel size, and vessel density in the melasma skin compared with the perilesional normal skin [41].

The elevated expression of vascular endothelial growth factor (VEGF) in keratinocytes has led to the hypothesis that VEGF may play a role in the behavior of the melanocytes in the skin, because the functioning VEGF receptors were demonstrated in melanocytes in vitro [44]. Elevations in the levels of c-kit, SCF, and inducible nitric oxide synthase have also been observed, which could affect vascularization [5, 45]. Moreover, blood vessels or endothelial cells modified by UV irradiation may release cytokines and soluble factors, such as plasminogen, which is a possible cause of hyperpigmentation in melasma [46].

Tranexamic acid (TXA) inhibits plasmin, a key molecule involved in angiogenesis that converts extracellular matrix-bound VEGF into its free forms [47]. TXA has also been reported to suppress neovascularization-induced bFGF [48]. In a recent clinical trial that evaluated the efficacy of systemic TXA in the treatment of melasma, we demonstrated significant decreases in the lesional melanin index and in the erythema index after the oral administration of 250 mg TXA, three times per day, for 8 weeks [49]. A histologic analysis showed significant reductions in the level of epidermal pigmentation and vessel numbers (Fig. 4.2a–d). These findings suggest that the interactions between increased levels of vascularization and melanocytes may have an influence on the development of hyperpigmentation.

4.3.2.5 Mast Cell Prevalence

Mast cells are observed more frequently in the melasma skin than in the nonlesional skin, especially in the dermal elastotic areas (Fig. 4.2e, f) [49]. The median prevalence of dermal mast cells was significantly higher in the melasma skin than in the perilesional normal skin (173 ± 57 % vs. 145 ± 57 %, $p = 0.04$) [35]. Using an antitryptase antibody, the number of mast cells was 58 ± 39.9 cells/mm^2 in the melasma skin compared with 37 ± 28.8 cells/mm^2 in the perilesional normal skin ($p < 0.04$) [36].

The role of mast cells in the development of melasma has not been elucidated. Since repetitive UV irradiation induces the production of mast cell tryptase, which degrades type IV collagen, elevated mast cell numbers and tryptase levels could weaken the basement membrane in the melasma skin [50]. Mast cells could trigger

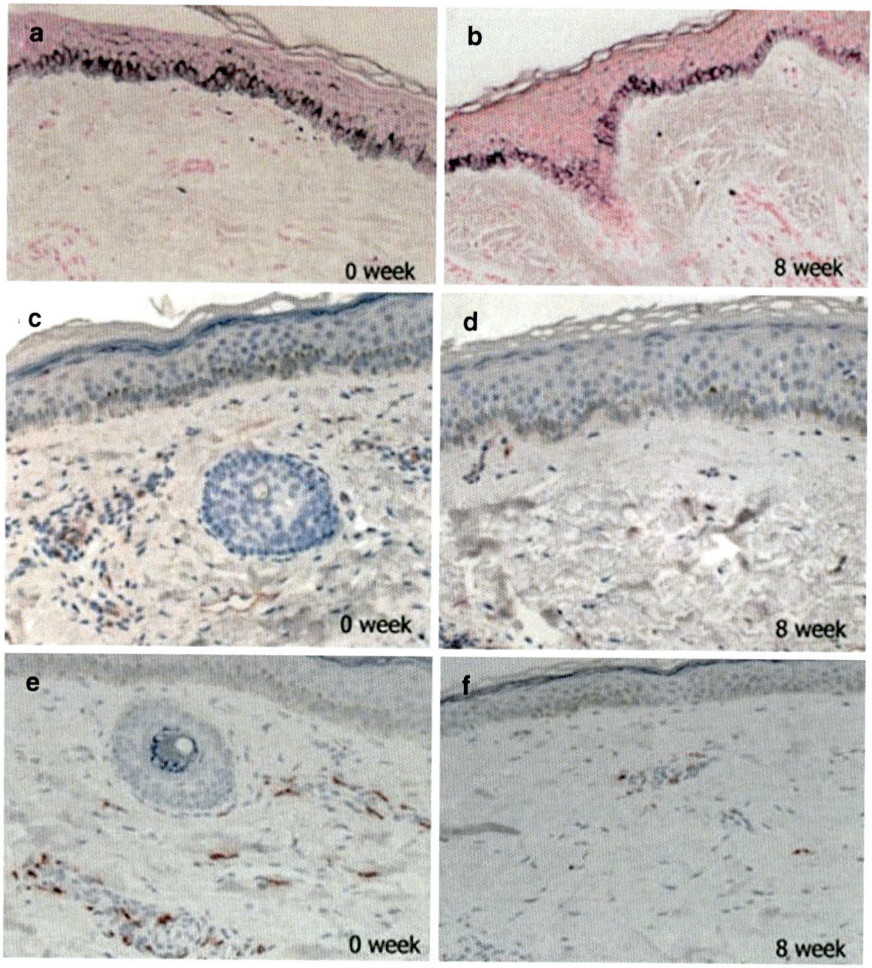

Fig. 4.2 Histologic changes after 8 weeks of treatment with tranexamic acid. (**a**, **b**) Fontana-Masson staining shows reduced epidermal pigmentation (×100). (**c**, **d**) Anti-CD31 staining shows reduced levels of vascularity (×100). (**e**, **f**) Antitryptase staining shows reduced mast cell numbers (×100) [49]

solar elastosis by inducing the production of elastin by fibroblasts, either directly or via other cell types or cytokines [51, 52]. Solar elastosis did not develop in mast cell-deficient mice that were repeatedly irradiated with UV [53]. The elevated numbers of mast cells, together with the presence of infiltrating leukocytes and dilated blood vessels, might reflect chronic skin inflammation that underlies the development of melasma [35]. Mast cells can also induce vascular proliferation by secreting angiogenic factors, including VEGF, fibroblast growth factor-2, and transforming growth factor-β [54].

4.4 Conclusion

In addition to the genetic background and exposure to ultraviolet radiation, there may be an association between female sex hormones/hormonal receptors and melasma. Furthermore, a gene profiling study showed that melasma might be associated with changes in gene expression, which are related with melanogenesis, Wnt signaling pathway, and lipid metabolism. Although melasma is characterized by epidermal pigmentation, there are distinctive histologic findings in melasma, such as epidermal hyperpigmentation, basement membrane disruption, solar elastosis, increased vascularization, and high prevalence of mast cells. Such findings suggest that these have important and interactive roles in the pathogenesis of melasma.

References

1. Pathak MA, Riley FC, Fitzpatrick TB. Melanogenesis in human skin following exposure to long-wave ultraviolet and visible light. J Invest Dermatol. 1962;39:435–43.
2. Grimes PE. Melasma. Etiologic and therapeutic considerations. Arch Dermatol. 1995;131:1453–7.
3. Ortonne JP, Arellano I, Berneburg M, Cestari T, Chan H, Grimes P, et al. A global survey of the role of ultraviolet radiation and hormonal influences in the development of melasma. J Eur Acad Dermatol Venereol. 2009;23:1254–62.
4. Resnik S. Melasma induced by oral contraceptive drugs. JAMA. 1967;199:601–5.
5. Kang HY, Hwang JS, Lee JY, Ahn JH, Kim JY, Lee ES, Kang WH. The dermal stem cell factor and c-kit are overexpressed in melasma. Br J Dermatol. 2006;154:1094–9.
6. Lee DJ, Park KC, Ortonne JP, Kang HY. Pendulous melanocytes: a characteristic feature of melasma and how it may occur. Br J Dermatol. 2012;166:684–6.
7. Lee J, Jung E, Huh S, Boo YC, Hyun CG, Kim YS, Park D. Mechanisms of melanogenesis inhibition by 2,5-dimethyl-4-hydroxy-3(2H)-furanone. Br J Dermatol. 2007;157:242–8.
8. Hexsel D, Arellano I, Rendon M. Ethnic considerations in the treatment of Hispanic and Latin-American patients with hyperpigmentation. Br J Dermatol. 2006;156(S1):7–12.
9. Miot LD, Miot HA, Silva MG, Marques ME. Physiopathology of melasma. An Bras Dermatol. 2009;84:623–35.
10. Hughes BR. Melasma occurring in twin sisters. J Am Acad Dermatol. 1987;17:841.
11. Werlinger KD, Guevara IL, Gonzalez CM, Rincon ET, Caetano R, Haley RW, Pandya AG. Prevalence of self-diagnosed melasma among premenopausal Latino women in Dallas and Fort Worth Tex. Arch Dermatol. 2007;143:424–5.
12. Sivayathorn A. Melasma in orientals. Clin Drug Invest. 1995;10(S 2):34–40.
13. Verdier-Sevrain S, Bonte F, Gilchrest B. Biology of estrogens in skin: implications for skin aging. Exp Dermatol. 2006;15:83–94.
14. Moin A, Jabery Z, Fallah N. Prevalence and awareness of melasma during pregnancy. Int J Dermatol. 2006;45:285–8.
15. Cestari T, Arellano I, Hexsel D, Ortonne JP. Melasma in Latin America: options for therapy and treatment algorithm. J Eur Acad Dermatol Venereol. 2009;23:760–72.
16. Kippenberger S, Loitsch S, Solano F, Bernd A, Kaufmann R. Quantification of tyrosinase, TRP-1, and Trp-2 transcripts in human melanocytes by reverse transcriptase-competitive multiplex PCR--regulation by steroid hormones. J Invest Dermatol. 1998;110:364–7.
17. McLeod SD, Ranson M, Mason RS. Effects of estrogens on human melanocytes in vitro. J Steroid Biochem Mol Biol. 1994;49:9–14.

18. Jang YH, Lee JY, Kang HY, Lee ES, Kim YC. Oestrogen and progesterone receptor expression in melasma: an immunohistochemical analysis. J Eur Acad Dermatol Venereol. 2010;24:1312–6.
19. Luger TA, Schwarz T. Evidence for an epidermal cytokine network. J Invest Dermatol. 1990;95:S100–4.
20. Imokawa G, Miyagishi M, Yada Y. Endothelin-1 as a new melanogen: coordinated expression of its gene and the tyrosinase gene in UVB-exposed human epidermis. J Invest Dermatol. 1995;105:32–7.
21. Schauer E, Trautinger F, Kock A, Schwarz A, Bhardwaj R, Simon M, et al. Proopiomelanocortin-derived peptides are synthesized and released by human keratinocytes. J Clin Invest. 1994;93:2258–62.
22. Smit N, Le Poole I, Van Den Wijngaard R, Tigges A, Westerhof W, Das P. Expression of different immunological markers by cultured human melanocytes. Arch Dermatol Res. 1993;285:356–65.
23. Tomita Y, Iwamoto M, Masuda T, Tagami H. Stimulatory effect of prostaglandin E2 on the configuration of normal human melanocytes in vitro. J Invest Dermatol. 1987;89:299–301.
24. Imokawa G, Yada Y, Morisaki N, Kimura M. Biological characterization of human fibroblast-derived mitogenic factors for human melanocytes. Biochem J. 1998;330(Pt 3):1235–9.
25. Grichnik JM, Burch JA, Burchette J, Shea CR. The SCF/KIT pathway plays a critical role in the control of normal human melanocyte homeostasis. J Invest Dermatol. 1998;111:233–8.
26. Kang HY, Suzuki I, Lee DJ, Ha J, Reiniche P, Aubert J, et al. Transcriptional profiling shows altered expression of wnt pathway- and lipid metabolism-related genes as well as melanogenesis-related genes in melasma. J Invest Dermatol. 2011;131:1692–700.
27. Takeda K, Yasumoto K, Takada R, Takada S, Watanabe K, Udono T, et al. Induction of melanocyte-specific microphthalmia-associated transcription factor by Wnt-3a. J Biol Chem. 2000;275:14013–6.
28. Chien AJ, Conrad WH, Moon RT. 2009. A Wnt survival guide: from flies to human disease. J Invest Dermatol. 2009;129:1614–27.
29. Park TJ, Kim M, Kim H, Park SY, Park KC, Ortonne JP, Kang HY. Wnt inhibitory factor (WIF)-1 promotes melanogenesis in normal human melanocytes. Pigment Cell Melanoma Res. 2014;27:72–81.
30. Kim NH, Lee CH, Lee AY. H19 RNA downregulation stimulated melanogenesis in melasma. Pigment Cell Melanoma Res. 2010;23:84–92.
31. Gabory A, Ripoche MA, Yoshimizu T, Dandolo L. The H19 gene: regulation and function of a non-coding RNA. Cytogenet Genome Res. 2006;113:188–93.
32. Reese KJ, Bartolomei MS. Establishment and maintenance of H19 imprinting in the germline and preimplantation embryo. Cytogenet Genome Res. 2006;113:153–8.
33. Kang WH, Yoon KH, Lee ES, Kim J, Lee KB, Yim H, et al. Melasma: histopathological characteristics in 56 Korean patients. Br J Dermatol. 2002;146:228–37.
34. Grimes PE, Yamada N, Bhawan J. Light microscopic, immunohistochemical, and ultrastructural alterations in patients with melasma. Am J Dermatopathol. 2005;27:96–101.
35. Hernandez-Barrera R, Torres-Alvarez B, Castanedo-Cazares JP, Oros-Ovalle C, Moncada B. Solar elastosis and presence of mast cells as key features in the pathogenesis of melasma. Clin Exp Dermatol. 2008;33:305–8.
36. Torres-Alvarez B, Mesa-Garza IG, Castanedo-Cazares JP, Fuentes-Ahumada C, Oros-Ovalle C, Navarrete-Solis J, Moncada B. Histochemical and immunohistochemical study in melasma: evidence of damage in the basal membrane. Am J Dermatopathol. 2011;33:291–5.
37. Miot LD, Miot HA, Polettini J, Silva MG, Marques ME. Morphologic changes and the expression of alpha-melanocyte stimulating hormone and melanocortin-1 receptor in melasma lesions: a comparative study. Am J Dermatopathol. 2010;32:676–82.
38. Kwon SH, Park KC. Clues to the pathogenesis of melasma from its histologic findings. Pigmentary Disorders. 2014;1:141.

39. Sanchez NP, Pathak MA, Sato S, Fitzpatrick TB, Sanchez JL, Mihm MCJ. Melasma: a clinical, light microscopic, ultrastructural, and immunofluorescence study. J Am Acad Dermatol. 1981;4:698–710.
40. Inomata S, Matsunaga Y, Amano S, Takada K, Kobayashi K, Tsunenaga M, et al. Possible involvement of gelatinases in basement membrane damage and wrinkle formation in chronically ultraviolet B-exposed hairless mouse. J Invest Dermatol. 2003;120:128–34.
41. Kim EH, Kim YC, Lee ES, Kang HY. The vascular characteristics of melasma. J Dermatol Sci. 2007;46:111–6.
42. Kang HY, Bahadoran P, Suzuki I, Zugaj D, Khemis A, Passeron T, et al. In vivo reflectance confocal microscopy detects pigmentary changes in melasma at a cellular level resolution. Exp Dermatol. 2010;19:e228–33.
43. Passeron T. Long-lasting effect of vascular targeted therapy of melasma. J Am Acad Dermatol. 2013;69:e141–2.
44. Kim EJ, Park HY, Yaar M, Gilchrest BA. Modulation of vascular endothelial growth factor receptors in melanocytes. Exp Dermatol. 2005;14:625–33.
45. Jo HY, Kim CK, Suh IB, Ryu SW, Ha KS, Kwon YG, Kim YM. Co-localization of inducible nitric oxide synthase and phosphorylated Akt in the lesional skins of patients with melasma. J Dermatol. 2009;36:10–6.
46. Navid F, Kolbe L, Stab F, Korff T, Neufang G. UV radiation induces the release of angiopoietin-2 from dermal microvascular endothelial cells. Exp Dermatol. 2012;21:147–53.
47. Ferrara N. Binding to the extracellular matrix and proteolytic processing: two key mechanisms regulating vascular endothelial growth factor action. Mol Biol Cell. 2010;21:687–90.
48. Bastaki M, Nelli EE, Dell'era P, Rusnati M, Molinari-Tosatti MP, Parolini S, et al. Basic fibroblast growth factor-induced angiogenic phenotype in mouse endothelium. A study of aortic and microvascular endothelial cell lines. Arterioscler Thromb Vasc Biol. 1997;17:454–64.
49. Na JI, Choi SY, Yang SH, Choi HR, Kang HY, Park KC. Effect of tranexamic acid on melasma: a clinical trial with histological evaluation. J Eur Acad Dermatol Venereol. 2013;27:1035–9.
50. Iddamalgoda A, Le QT, Ito K, Tanaka K, Kojima H, Kido H. Mast cell tryptase and photoaging: possible involvement in the degradation of extra cellular matrix and basement membrane proteins. Arch Dermatol Res. 2008;300(S1):S69–76.
51. Lavker RM, Kligman AM. Chronic heliodermatitis: a morphologic evaluation of chronic actinic dermal damage with emphasis on the role of mast cells. J Invest Dermatol. 1988;90:325–30.
52. Grimbaldeston MA, Simpson A, Finlay-Jones JJ, Hart PH. The effect of ultraviolet radiation exposure on the prevalence of mast cells in human skin. Br J Dermatol. 2003;148:300–6.
53. Gonzalez S, Moran M, Kochevar IE. Chronic photodamage in skin of mast cell-deficient mice. Photochem Photobiol. 1999;70:248–53.
54. Crivellato E, Nico B, Ribatti D. Mast cells and tumour angiogenesis: new insight from experimental carcinogenesis. Cancer Lett. 2008;269:1–6.

Chapter 5
Classification and Clinical Presentations of Melasma in Brown Skin

Filomena Legarda-Montinola

5.1 Introduction

The color tone of brown (brown racial classification) is predominantly seen among Asians, Latinos, Latin Americans, American Indians, Middle Eastern population, Mediterranean-Africans, and South African population. Melanin deciphers the skin color of the skin. There are various interracial tones of brown skin. The density of the melanocytes and their location, activity, and function are an important focus in the study and treatment of melasma. Every effort is directed to improve methods to locate that specific melanocyte as well as investigate the many factors that may influence its activity. This unique interplay of location, number, and activity may vary from one skin type to another. The typical brown skin tone patient affected with melasma is usually from Fitzpatrick skin types III, IV, and V, sometimes VI. Factors such as sun exposure and hormones are known triggers exacerbating this condition. Equally important are the genetic and hormonal factors in combination with UV radiation [1]. A study of 324 patients in nine centers globally showed significant relationship with a positive family history of at least one relative with melasma, 97 % of which were first-degree relatives [2–4].

The classification of melasma has been categorized by different methods. Clinical presentation, in reference to the anatomical location of the hyperpigmentation, is the most commonly used classification method. Another is by grading the severity of melasma as mild, moderate, and severe. This is a quick glance simple terminology serving more as a rapid descriptive assessment in reference to the overall clinical picture. Classification can also be done using aids such as Wood's light, histopathology, dermoscopy, and confocal microscopy. The Melasma Area and

F. Legarda-Montinola
Asian Hospital and Medical Center, Muntinlupa, Philippines
e-mail: pitmontinola@gmail.com

E.B. Handog, M.J. Enriquez-Macarayo (eds.), *Melasma and Vitiligo in Brown Skin*,
DOI 10.1007/978-81-322-3664-1_5

Severity Index (MASI) score and the Melasma Quality of Life Scale (MELASQol) are additional objective and subjective classification methods useful in research and treatment protocols [2]. These are all discussed in the succeeding chapters.

5.2 Clinical Presentations

The clinical feature of melasma is described as an acquired symmetrical hyperpigmentation occurring in exclusively photo-exposed areas, commonly on the face. Other sun-exposed areas such as the extensors of the forearms and upper mid-chest may also be involved. It is most common in women but may occur in men in about 10 % of cases [5, 6]. This hyperpigmentation varies from light to dark brown or brown-gray patches with irregular borders which may coalesce in a reticular pattern. On closer look, one notices some areas to be more homogenous or darker in tone in contrast to other areas. This detail, together with percentage involvement, is an important point of reference when doing clinical research in melasma.

Melasma is commonly referred to as "chloasma" or the "mask of pregnancy." The name is derived from the Latin word "chloos" and the Greek "cloazein" to mean green and "melas" to mean black. Areas of hypermelanosis tend to disappear or diminish after parturition, but in brown or darker skin tone, this may persist for long periods of time [4].

5.3 Classifications

5.3.1 *Classification of Melasma According to Location and Clinical Presentation*

Classification of melasma is of utmost importance as this can signify prognosis and assist in the search for treatment which at present remains unsatisfactory.

Classification according to location and clinical presentation (Fig. 5.1a–e) is the most commonly used in practice as this delineates the specific location of the hypermelanosis at a glance. The most frequent site is the *centrofacial area* (63 %) involving the forehead, cheeks, nose, upper lip (except the philtrum), and the chin (Fig. 5.2a). Onset of this type occurs in the childbearing years at an average of 29 years old. The *malar* type involves the cheek and nose (21 %) (Fig. 5.2b). *Mandibular* melasma (16 %) is a clinical presentation where the hyperpigmentation is along the mandibular ramus or jaw area (Fig. 5.2c). This type may involve the lateral aspect of the face and may even extend to the neck [5, 7].

Studies done on middle-aged women of Puerto Rican descent (average 44 years old) have shown melasma to be aggravated by sunlight with severe sun damage and epidermal hyperpigmentation on histopathology. Almost all patients had melanophages or melanin in the papillary dermis [8]. Patients with mandibular

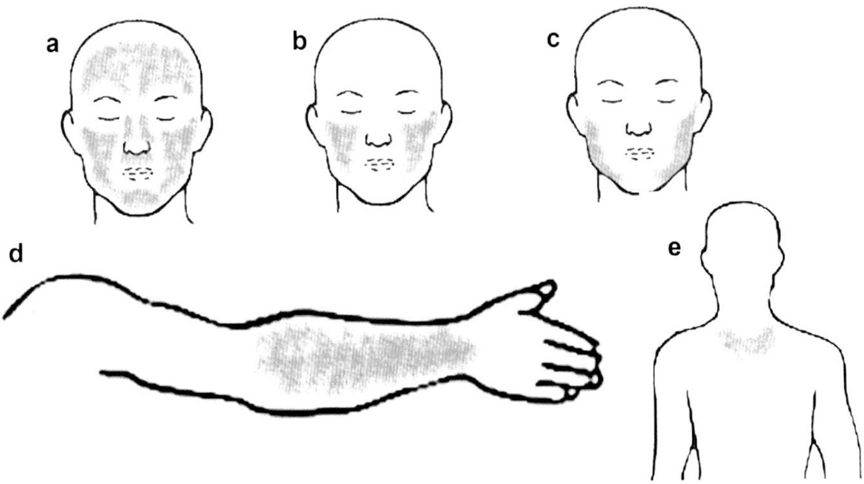

Fig. 5.1 (**a**–**e**) Sites of predilection of melasma: centrofacial (**a**), malar (**b**), mandibular (**c**), forearm extensor (**d**), upper chest (**e**)

melasma showed no association with the use of estrogen and progesterone supplements, oral contraceptives, or pregnancy. Most of these patients were of perimenopausal age. Studies suggest that mandibular melasma may be a subset of poikiloderma of Civatte [8].

Melasma of the forearms appears to be a common occurrence and appear in postmenopausal women receiving estrogen supplements. It is observed as sharply demarcated patches with a tinge of erythema. The pigmentation may be macular, speckled, scattered, or confluent. It is postulated that the outer forearm melasma pattern may be due to the higher melanocyte population in this area [9]. The melasma in the mid-upper chest may be observed in combination with facial lesions.

5.3.2 *Classification of Melasma According to Severity on Physical Examination*

For the purpose of simplicity, melasma presentation in our daily outpatient clinic can be graded as mild (Fig. 5.3a), moderate (Fig. 5.3b), and severe (Fig. 5.3c), using the Melasma Severity Scale (MSS). It rates melasma into four grades: 0 = melasma lesions almost equivalent to the surrounding normal skin or with minimal residual pigmentation; 1 = mild, slightly darker than the surrounding normal skin; 2 = moderate, moderately darker than the surrounding normal skin; and 3 = severe, markedly darker than the surrounding normal skin [10, 11].

Other grading/scoring systems have been in use such as the Melasma Area and Severity Index (MASI) and modified MASI (mMASI). Lately, a Melasma Severity Index (MSI) has been proposed as a new and more practical office-based scoring system [12].

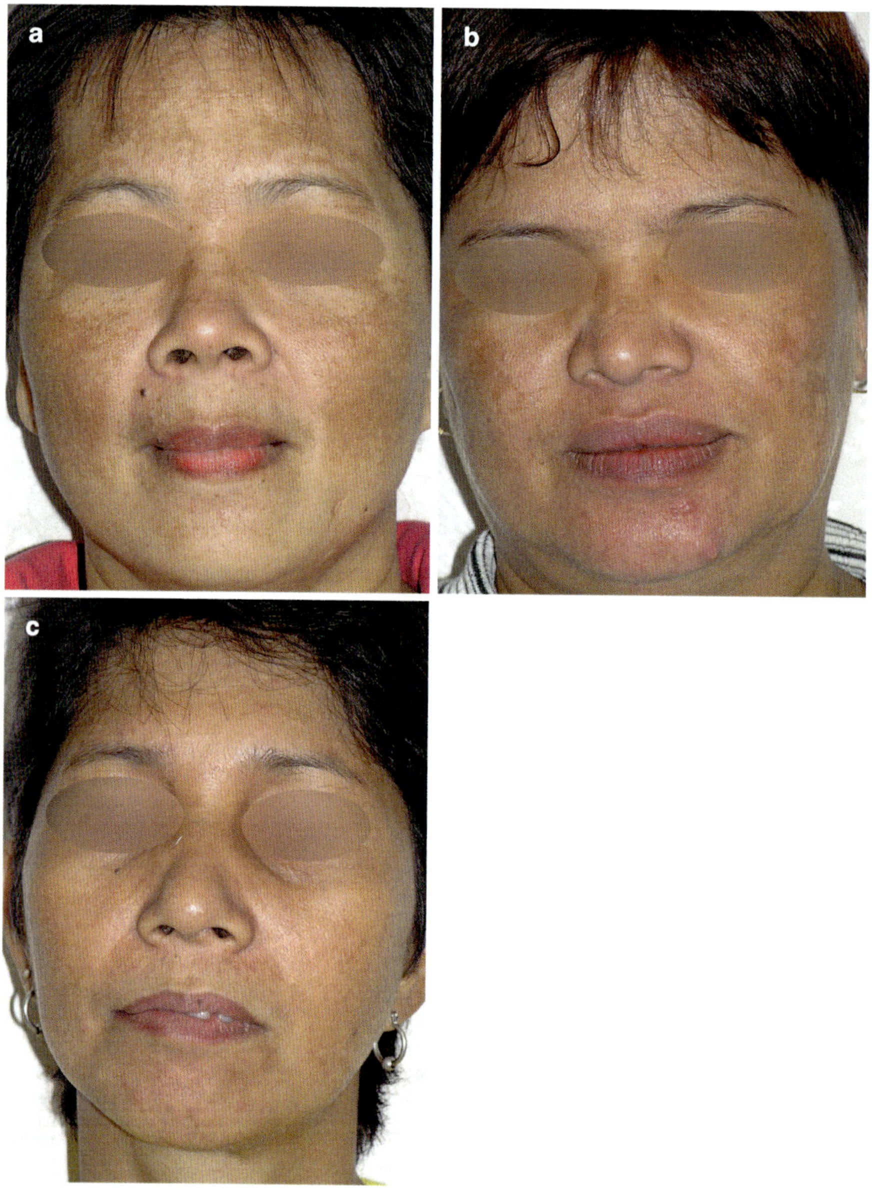

Fig. 5.2 (**a**) Centrofacial melasma, (**b**) malar melasma, (**c**) mandibular melasma

5.3.3 *Classification of Melasma Using Diagnostic Tools*

5.3.3.1 Light Examination

Under the natural visible light, *epidermal*, *dermal, and mixed* pigmentation appears light brown, blue-gray, and deep brown, respectively. Visualization by ordinary

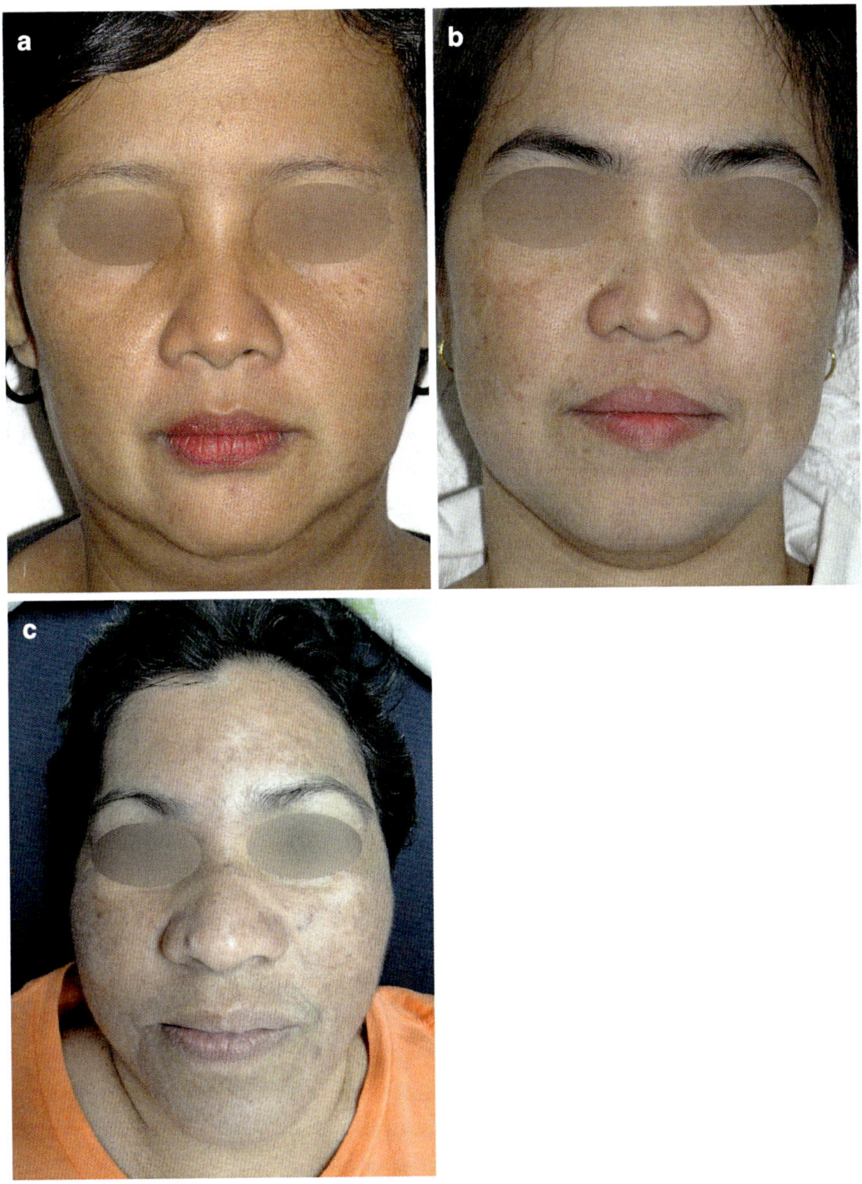

Fig. 5.3 Melasma: (a) mild, (b) moderate, (c) severe

visible light is limited and highly subjective. With Wood's light, the visualization of melasma pigmentation is clearer.

Wood's light, developed for military use by Dr. Walter Wood in 1903, has found its niche in dermatology practice for cases such as tinea capitis, erythrasma, pseudomonas infections, and porphyria cutanea tarda. For melasma, it has been a practical device to calculate the histological classification of the hyperpigmentation.

Under Wood's light, the contrast in pigmentation is increased if melasma is of the epidermal type, decreased when it is a dermal type, and subtle or slightly perceptible if it is a mixed type of melasma [13]. In patients with very dark skin, contrast is unnoticeable. The abundance of melanin in patients with phototypes V and VI allows absorption of most of the light. The skin appears dark as a whole since only a small amount of light returns back to the eye of the examiner [9]. In recent years, however, studies are being conducted assessing this instrument's sensitivity, specificity, and accuracy as compared to histopathology, dermoscopy, and confocal microscopy [14].

5.3.3.2 Dermoscopy

The use of dermoscopy in melasma has been gaining interest in the past few years. It is a noninvasive technique where the optimal equipment permits a variable magnification from 6× to 400×. Some authors consider the dermoscope as more suitable than Wood's light in determining the depth of melasma, as the pigment deposition is visualized in an objective manner.

Epidermal melasma shows a brownish hue with regular pigmentary network on dermoscopy. Dermal melasma, on the other hand, presents with a bluish-gray hue with a pigment network that is irregular. Mixed-type melasma shows features compatible to both types. Additional findings such as vascular proliferation have also been appreciated [15, 16]. This is fully discussed in the succeeding chapters.

5.3.3.3 In Vivo Reflectance Confocal Microscopy

This method allows an in vivo evaluation of melasma areas through a direct and noninvasive manner. The enlarged melanocytes are detected by high resolution, and melanin is detected in all the layers of the epidermis and dermis. Studies are favoring for in vivo focal reflectance microscopy to be closely coordinated with histopathology results. This method is gaining ground as a basis for future classification of melasma [17–19].

5.3.3.4 Basic Light Microscopy

Histopathology (Table 5.1) studies suggest that melasma is characterized by epidermal hyperpigmentation and probably secondary to increased number of melanocytes and increased activity of melanogenic enzymes overlying dermal changes caused by solar radiation [20]. A detailed discussion on histopathology classification is on Chap. 7.

Table 5.1 Classification of melasma according to basic light microscopy

	Findings
Epidermal type	Predominant melanin deposition located in the basal cell and suprabasal layers, occasionally throughout the stratum malpighii and the stratum corneum
Dermal type	Presence of melanin-laden macrophages around blood vessels both in the superficial and deep dermis
Combination	Presence of melanin in both the epidermis and dermis
Indeterminate type	Seen in individuals with Fitzpatrick types V and VI; Wood's light examination not helpful

5.4 Conclusion

The very complex world of melasma remains a challenge. Research studies continue throughout the world. We now have newer diagnostic tools with relevant findings. The present classification of melasma today will need to be expanded to include results of all these significant studies.

References

1. Sheth VM, Pandya SG. Melasma: a comprehensive update part I. J Am Acad Dermatol. 2001;65:689–97.
2. Sheth VM, Pandya SG. Melasma: a comprehensive update part II. J Am Acad Dermatol. 2001;65:699–714.
3. Ortonne JP, Arellano I, Berneburg M, Cestari T, Chan H, Grimes P, et al. A global survey of the role of ultraviolet radiation and hormonal influences in the development of melasma. J Eur Acad Dermatol Venereol. 2009;23:1254–64.
4. Handel AC, Miot LDB, Miot HA. Melasma: a clinical and epidemiological review. An Bras Dermatol. 2014;89(5):771–82.
5. Sanchez NP, Pathak MA, Sato S, Fitzpatrick TB, Sanchez JL, Mihm Jr MC. Melasma: a clinical, light microscopic, ultrastructural and immunofluorescence study. J Am Acad Dermatol. 1981;4:698–710.
6. Vasquez M, Maldonado H, Benaman C, Sanchez JL. Melasma in men: a clinical and histologic study. Int J Dermatol. 1988;27:25–7.
7. Ingber A, editor. Obstetric dermatology: a practical guide. Springer: Berlin Heideberg; 2009. p. 7–18.
8. Pagan RM, Sanchez JL. Clinical studies, Mandibular melasma. PRHSJ. 2000;19(3):231–4.
9. O'Brien TJ, Dyall-Smith D, Hall AP. Melasma of the forearms. Aust J Dermatol. 1997;38:35–7.
10. Taylor SC, Torok H, Jones T, Lowe N, Rich P, Tschen E, et al. Efficacy and safety of a new triple-combination agent for the treatment of facial melasma. Cutis. 2003;72:67–72.
11. Pandya A, Berneburg M, Ortonne JP, Picardo M. Guidelines for clinical trials in melasma. Br J Dermatol. 2007;156(S1):21–8.
12. Majid I, Haq I, Imran S, Keen A, Aziz K, Arif T. Proposing melasma severity index: a new, more practice, office-based scoring system for assessing the severity of melasma. Ind J Dermatol. 2016;16(1):39–44.

13. Gilchrest BA, Fitzpatrick TB, Anderson RR, Parrish JA. Localization of melanin pigmentation in the skin with woods light. Br J Dermatol. 1977;96:245–8.
14. Tamler C, Fonseca RMB, Pereira FBC, Barcaul CB. Classification of melasma by dermoscopy: comparative study with Woods lamp. Surg Cosm Dermatol. 2009;1(3):115–9.
15. Stolz W, Schiffner R, Burgdorf WHC. Dermoscopy for facial pigmented skin lesions. Clin Dermatol. 2009;20:276–8.
16. Liu H, Lin Y, Nie X, Chen S, Chen X, Shi B, Tian H. Histologic classification of melasma with reflectance confocal microscopy: a pilot study in Chinese patients. Skin Res Tech Hol. 2011;17(4):398–403.
17. Costa MC, Eljaiek HV, Abraham LS, Azulay-Abulafia L, Ardigo M. In vivo reflectance confocal Microscopy in a typical case of melasma. An Bras Dermatol. 2012;87(5):782–4.
18. Kang HY, Ortonne JP. What should be considered in treatment of melasma. Ann Dermatol. 2010;22(4):373–8.
19. Melasma. The BMJ Best Practice. us.bestpractice.bmj.com/best-practice/monograph/627.html Accessed 12 Dec 2015.
20. Kang WH, Yoon KH, Lee ES, Kim J, Lee KB, Yim H. Melasma: histopathological characteristics in 56 Korean patients. Br J Dermatol. 2002;146:228–37.

Chapter 6
Diagnosis of Melasma in Brown Skin: Wood's Lamp, Dermoscopy, and Confocal Microscopy

Sai Yee Chuah and Tien Guan Steven Thng

6.1 Introduction

The diagnosis of melasma is usually made clinically due to its characteristic appearance. In addition to the clinical classification based upon distribution pattern (Fig. 6.1a–c), melasma has also been subdivided into four subtypes based on different depths of melanin pigment [1]. The use of additional tools such as Wood's lamp, dermoscopy, and reflectance confocal microscopy (RCM) can help in the classification of melasma into epidermal, dermal, mixed, and indeterminate subtype. These classifications aid in prognosis and prediction of the therapeutic outcome [2–4]. In general, epidermal type of melasma responds slightly better to treatment than those with dermal type of melasma [5].

6.2 Wood's Lamp

Wood's lamp is an ultraviolet light A of long wavelength which emits wavelength between 340 and 400 nm with a peak at 365 nm [6, 7]. It is the most widely used method of melasma classification by highlighting the difference in pigmentation of the affected skin into four subtypes: epidermal, dermal, mixed, and indeterminate [2, 3, 8].

S.Y. Chuah (✉) • T.G.S. Thng
Department of Dermatology, National Skin Centre,
1 Mandalay Road, Singapore 308205, Singapore
e-mail: sychuah@nsc.com.sg; steventhng@nsc.com.sg

E.B. Handog, M.J. Enriquez-Macarayo (eds.), *Melasma and Vitiligo in Brown Skin*,
DOI 10.1007/978-81-322-3664-1_6

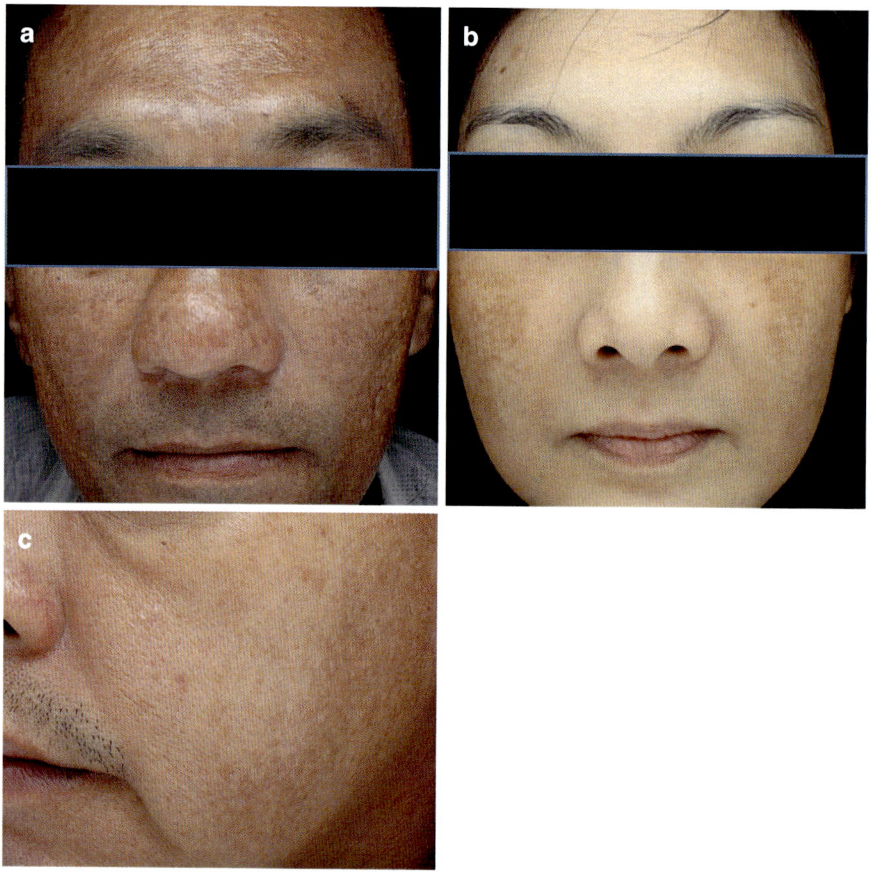

Fig. 6.1 Clinical Classification of melasma based on distribution pattern. (**a**) Centrofacial melasma, (**b**) malar melasma, and (**c**) mandibular melasma

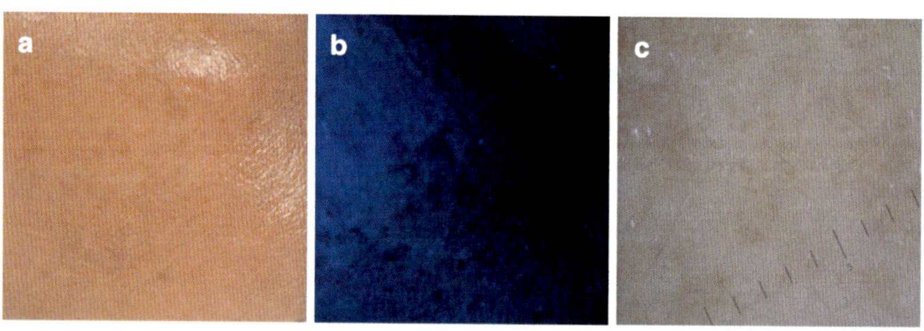

Fig. 6.2 (**a**) Epidermal melasma on the right cheek. (**b**) Wood's lamp showed enhanced pigmented areas. (**c**) Dermoscopy showing dispersed reticular brown pigmentation

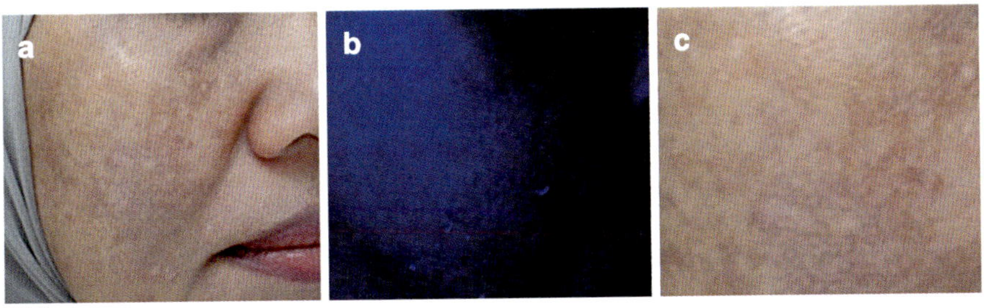

Fig. 6.3 (**a**) Dermal melasma on the right cheek. (**b**) Wood's lamp showed non-enhanced pigmented areas. (**c**) Dermoscopy showing diffuse dark brown to grayish pseudoreticular pigmentation

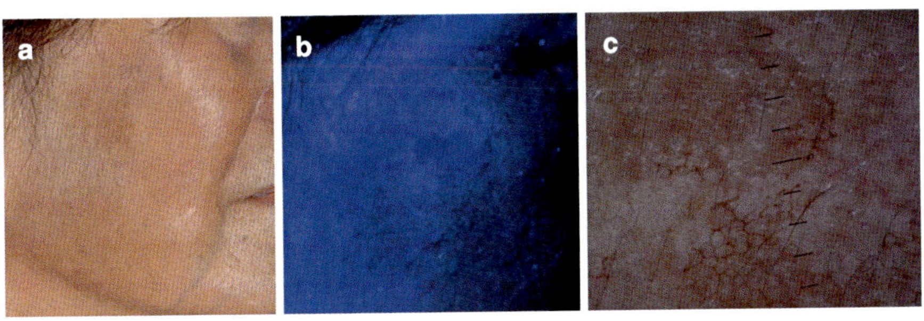

Fig. 6.4 (**a**) Mixed type of melasma on the right cheek. (**b**) Wood's lamp showed both enhanced and non-enhanced pigmented areas. (**c**) Dermoscopy showing both diffuses reticular brown pigmentation with sparing of follicular openings and diffuses dark brown to grayish pseudoreticular pigmentation

The pigmented areas that are enhanced when viewed under a Wood's lamp imply increased epidermal melanin content (epidermal subtype) (Fig. 6.2b), whereas those that are not enhanced imply an increased in dermal melanin content (dermal subtype) (Fig. 6.3b). The pigmented areas that have both enhancing and non-enhancing areas imply a mixed subtype of melasma (Fig. 6.4b). For those with darker skin type V and VI, their melasma will not be evident under Wood's lamp examination, and hence, this is classified as indeterminate subtype. Many patients have a mixture of these subtypes of melasma [1–3].

Recent histopathological studies suggested that Wood's light examination may not be accurate in determining the depth of pigment [2, 8–10]. Despite Wood's lamp evaluation indicating epidermal melasma in some patients, the biopsy specimens from both the lesional and perilesional skin examined by Grimes et al. and Kang et al. showed that there was increased melanin deposition in both epidermis and dermis. Therefore, patients with apparent epidermal melasma after a Wood's lamp examination may have significant melanin in the dermis. The presence of dermal melanin and melanophages in these studies may explain the difficulty in treating patients with apparent epidermal melasma [1, 2, 9, 10].

6.3 Dermoscopy

Dermoscopy is a noninvasive optical equipment that permits a variable magnification from 6 to 400 times. It is a proven reliable tool for direct visualization of skin pigmentation including melasma as it has been shown to be useful to observe pigment components as well as their position on the skin layers [11–14]. The color intensity of melanin and the regularity of the pigment network depend on the quantity or density and the location of melanin.

When the melanin is located in the stratum corneum, it appears as black or dark brown in color with well-defined network. When the melanin is located in the lower layers of the epidermis, the color will appear as shades of light brown, and the pigment network will appear irregular. Dermoscopy of melanin located in the dermis will appear blue or bluish-gray color with pseudoreticular network. The follicular openings are spared throughout the level of pigmentation [12–15]. Therefore, melasma is considered epidermal when a regular pigment network, with a brownish homogeneous pigmentation, is observed (Fig. 6.2c), and it is considered dermal when an irregular and mixed network with bluish-gray pigmentation is observed (Fig. 6.3c). Finally, the melasma is considered a mixed subtype when the areas show both features (Fig. 6.4c).

Additionally, dermoscopy allows observation of a vascular component (Fig. 6.5), which is present in many patients with melasma, as reported in recent literature [15–17]. An immunohistochemistry study demonstrated a significant increase in the number and size of dermal blood vessels in the lesional skin of melasma [16]. It has also been suggested that the number of vessels is positively related to the degree of pigmentation, which is also reported in other studies which state that the deoxyhemoglobin contributes significantly to the skin color [16–18].

Based on the principles of dermoscopic examination, some dermatologists may consider this method more appropriate and helpful for routine diagnosis, assessment,

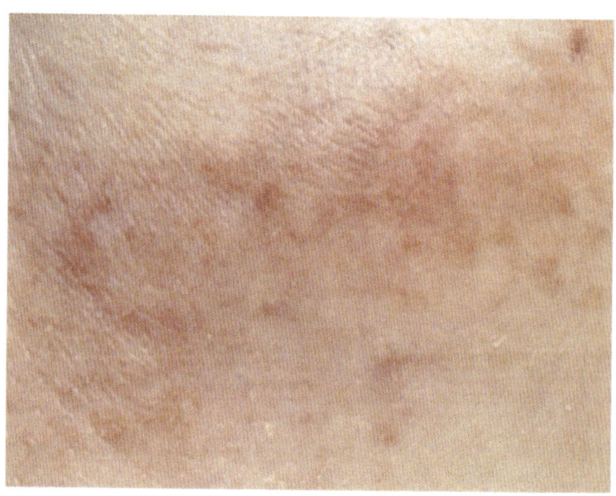

Fig. 6.5 Epidermal melasma with vascular component. Dermoscopy on the left cheek melasma showing diffuse brown pigmentation with fine telangiectasias

and monitoring of patients with melasma when compared to Wood's lamp examination. This may be due to the fact that dermoscopy examination allows an objective classification of melasma by providing an accurate observation of the color of melanin which is not affected by factors such as the patient's skin phototype, vascular and collagen changes, or the use of topical products [15].

6.4 Reflectance Confocal Microscopy

In the recent years, various noninvasive imaging tools such as high-frequency ultrasonography, optical coherence tomography, magnetic resonance imaging, and reflectance confocal microscopy (RCM) have been developed to provide additional information that is not readily available through mere clinical inspection. All these imaging tools are noninvasive and can provide both real-time diagnostics and also the possibility of following the progression of skin lesions or conditions over time.

Among these new techniques, RCM has emerged to be a novel noninvasive imaging technique that can provide real-time in vivo examination of the skin up to the level of the papillary dermis while providing a cellular resolution comparable with histology. In a confocal microscope, near-infrared light from a diode laser (830 nm) is focused on a microscopic skin target. As this light passes between cellular structures with different refraction indexes generated mainly by keratin, melanin, hemoglobin, and cellular organelles, it is naturally reflected, captured, and recomposed into a two-dimensional gray scale image by computer software [19–21]. This technique has been used for the evaluation of several inflammatory, neoplastic, and melanocytic skin conditions and may constitute an excellent alternative to invasive skin biopsy in the diagnosis of several skin disorders [22–26].

As melanin is the best endogenous contrast agent in the pigmented skin, which causes strong backscattering, this would allow precise identification of melanocytes, pigmented keratinocytes, and melanophages. A few studies reported the role of RCM in the classification of melasma and found good correlation with histology [27–30]. The distributions of melanin were found to be located at all the different levels of the melasma lesion (epidermis, dermoepidermal junction (DEJ), and upper dermis). At the level of the epidermis, increased pigmentation or melanin was observed as highly refractile keratinocytes distributed within the spinous layer and basal layer. At the DEJ, the presence of strongly visible papillary rings around the dermal papillae composed by a sequence of bright cellular structures was observed, corresponding to activated melanocytes and junctional keratinocytes receiving packed melanosomes. At the superficial dermis, an abnormal presence of round or polygonal refractile structures within dermal collagen bundles was observed. These structures were consistent with melanophages filled with melanin originating in the DEJ [27, 29, 30].

Based on the distribution of melanin, RCM has classified melasma into epidermal type if the distribution of increased melanin was observed only in the epidermis (Fig. 6.6a, b) and mixed type if the distribution of increased melanin was observed

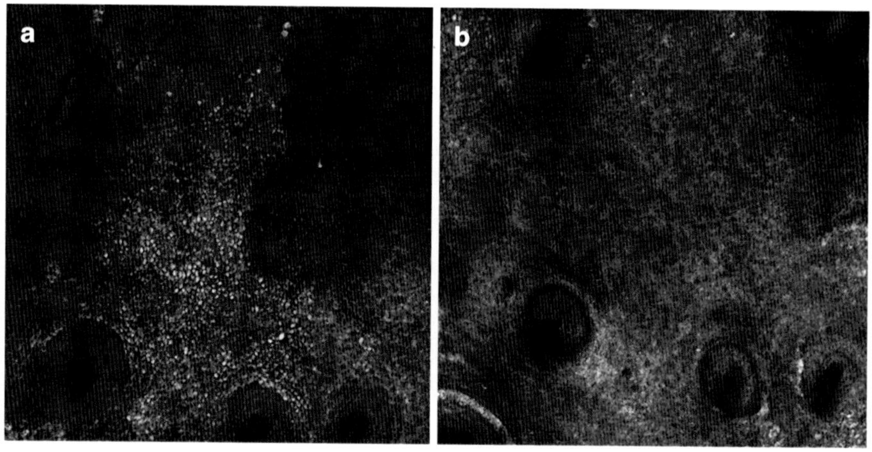

Fig. 6.6 RCM showing epidermal type of melasma. (**a**) RCM showing highly refractile keratinocytes with cobblestone pattern distributed within the spinous layer and basal layer. (**b**) There are no plump bright cells seen at the dermal layer

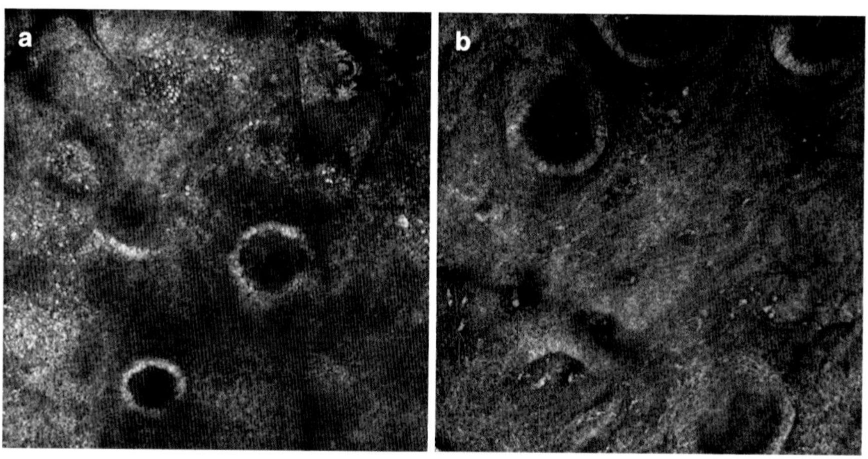

Fig. 6.7 RCM showing mixed type of melasma. (**a**) There are highly refractile keratinocytes with cobblestone pattern distributed within the spinous layer and basal layer. (**b**) There were scattered plump bright cells at the dermal layer (*red arrow*)

in both epidermis and dermis (Fig. 6.7a, b). No genuine dermal type of melasma has been found in RCM studies [27, 29, 30]. This differs from the traditional Wood's lamp classification of epidermal, dermal, mixed, and indeterminate subtypes. Wood's lamp technique is not microscopic, but based on the quantification of the different levels of fluorescence according to the depth of the pigment, and does not take into account the contributions of different layers. Hence, it has been shown to have questionable accuracy when compared histologically [2, 8–10, 27]. Ardigo et al. also found no correlation between the classification of melasma using Wood's lamp and RCM [27]. For example, there were cases classified as an epidermal melasma using the Wood's lamp, but RCM imaging revealed pigmentation both in the epidermis and dermis.

Treatment of melasma is challenging. As lightening creams such as hydroquinone target epidermal melanin, determination of pigment depth is helpful to predict the outcome. With more accurate classification of melasma using RCM, this can help in refining the prognosis of melasma. Furthermore, the ability to evaluate large areas of melasma noninvasively has made this tool useful in monitoring response to therapy more objectively [27, 29–32].

6.5 Conclusions

The classification of melasma is important not only to prognosticate melasma but to aid clinicians to decide on the management plans and to predict the therapeutic outcome. Traditionally, Wood's lamp is used to classify melasma into four subtypes: epidermal, dermal, mixed, and indeterminate. However, recent histopathological studies suggested that Wood's lamp examination may not be accurate in determining the depth of pigment.

Dermoscopy examination allows an objective classification of melasma by providing an accurate observation of the color of melanin. The color intensity of melanin and the regularity of the pigment network depend on the quantity or density and the location of melanin. Additionally, dermoscopy allows observation of a vascular component, which has been reported to be present in some cases of melasma. Some dermatologists may consider this method more appropriate and helpful for routine diagnosis, assessment, and monitoring of patients with melasma when compared to Wood's lamp examination.

Recently, RCM has been shown to be an invaluable noninvasive imaging tool that can provide real-time in vivo examination of melasma lesion with good correlation with histology. RCM classifies melasma into epidermal and mixed subtype with no true dermal subtype being observed. It has proven to be accurate in melasma classification and, hence, bears promise for the noninvasive management, follow-up, and monitoring of the response to therapy. However, one needs training to analyze the RCM image, and this tool may not be available in all dermatological centers.

References

1. Sanchez NP, Pathak MA, Sato S, Fitzpatrick TB, Sanchez JL, Mihm Jr MC. Melasma: a clinical, light microscopic, ultrastructural, and immunofluorescence study. J Am Acad Dermatol. 1981;4:698–709.
2. Sheth VM, Pandya AG. Melasma: a comprehensive update: part I. J Am Acad Dermatol. 2011;65(4):689–97.

3. Sarkar R, Arora P, Garg VK, Sonthalia S, Gokhale N. Melasma update. Indian Dermatol Online J. 2014;5(4):426–35.
4. Handel AC, Miot LD, Miot HA. Melasma: a clinical and epidemiological review. An Bras Dermatol. 2014;89(5):771–82.
5. Goh CL, Dlova CN. A retrospective study on the clinical presentation and treatment outcome of melasma in a tertiary dermatological referral centre in Singapore. Singapore Med J. 1999; 40:455–8.
6. Gilchrest BA, Fitzpatrick TB, Anderson RR, Parrish JA. Localization of melanin pigmentation in the skin with Wood's lamp. Br J Dermatol. 1977;96:245–8.
7. Asawanonda P, Taylor CR. Wood's light in dermatology. Int J Dermatol. 1999;38:801–7.
8. Katsambas A, Antoniou C. Melasma. Classification and treatment. J Eur Acad Dermatol Venereol. 1995;4:217–23.
9. Grimes PE, Yamada N, Bhawan J. Light microscopic, immunohistochemical, and ultrastructural alterations in patients with melasma. Am J Dermatopathol. 2005;27:96–101.
10. Kang WH, Yoon KH, Lee ES, Kim J, Lee KB, Yim H, et al. Melasma: histopathological characteristics in 56 Korean patients. Br J Dermatol. 2002;146:228–37.
11. Stolz W, Schiffner R, Burgdorf WHC. Dermatoscopy for facial pigmented skin lesions. Clin Dermatol. 2002;20:276–8.
12. Braun RP, Rabinovitz HS, Oliviero M, Kopf AW, Saurat JH. Dermoscopy of pigmented skin lesions. J Am Acad Dermatol. 2005;52:109–21.
13. Weismann K, Lorentzen HF. Dermoscopic color perspective. Arch Dermatol. 2006;142:1250.
14. Piccolo D, Fargnoli MC, Ferrara G, Lozzi GP, Altamura D, Ventura T, et al. Hypoepiluminescence microscopy of pigmented skin lesions: new approach to improve recognition of dermoscopic structures. Dermatol Surg. 2006;32:1391–97.
15. Tamler C, Fonseca RMR, Pereira FBC, Barcaui CB. Classification of melasma by dermoscopy: comparative study with Wood's lamp. Surg Cosmetic Dermatol. 2009;1(3):115–9.
16. Kim EH, Kim YC, Lee ES, Kang HY. The vascular characteristics of melasma. J Dermatol Sci. 2007;46(2):111–6.
17. Stamatas GN, Kollias N. Blood stasis contributions to the perception of skin pigmentation. J Biomed Opt. 2004;9(2):315–22.
18. Kim EJ, Park HY, Yaar M, Gilchrest BA. Modulation of vascular endothelial growth factor receptors in melanocytes. Exp Dermatol. 2005;14:625–33.
19. Gonzalez S, Gilaberte-Calzada Y. In vivo reflectance-mode confocal microscopy in clinical dermatology and cosmetology. Int J Cosmet Sci. 2008;30:1–17.
20. Rajadhyaksha M, Gonzalez S, Zavislan JM, Anderson RR, Webb RH. In vivo confocal scanning laser microscopy of human skin II: advances in instrumentation and comparison with histology. J Invest Dermatol. 1999;113:293–303.
21. Rajadhyaksha M, Grossman M, Esterowitz D, Webb RH, Anderson RR. In vivo confocal scanning laser microscopy of human skin: melanin provides strong contrast. J Invest Dermatol. 1995;104:946–52.
22. Ardigo M, Malizewski I, Cota C, Scope A, Sacerdoti G, Gonzalez S, et al. Preliminary evaluation of in vivo reflectance confocal microscopy features of discoid lupus erythematosus. Br J Dermatol. 2007;156:1196–203.
23. Ardigo M, Malizewski I, Dell'anna ML, Berardesca E, Picardo MI. Preliminary evaluation of vitiligo using reflectance confocal microscopy. J Eur Acad Dermatol Venereol. 2007;21:1344–50.
24. Pellacani G, Longo C, Malvehy J, Puig S, Carrera C, Sequra S, et al. In vivo confocal microscopic and histopathologic correlations of dermoscopic features in 202 melanocytic lesions. Arch Dermatol. 2008;144:1597–608.
25. Middelkamp-Hup MA, Park HY, Lee J, Gilchrest BA, Gonzalez S. Detection of UV-induced pigmentary and epidermal changes over time using in vivo reflectance confocal microscopy. J Invest Dermatol. 2006;126:402–7.
26. Gonzalez S, Rajadhyaksha M, Rubinstein G, Anderson RR. Characterization of psoriasis in vivo by reflectance confocal microscopy. J Med. 1999;30:337–56.

27. Ardigo M, Cameli N, Berardesca E, Gonzalez S. Characterization and evaluation of pigment distribution and response to therapy in melasma using in vivo reflectance confocal microscopy: a preliminary study. J Eur Acad Dermatol Venereol. 2010;24:1296–303.
28. Kang HY, Bahadoran P, Suzuki I, Zugai D, Khemis A, Passeron T, et al. In vivo reflectance confocal microscopy detects pigmentary changes in melasma at a cellular level resolution. Exp Dermatol. 2010;19:e228–33.
29. Liu H, Lin Y, Nie X, Chen S, Chen X, Shi B, et al. Histological classification of melasma with reflectance confocal microscopy: a pilot study in Chinese patients. Skin Res Technol. 2011;17:398–403.
30. Kang HY, Bahadoran P. Application of in vivo reflectance confocal microscopy in melasma classification. J Am Acad Dermatol. 2012;67:157.
31. Costa MC, Eljaiek HV, Abraham LS, Azulay-Abulafia L, Adigo M. In vivo reflectance confocal microscopy in a typical case of melasma. An Bras Dermatol. 2012;87:782–4.
32. Funasaka Y, Mayumi N, Ayasama S, Takayama R, Kosaka M, Kato T, et al. In vivo reflectance confocal microscopy for skin imaging in melasma. J Nippon Med Sch. 2013;80(3):172–3.

Chapter 7
The Histopathology of Melasma in Brown Skin

Johannes F. Dayrit

7.1 Histopathology of Melasma

Racial variations exist in terms of epidermal melanin content and melanosome distribution in pigmented skin compared with fair-skinned individuals [1]. Melanosomes in darker skin types are distributed throughout the entire epidermis with dense clusters in the basal layer [2–4]. In contradistinction, fewer melanosomes in the basal cell layer are observed in fair-skinned individuals [5, 6]. It has been established, however, that there are no differences in melanocyte density among races [7].

Histopathological studies of Grimes et al. [8] and Kang et al. [9] demonstrated an increased amount of melanin in all epidermal layers in melasma skin (Figs. 7.1 and 7.2). A 61 % and 83 % increase in epidermal hyperpigmentation were demonstrated in lesional skin of 11 patients with Fitzpatrick skin types IV to VI and 56 Korean melasma patients, respectively [8, 9]. Fontana-Masson and an immunohistochemical stain NK1-beteb were both utilized to highlight epidermal hyperpigmentation and detect melanocytes present in the epidermis and dermis [8, 9]. The intensity of staining and number of epidermal melanocytes are increased in melasma lesions in contrast to perilesional normal skin. No difference in melanocyte number between lesional and non-lesional skin was observed which validates the findings of Szabo [7]. Ultrastructurally, lesional melanocytes had more mitochondria, Golgi apparatus, rough endoplasmic reticulum, and ribosomes in

J.F. Dayrit (✉)
Department of Dermatology, Research Institute for Tropical Medicine, Muntinlupa, Philippines

Department of Internal Medicine, De La Salle University Medical Center, Dasmariñas, Philippines
e-mail: yohannmdderm@gmail.com

E.B. Handog, M.J. Enriquez-Macarayo (eds.), *Melasma and Vitiligo in Brown Skin*, DOI 10.1007/978-81-322-3664-1_7

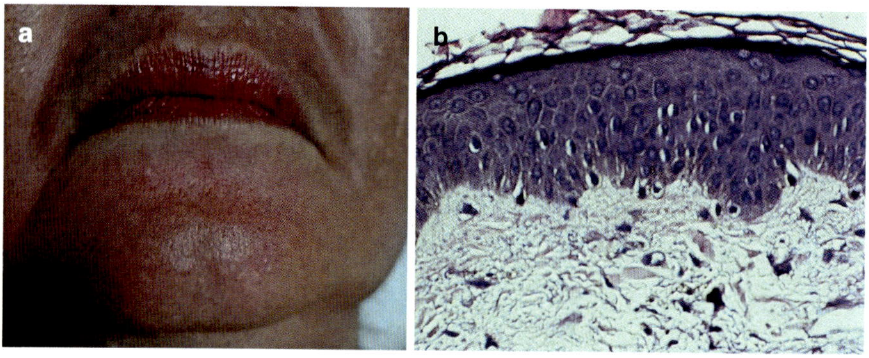

Fig. 7.1 Clinical picture of melasma where biopsy was performed (**a**) and histopathology (**b**) showing larger melanocytes in the epidermis accompanied by solar elastosis, sparse lymphocytic infiltrate, and few pigment-laden macrophages in the dermis (H&E, ×400)

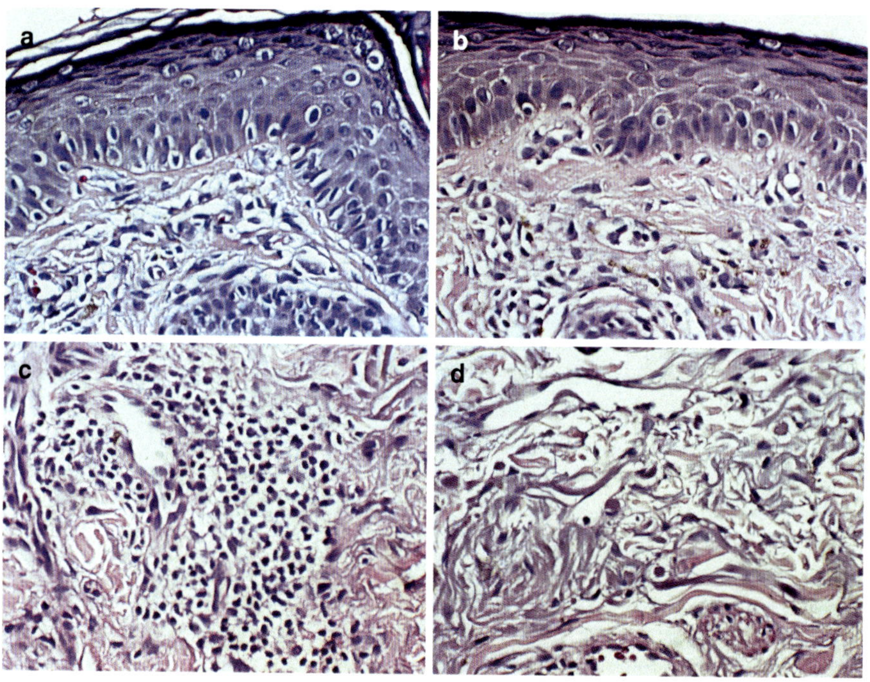

Fig. 7.2 Histopathological findings of melasma characterized by (**a**) large melanocytes in the epidermis, (**b**) pigment-laden macrophages in the papillary dermis, (**c**) perivascular lymphocytic infiltrate, and (**d**) solar elastosis (H&E ×400)

their cytoplasm [9]. The melanocytes in the hyperpigmented areas were larger intensely stained cells with very prominent dendrites (Fig. 7.3) [8, 9].

Electron microscopy revealed more melanosomes in keratinocytes, melanocytes, and dendrites in the involved skin, in comparison to the uninvolved skin. Miot et al.

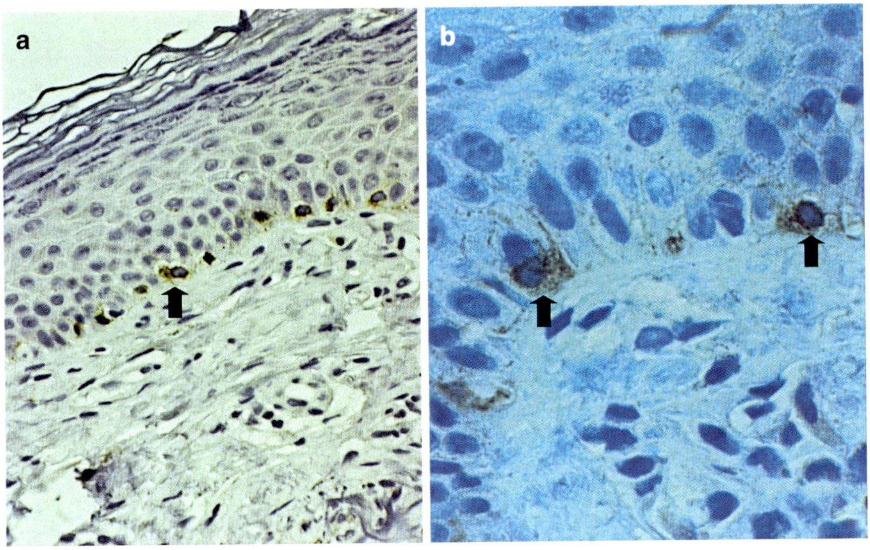

Fig. 7.3 Immunohistochemical marker Melan-A highlights larger, intensely staining melanocytes (*arrow*) in the basal cell layer (H&E ×400 (**a**), H&E ×1000 (**b**))

[10] demonstrated similar findings of greater epidermal melanin in the epidermis. In addition, dermal findings include a mild lymphohistiocytic infiltrate and solar elastosis in lesional melasma skin. A mild lymphohistiocytic infiltrate in 75 % of hyperpigmented areas was likewise observed by Grimes et al. [8]. Pigment-laden macrophages were present both in melasma lesional and perilesional normal skin in 36 % of Korean patients and in all 11 melasma patients of Fitzpatrick skin types IV to VI [8, 9]. The degrees of basement membrane damage and vascularization have not been extensively studied and warrant further investigation.

Presently, few conclusions can be drawn from evaluating all light microscopic, immunohistochemical, and ultrastructural alterations in patients with melasma: (1) that melasma is a consequence of specific hyperfunctional melanocytes that cause excessive melanin deposition in the epidermis and dermis and (2) that melasma is characterized by epidermal hyperpigmentation with or without melanophages and raising the question if there is indeed a "dermal variant" [7–9].

7.2 Histopathology of Ochronosis

Two cases of hydroquinone-induced ochronosis in two Filipinos with Fitzpatrick skin type IV showed on histology numerous fragmented reddish-brown fibers in various configurations, some of which appear crescentic or "banana shaped." Swelling and homogenization of collagen bundles are seen in the papillary and reticular dermis. The blood vessels are telangiectatic and mild solar elastosis is seen (Fig. 7.4) [11, 12].

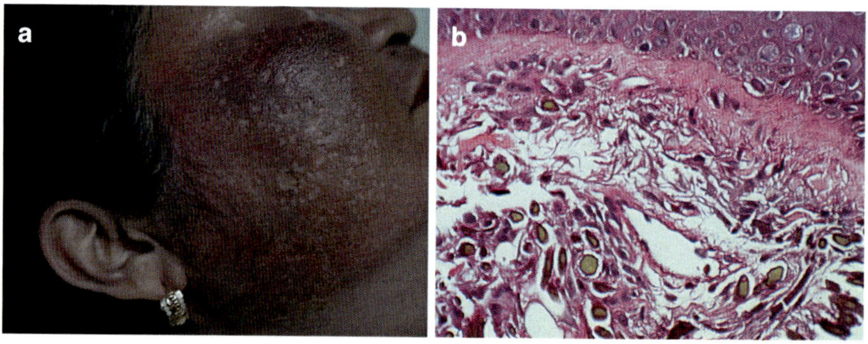

Fig. 7.4 Hydroquinone-induced ochronosis in a Filipino (**a**) and histopathological findings (**b**) of yellowish-brown-colored material in the dermis accompanied by solar elastosis, mild lymphocytic infiltrate, and pigment-laden macrophages (H&E ×400)

Early lesions show basophilic and swollen collagen fibers before developing the characteristic yellow ochronotic morphology. Fully developed lesions are characterized by focal collections of refringent, yellow-brown, sharply defined, irregularly shaped, and frequently fragmented fibers in the superficial dermis. There is often coexisting mild solar elastosis [13, 14]. Depigmentation of epidermal melanocytes is usually associated with pigment-laden macrophages in the papillary dermis [15]. Pigment granules are often present in the epithelium and basement membrane of sweat glands, in endothelial cells, and within dermal macrophages [16]. In chronic lesions, large amorphous eosinophilic granules may develop, resembling colloid milium [17]. An infiltrate of histiocytes is present focally in relation to some of the deposits [14]. The granulomatous reaction is believed to contain and selectively destroy the fragments of ochronotic fibers. Occasionally ochronotic material can be identified in giant cells [18].

Electron microscopic studies have shown electron-dense ochronotic bodies embedded in a granular material infiltrating the adjacent collagen bundles. The swollen collagen fibrils characteristically lose their banding pattern, subsequently degenerate, and are replaced by amorphous ochronotic pigments. The fibrils rupture and the pigments scatter free in the dermis. These pigments are phagocytosed later on by macrophages and giant cells [18–20].

7.3 Histopathology of Dermal Melanocytosis (Acquired Bilateral Nevus of Ota-Like Macules (ABNOM) or Hori's Macules, Nevus of Ota, and Sun's Nevus)

Dermal melanocytoses comprise a variety of congenital and acquired conditions characterized by a sparse population of intradermal dendritic, variably pigmented, spindle-shaped melanocytes, with or without the presence of dermal melanophages. These forms of facial melanoses are most commonly found in the skin of Asians and

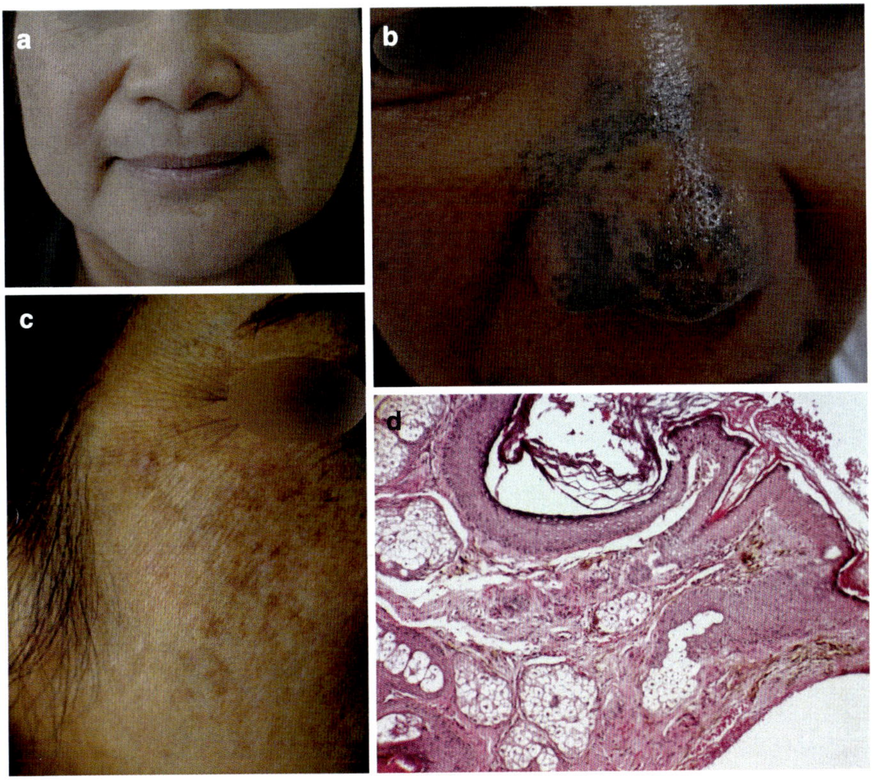

Fig. 7.5 Clinical photos of ABNOM (**a**, **b**), acquired nevus of Ota/dermal melanocytosis, (**c**) and histopathological findings (**d**) of heavily pigmented, spindle-shaped melanocytes in the dermis (H&E ×100)

other darkly pigmented people. Nevus of Ota, acquired bilateral nevus of Ota-like macules (ABNOM), and acquired unilateral nevus of Ota, also known as Sun's nevus, represent distinct types of dermal melanocytosis occurring on the face [21, 22].

ABNOM shares similarities to melasma with regard to clinical features, including female preponderance, acquired onset, and principal involvement of the malar area [23]. However, the histopathological elements are distinct. Controversy still exists whether what was previously thought of as dermal melasma is actually ABNOM or other forms of dermal melanocytoses.

Lee et al. [24] compared the histopathological characteristics of ABNOM with nevus of Ota using hematoxylin and eosin, GP-100 (NK1-beteb), and Fontana-Masson stains. In the epidermis, there was no difference in the density of melanocytes and pigments between ABNOM and nevus of Ota. In the dermis, the differences between ABNOM and nevus of Ota have been documented. The spindle-shaped melanocytes in ABNOM were concentrated perivascularly in the superficial dermis. In contradistinction, the spindle-shaped melanocytes in nevus of Ota were more numerous and distributed interstitially in both the superficial and deep dermis. The long axis of these melanocytes was oriented parallel to the collagen bundles (Fig. 7.5).

Lee et al. [23] also demonstrated that solar elastosis is slightly more prominent in the lesional skin of ABNOM. The increased dermal expression of stem cell factor (SCF) and c-kit in ABNOM may suggest a possible role in the pathogenesis of this pigmentary disorder.

The degree of melanin pigmentation and number and distribution of melanocytes per unit area in the epidermis and dermis were not significantly different in ABNOM as compared to extrafacial forms of acquired dermal melanocytosis suggesting that both diseases form part of the same disease spectrum [25].

7.4 Histopathology of Ashy Dermatosis, Erythema Dyschromicum Perstans, and Lichen Planus Pigmentosus

Ashy dermatosis (AD), erythema dyschromicum perstans (EDP), and lichen planus pigmentosus (LPP) present as acquired macules and patches of hyperpigmentation. The etiology and pathogenesis of each disease remains an enigma; thus, there is no effective widely accepted treatment. The clinical features overlap and racial variations may exist. The diseases share common histological features but subtle differences have been noted.

Salient histological features of ashy dermatosis from the original study of Ramirez [26, 27] were liquefaction degeneration of the basal layer with a perivascular infiltrate of histiocytes, some lymphocytes, and melanin-laden macrophages (Fig. 7.6). A lichenoid tissue reaction pattern was likewise observed in "erythema dyschromicum perstans" when the disease was introduced by Convit et al. in 1961 [28].

Bhutani et al. [29] reported 40 cases in India with lesions similar to those described by Ramirez. However, clinical and histological findings in one-third of patients had association with lichen planus; they named them lichen planus pigmentosus. It is believed to be a macular variant of lichen planus and more recent observations show that it usually starts on the face, neck, and earlobes. It is usually associated with pruritus and oral mucosal involvement is seen [30]. The histopathological findings have similarities to lichen planus (Fig. 7.7).

Controversy exists regarding the relationship of AD, EDP, and LPP based on clinical and histopathological features. Pinkus [31, 32] included ashy dermatosis and atrophic lichen planus in the same section of his classification of "lichenoid tissue patterns" because of their histologic similarities. Novick and Phelps [33] suggested that EDP is a variant of lichen planus. On the other hand, Vega et al. [34] reviewed 20 cases of AD and 11 cases of LPP in 1992. They distinguished these two entities despite similar histopathologic findings and believed that ashy dermatosis predominates in type IV skin, and there are probably some undefined ecological and nutritional conditions that are not applicable to other races or countries in North America and Europe.

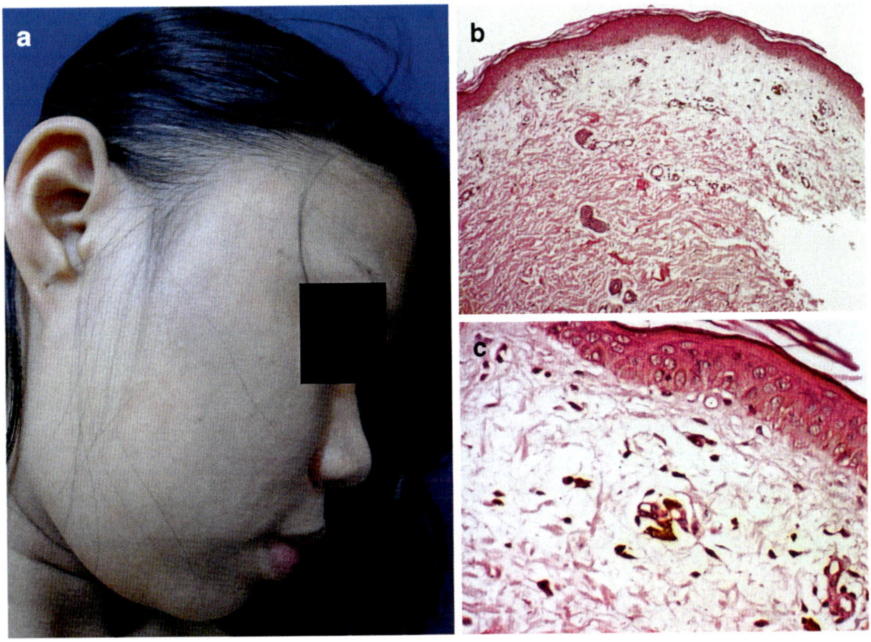

Fig. 7.6 Ashy dermatosis in a Filipino (**a**) and histopathological findings (**b**, **c**) of subtle vacuolar change in the basal layer and prominent pigment incontinence in the dermis (H&E ×100 (**b**), ×400 (**c**))

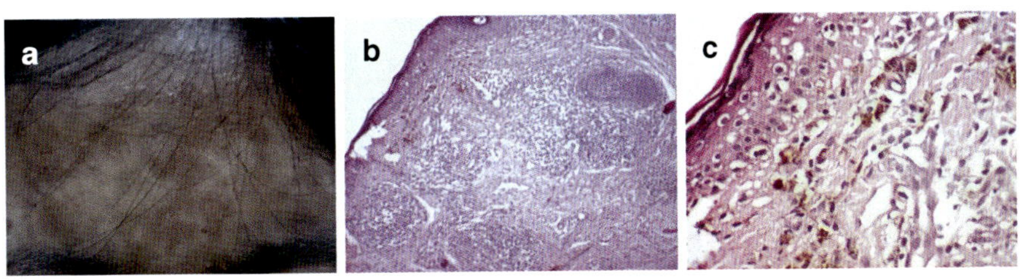

Fig. 7.7 Lichen planus pigmentosus in a Filipino (**a**) and histopathological findings of (**b**) a lichenoid and periadnexal dermal infiltrate (H&E ×100), (**c**) prominent vacuolar alteration of the basal layer with Civatte bodies, and numerous pigment-laden macrophages (H & E ×400)

To differentiate AD from EDP, Weedon [35] recently proposed that the term EDP should be used in cases where lesions have or have previously had an erythematous border, while AD should be used for other cases where the "erythematous feature" is lacking. Histologically, EDP shows a patchy vacuolar alteration of the epidermis, pigment incontinence, and moderately dense lymphocytic infiltrate of lymphocytes. In contrast, AD reveals atrophy of the epidermis with subtle vacuolar alteration of the basal cell layer, marked melanin incontinence, and mild infiltrate referred to as "burnt-out" appearance [35]. The "burnt-out" appearance is commonly used to describe post-inflammatory pigmentary alteration following interface dermatitis such as in lichen planus, lupus erythematosus, erythema multiforme, and lichenoid drug eruptions.

The erythematous component of EDP demonstrates a vacuolar alteration of the basal cell layer, the presence of occasional colloid bodies, pigment-laden macrophages, and a perivascular infiltrate of lymphocytes and histiocytes. In the hyperpigmented macules and patches, pigment incontinence is a more prominent histological finding, while the vacuolar change in the basal cell layer and the lymphohistiocytic infiltrate in the dermis may only be mild or absent [36].

The histopathological findings of LPP is characterized by an atrophic epidermis with vacuolar alteration of the basal layer; a scarce lymphohistiocytic or lichenoid infiltrate with incontinence of pigment and the presence of melanophages are seen in the dermis [34].

For LPP, a biopsy of a raised lesion shows typical lichen planus pathology characterized by saw toothing of the rete ridges, wedge-shaped hypergranulosis, vacuolar alteration of the basal layer, Civatte bodies, and lichenoid lymphocytic infiltrate. A biopsy of a macule, on the other hand, reveals a relatively flat epidermis with loss of the rete pattern, focal vacuolar change with occasional necrotic keratinocytes and Civatte bodies, dermal melanophages, and lymphocytic infiltrate [33]. The lichenoid inflammatory infiltrate, which is often focal and peri-infundibular, is a helpful histological feature which may differentiate LPP from either EDP or AD.

7.5 Histopathology of Riehl's Melanosis/Pigmented Contact Dermatitis

Riehl's melanosis is a nonpruritic brownish-gray pigmentation that develops rapidly over the face, more intense on the forehead and the temples. It often has a reticulated pattern. The condition is believed to be associated with contact sensitivity to cosmetics or to a photocontact dermatitis resulting from fragrances in cosmetics. Musk ambrette, lemon oil, and some bactericidal compounds present in cosmetics have been known to cause "pigmented cosmetic dermatitis" in Japan, which is similar to Riehl's melanosis [37, 38]. Optical whiteners from detergents, formaldehyde, and azo dyes have also been implicated in occupationally related pigmented contact dermatitis. Most patients presented with no preceding eczematous lesions [39, 40].

Histopathological findings from Riehl's melanosis reveal epidermal atrophy, vacuolar alteration of the basal cell layer, pigment incontinence, and dermal lymphohistiocytic infiltrate. Spongiosis is absent and periodic acid Schiff stain shows a thickened basal layer (Fig. 7.8) [37, 41].

7.6 Histopathology of Minocycline-Induced Hyperpigmentation

Minocycline hyperpigmentation presents in patients on long-term treatment for acne, rosacea, or leprosy. Three distinct types occur: *type I*, blue-black macules on areas of current or previous inflammation; *type II*, blue-gray pigment on the shins and forearms; and *type III*, diffuse muddy-brown discoloration sun-exposed areas [42–44].

The histopathological features of the three different types of minocycline pigmentation are variable (Fig. 7.9). *Types I* and *II* show normal density of melanin pigmentation in the epidermal melanocytes. *Type III* shows more pronounced

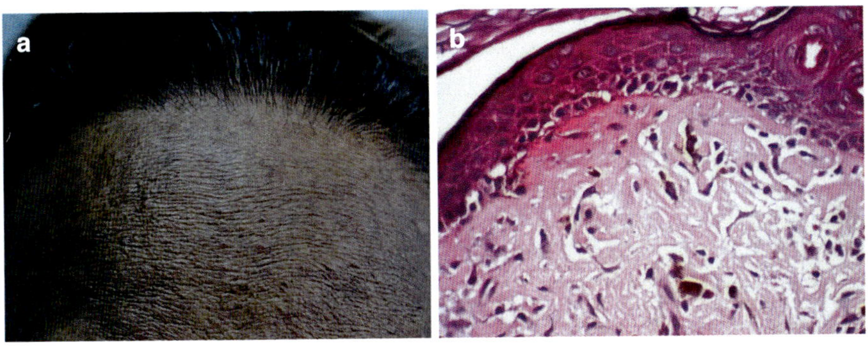

Fig. 7.8 Shows reticulated hyperpigmentation in a Filipino with known cosmetic allergy (**a**) and histopathology (**b**) showing vacuolar alteration of the basal cell layer, pigment incontinence, and dermal lymphocytic infiltrate

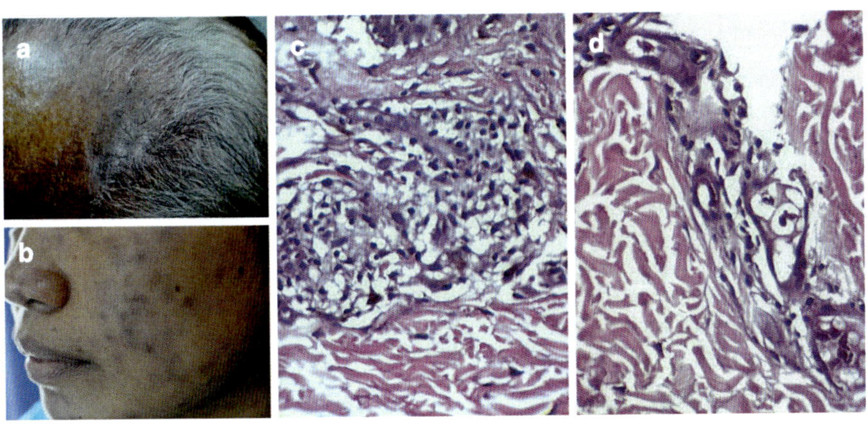

Fig. 7.9 Hyperpigmented patches in two patients with Hansen's disease after treatment with minocycline (**a**, **b**) and histopathological features of perivascular (**c**) and periadnexal (**d**) brown-black granules (H&E ×400)

melanin pigmentation in the basal cell layer [45]. In the dermis, golden-brown to brown-black pigment granules within macrophages surround blood vessels and eccrine coils. *Type I* and *type III* pigments stain for hemosiderin and melanin, respectively. *Type II* pigments stain for both hemosiderin and melanin [46, 47].

Hu et al. [47] reported two leprosy patients who developed minocycline pigmentation on preexisting leprosy lesions. Skin biopsies revealed brownish-black pigments within macrophages which stained positively for both hemosiderin and melanin. On the other hand, a case of minocycline pigmentation in a patient with acne vulgaris revealed brown-black pigments within macrophages located throughout the interstitial dermis. The pigment was identified by immunohistochemistry as a calcium-containing melanin-like substance hypothesized to be an insoluble drug metabolite-protein complex chelated with calcium [48].

References

1. Taylor SC. Skin of color: biology, structure, function, and implications for dermatologic disease. J Am Acad Dermatol. 2002;46(S2):S41–62.
2. Montagna W, Carlisle K. The architecture of black and white facial skin. J Am Acad Dermatol. 1991;24:929–37.
3. Herzberg AJ, Dinehart SM. Chronologic aging in black skin. Am J Dermatopathol. 1989;11: 319–28.
4. Kotrajaras R, Kligman AM. The effect of topical tretinoin on photo damaged facial skin: the Thai experience. Br J Dermatol. 1993;129:302–9.
5. Toda K, Patnak MA, Parrish A, Fitzpatrick TB. Alteration of racial differences in melanosome distribution in human epidermis after exposure to ultraviolet light. Nat New Biol. 1972;236:143–4.
6. Goldschmidt H, Raymond JZ. Quantitative analysis of skin colour from melanin content of superficial skin cells. J Forensic Sci. 1972;17:124.
7. Szabo G. The number of melanocytes in human epidermis. Br Med J. 1954;1(4869):1016–7.
8. Grimes PE, Yamada N, Bhawan J. Light microscopic, immunohistochemical, and ultrastructural alterations in patients with melasma. Am J Dermatopathol. 2005;27:96–101.
9. Kang WH, Yoon KH, Lee ES, Kim J, Lee KB, Yim H, et al. Melasma: histopathological characteristics in 56 Korean patients. Br J Dermatol. 2002;146:228–37.
10. Miot LD, Miot HA, Polettini J, Silva MG, Marques ME. Morphological changes and the expression of alpha-melanocyte stimulating hormone and melanocortin-1 receptor in melasma lesions: a comparative study. Am J Dermatopathol. 2010;32(7):676–82.
11. Dayrit J, Manuel M. Hydroquinone-induced ochronosis. Dermatopathology: practical and conceptual. 2007 [cited 2015];13(1):[about 4p]. Available from: http://www.derm101.com/dpc-archive/january-march-2007-volume-13-no.1/dpc1301a12-hydroquinone-induced-ochronosis/.
12. Sutantoyo C, Mendoza CB, Dayrit JF, Handog EB. Endogenous ochronosis presenting as recalcitrant facial hyperpigmentation aggravated with prolonged use of topical hydroquinone 2%. Glob Dermatol. 2015;2(2):87–99.
13. Lawrence N, Bligard CA, Reed R, Perret WJ. Exogenous ochronosis in the United States. J Am Acad Dermatol. 1988;18:1207–11.
14. Dogliotti M, Leibowitz M. Granulomatous ochronosis-a cosmetic-induced skin disorder in blacks. S Afr Med J. 1979;56:757–60.
15. Hardwick N, Van Gelder LW, Van der Merwe CA, Van der Merwe MP. Exogenous ochronosis: an epidemiological study. Br J Dermatol. 1989;120:229–38.
16. Jordaan HF, Van Niekerk DJT. Transepidermal elimination in exogenous ochronosis: a report of two cases. Am J Dermatopathol. 1991;13:418–24.

17. Phillips JI, Isaacson C, Carman N. Ochronosis in black South Africans who used skin lighteners. Am J Dermatopathol. 1986;8:14–21.
18. Findlay GH. Ochronosis and colloid milium from hydroquinone in man: 50 cases with pathology and electron microscopy. Br J Dermatol. 1975;93(Supp II):9.
19. Tidman MJ, Horton JJ, Mac Donald DM. Hydroquinone induced ochronosis: light and electron microscopic features. Clin Exp Dermatol. 1985;11:224–8.
20. Gaines Jr JJ. The pathology of alkaptonuric ochronosis. Hum Pathol. 1989;20:40–6.
21. Harrison-Balestra C, Gugic D, Vincek V. Clinically distinct form of acquired dermal melanocytosis with review of published work. J Dermatol. 2007;34(3):178–82.
22. Matais J, Lopez N, Haro R, Gonzalez E, Angulo J, Requena L. Late-onset Ito's nevus: an uncommon acquired dermal melanocytosis. J Cutan Pathol. 2007;34(8):640–3.
23. Lee JY, Kim EH, Kim KH, Kang HY, Lee ES, Kim YC. Acquired bilateral naevus of Ota-like macules: an immunohistological analysis of dermal melanogenic paracrine cytokine networks. Br J Dermaol. 2011;164(3):580–5.
24. Lee B, Kim YC, Kang WH, Lee E. Comparison of characteristics of acquired bilateral nevus of Ota-like macules and nevus of Ota according to therapeutic outcome. J Korean Med Sci. 2004;19(4):554–9.
25. Lee JY, Lee JS, Kim YC. Histopathological features of acquired dermal melanocytosis. Eur J Dermatol. 2010;20(3):345–8.
26. Ramirez CO. Los Cenicientos: Problema Clinico. In: Report of the First Central American Congress of Dermatology, San Salvador, December 5–8, 1957. San Salvador: Publisher. 1957, p. 122–30.
27. Ramirez CO. The ashy dermatosis (erythema dyschromicum perstans). Epidemiological study and report of 139 cases. Cutis. 1967;3:244–7.
28. Convit J, Kerdel-Vegas F, Rodriguez G. Erythema dyschromicum perstans. A hitherto undescribed skin disease. J Invest Dermatol. 1961;36:457–62.
29. Bhutani LK, Bedi TR, Pandhi RK. Lichen planus pigmentosus. Dermatologica. 1974;149:43–50.
30. Kanwar AJ, Dogra S, Handa S, Parsad D, Radotra BD. A study of 124 Indian patients with lichen planus pigmentosus. Clin Exp Dermatol. 2003;28:481–5.
31. Knox JM, Dodge BG, Freeman RG. Erythema dyschromicum perstans. Arch Dermatol. 1968;97:262–72.
32. Pinkus H. Lichenoid tissue reactions. A speculative review of the clinical spectrum of epidermal basal cell damage with special reference to erythema dyschromicum perstans. Arch Dermatol. 1973;107:840–6.
33. Novick NL, Phelps R, Tom C. Erythema dyschromicum perstans. Int J Dermatol. 1985;24(10):630–3.
34. Vega ME, Waxtein L, Arenas R, Hodyo M, Dominguez-Soto L. Ashy dermatosis and lichen planus pigmentosus: a clinicopathologic study of 31 cases. Int J Dermatol. 1992;31:90–4.
35. Weedon D. Weedon's skin pathology. 2nd ed. London: Churchill Livingstone Elsevier; 2002. p. 37.
36. Sanchez NP, Pathak MA. Circumscribed dermal melanosis: classification, light, histochemical and electron microscopic studies on 3 patients with erythema dyschromicum perstans. Int J Dermatol. 1985;24:630.
37. Rorsman H. Riehl's melanosis. Int J Dermatol. 1982;21:75–80.
38. Nakayama H, Matsuo S, Hayakawa K, Takhashi K, Shigematsu T. Pigmented cosmetic dermatitis. Int J Dermatol. 1984;23:299–305.
39. Kozuka T, Tashiro M, Sano S, Fujimoto K, Nakamura Y, Hashimoto S, et al. Brilliant Lake Red R as a cause of pigmented contact dermatitis. Contact Dermatitis. 1979;5:297.
40. Fujimoto K, Hashimoto S, Kozuka T, Tashiro M, Sano S. Occupational pigmented contact dermatitis from azo dyes. Contact Dermatitis. 1985;12:15–7.
41. Serrano G, Pujol C, Cuadra J, Gallo S, Aliaga A. Riehl's melanosis: pigmented contact dermatitis caused by fragrances. J Am Acad Dermatol. 1989;5(2):1057–60.

42. Fenske NA, Millns JL. Cutaneous pigmentation due to minocycline hydrochloride. J Am Acad Dermatol. 1980;3:308–11.
43. Argenyi ZB, Finelli L, Bergfeld WF, Tuthill RJ, McMahon JT, Ratz JL, et al. Minocycline-related cutaneous pigmentation as demonstrated by light microscopy, electron microscopy and X-ray energy spectroscopy. J Cutan Pathol. 1987;14:176–80.
44. Okada N, Sato S, Sasou T. Characterization of pigmented granules in minocycline-induced cutaneous pigmentation: observations using fluorescent microscopy and high performance chromatography. Br J Dermatol. 1993;129:403–7.
45. Simons JJ, Morales A. Minocycline and generalized cutaneous pigmentation. J Am Acad Dermatol. 1980;3:244–7.
46. Geria AN, Tajirian AL, Kihiczak G, Schwartz RA. Minocycline-induced skin pigmentation: an update. Acta Dermatovenerol Croat. 2009;17(2):123–6.
47. Hu SW, Robinson MR, Newlove T, Meehan S, Levis WR, Patel RR. Minocycline-induced hyperpigmentation in multibacillary leprosy. Am J Dermatopathol. 2012;34(8):e114–8.
48. Mouton RW, Jordaan HF, Schneider JW. A new type of minocycline-induced cutaneous hyperpigmentation. Clin Exp Dermatol. 2004;29(1):8–14.

Chapter 8
The Scoring Aid: MASI and Modified MASI

Tien Guan Steven Thng and Sai Yee Chuah

8.1 Introduction

One of the challenges of dermatologists conducting clinical research in the management of melasma is to find ways to score the severity of melasma in a consistent, reproducible and accurate manner. Unlike other organ systems, there are no tests of clinical significance that can measure skin pigmentation in terms of extent and degree of pigmentation as compared to the patient's normal skin. While there are accurate quantitative point measurement devices like the chromameter, Mexameter and reflectance spectrophotometry, these however require the investigator to conduct measurement in exactly the same spot over time in order to get consistent result that can be used for comparison of severity of melasma over time. More importantly, these systems do not quantify the extent of involvement and as such are of limited use in monitoring the response to therapy and for evaluating the efficacy of new drugs.

Because of this lack of tests of clinical significance, early methods of evaluating the severity of melasma are often crude, subjective and have marked inter-individual and even intra-individual variations. As such, to maintain objectivity in assessing severity of melasma, scores like the melasma area and severity index (MASI) are used to evaluate the severity of the condition. Over the years, modification to the MASI scores has been proposed and adopted, and more recently, a computer algorithm has been developed to allow these scores to be calculated by a computer through digital image analysis. All these developments have greatly helped the cause of clinical practice and clinical research in melasma.

T.G.S. Thng, MBBS, MRCP (UK), FRCP (Edin) (✉) • S.Y. Chuah
Department of Dermatology, National Skin Centre,
1 Mandalay Road, Singapore 308205, Singapore
e-mail: steventhng@nsc.gov.sg; sychuah@nsc.gov.sg

E.B. Handog, M.J. Enriquez-Macarayo (eds.), *Melasma and Vitiligo in Brown Skin*,
DOI 10.1007/978-81-322-3664-1_8

8.2 Early Melasma Scoring Systems Using Point Scales

One of the earliest scoring systems adopted for assessment of treatment response for melasma is the physician and patient's global assessment scales [1, 2]. In this system, there is no attempt to score the severity of melasma before treatment; instead, these scales seek to quantify qualitatively the degree of improvement post therapeutic intervention. These are usually done through comparison of pre- and post-treatment photographs and scored via 3–5 graduations. For the physician global assessment, the investigator rates the improvement on a 3 point scale of 0 (completely clear), 1 (almost clear but still has evidence of melasma) and 2 (not clear, still has significant evidence of melasma) [2]. Patient's global assessment follows a similar 3 point scale of 1 (completely cleared), 2 (nearly cleared) and 3 (significant hyperpigmentation present) [2].

The melasma severity scale (MSS), on the other hand, attempts to score the severity of melasma before treatment on a 4 point scale and uses the changes in scale to determine degree of improvement. In the MSS, scores range from 0 (absence of melasma), 1 (mild melasma, where the colour of the affected area is just slightly darker than that of the surrounding normal skin), 2 (moderate melasma, where the affected area is moderately darker than the surrounding normal skin) and 3 (severe melasma, where the affected area is markedly darker than the surrounding normal skin) [2].

These early scoring systems are mainly qualitative in nature and require the physician to estimate the degree of darkness/improvement and as such is prone to inter-assessor variability. More importantly, they are usually one dimensional as they do not take into account both the area involved as well as the degree of pigmentation of melasma.

8.3 Melasma Area and Severity Index (MASI)

The melasma area and severity index (MASI), developed by Kimbrough-Green et al. [3] in 1994, was probably the first scoring system to try to objectively score and measure the response of melasma to treatment in a clinical trial by taking into account both the area involved, as well as the darkness of the melasma. The system was based on a similar scoring system devised for psoriasis and takes into account the extent and degree of pigmentation affected. There are three components used in the MASI system and they are: area (A) of involvement, darkness (D) and homogeneity (H).

For area (A) of involvement, the investigator has to estimate the areas affected, as compared to normal skin and assign a numeric value according to banding. A value of 0 implies no involvement; 1 when affected area is less than 10 %; 2 for 10–29 % affected; 3 for 30–49 % affected; 4 for 50–69 % affected; 5 for 70–89 % affected and 6 for 90 % or more affected.

The darkness (D) of the melasma is compared to the normal skin and graded on a scale of 0–4 as follows: 0 implies normal skin colour; 1 with barely visible hyperpigmentation; 2 if there is mild hyperpigmentation; 3 for moderate hyperpigmentation and 4 for severe hyperpigmentation. As the scoring is subjective, training picture library representing the various scores is given to ensure consistency of scores.

Similar to darkness, homogeneity (H) of the hyperpigmentation is also graded on a scale of 0–4: 0 implies normal skin colour without evidence of hyperpigmentation; 1 is given if there are specks of involvement; 2 if small patchy areas of involvement <1.5 cm diameter are noted; 3 is given if patches of involvement >2 cm diameter are noted and 4 for uniform skin involvement without any clear areas are noted.

The MASI calculation is then performed by scoring of these three components on the face, which is in turn divided into four main areas: the forehead (30 %), left malar (30 %), right malar (30 %) and the chin (10 %) (Fig. 8.1). The final MASI score is calculated by adding the sum of the severity ratings for darkness and homogeneity, multiplied by the value of the area of involvement, for each of the four facial areas:

$$
\text{MASI total score} = \left|\begin{aligned}
&0{:}3 \times A\ (\text{forehead}) \times (D + H)\ (\text{forehead}) + \\
&0{:}3 \times A\ (\text{left malar}) \times (D + H)\ (\text{left malar}) + \\
&0{:}3 \times A\ (\text{right malar}) \times (D + H)\ (\text{right malar}) + \\
&0{:}1 \times A\ (\text{chin}) \times (D + H)\ (\text{chin})
\end{aligned}\right.
$$

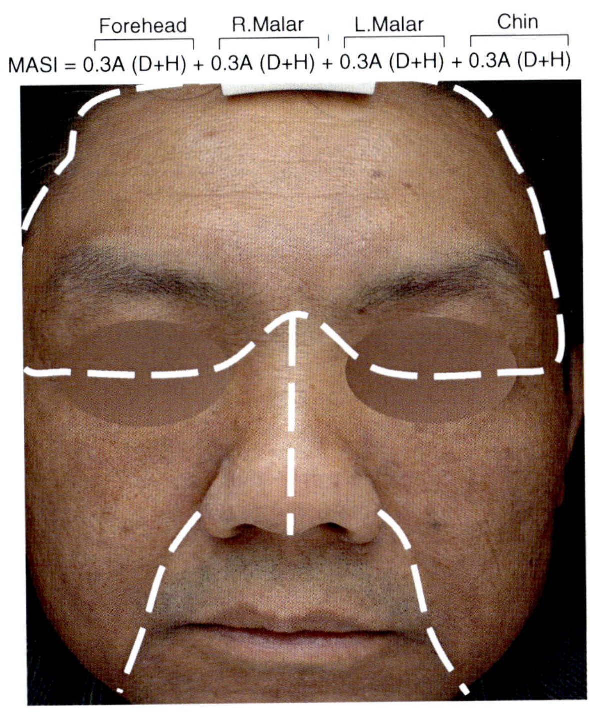

Fig. 8.1 Melasma area and severity index (MASI). *A* area, *D* darkness, *H* homogeneity

The MASI score range from 0 to 48, with 48 being the most severe. At first glance, the advantages of the MASI score is obvious as it takes into account both the area of involvement as well as the degree of pigmentation, two of the most important components that affects the patients adversely. In addition, as the MASI is a continuous score, it reflects changes much better than the old melasma severity scale, which is a categorical scale.

The MASI score has also been validated recently in a prospective study by Pandya, et al. [2]. In the study, the MASI score shows good reliability within raters on different days as well as between raters. It is important to note that all raters who participated in the study had some training and were given examples of different levels of area, darkness and homogeneity in aiding their scoring. This probably accounted for the consistency observed both within rater and inter-raters. The MASI scores were also compared with Mexameter readings as well as with melasma severity scale and showed good validity.

In actual practice, however, the MASI has its drawbacks. Firstly, consistency is difficult to achieve as MASI is based on subjective visual assessment of the three components of area of involvement, darkness and homogeneity which results in inter-assessor variability. Secondly, while the MASI score is a continuous score, the three components of area, darkness and homogeneity assessed are grouped in bands. This is not ideal as significant changes within each band will not be reflected, while small changes across bands result in a significant change in scores. Finally, MASI is rarely used outside clinical trials due to the complexity of calculations and is time-consuming in nature. As a result, modifications to the score have been made resulting in the simpler modified MASI score.

8.4 Modified Melasma Area and Severity Index (mMASI)

The modified melasma area and severity index (mMASI) was proposed by Pandya et al. [4] in 2011 after the team did a validation of the MASI score. In the study, despite training of the raters and providing them with examples of the different scales in the components of area, darkness and homogeneity, the study team still found assessing the different components of MASI problematic, particularly in the assessment of homogeneity. As such, the team proposed a modified MASI system with the removal of homogeneity component. In their study, removal of the homogeneity component did not affect the reliability or validity measures at all [4] and the authors suggested the removal of that component would result in a simpler, easier and more consistent scoring system. The modified MASI score is therefore calculated in the following manner:

$$
\begin{aligned}
\text{Modified MASI total score} = \; & 0{:}3 \times \text{A (forehead)} \times \text{D (forehead)} + \\
& 0{:}3 \times \text{A (left malar)} \times \text{D (left malar)} + \\
& 0{:}3 \times \text{A (right malar)} \times \text{D (right malar)} + \\
& 0{:}1 \times \text{A (chin)} \times \text{D (chin)}
\end{aligned}
$$

In addition, in order to improve consistency in assessment of the two components of area and darkness, the authors proposed that a training module as well as practice images be given so as to ensure reliability in mMASI scores. Since the introduction of mMASI in 2011, it has replaced MASI and is used in almost all of published clinical studies assessing treatment options for melasma. While the removal of the homogeneity component does help in making the mMASI simpler to perform, it still does not address the problems associated with MASI, which are mainly banding within the scale of each component, inter-observer variability and the need for training to ensure reliability. As such, a better scoring system is still needed to overcome the observed problems.

8.5 Automated Melasma Area and Severity Index (aMASI)

To address the problems noted in MASI and mMASI, a novel computer image analysis software system has recently been developed by Thng et al. [5] to derive the area and degree of hyperpigmentation in melasma. These scores are fed into the same formula used for mMASI scores cumulating in an automated MASI score (aMASI).

The software elegantly utilizes digital image analysis through extreme machine learning and thresholding method [6] to identify abnormal areas, calculate the areas involved as a percentage of the total surface and derive the degree of pigmentation in the abnormal area by comparing the abnormal with the normal in the *Lab* colour space. A detailed account of the technical details can be found in the paper by Liang et al. [6].

Briefly, the algorithm utilizes three main steps to derive the MASI score automatically from a set of three digital photographs. The first step involves defining the area that is affected by melasma. The algorithm automatically define the pixels of the eyebrows, eyes, nostrils and corner of mouth as non-skin set, and these are blackened out and are excluded from the analysis (Fig. 8.2). The identified areas are then segmented into forehead, left and right malar region and the chin, using the position of the eyes, nostrils and mouth as landmarks to determine the boundaries.

The frontal view of the photograph is used to define the forehead and the chin (Fig. 8.3), while the two lateral views are used to define the malar regions (Fig. 8.3). Thresholding is then performed by comparing the value of one pixel against the reference value of normal skin [6], and any area that is darker than the reference value would be considered as an area affected by melasma (Fig. 8.4).

The second step involves the calculation of degree of darkness of the identified melasma area as compared to the normal skin. This is done using the *Lab* colour space [7]. The difference between the *Lab* values of normal and affected skin will be calculated for each pixel and an average of the darkness of the pixels in areas affected by melasma will be used in the score to calculate the final MASI.

Finally, the percentage of area involved and darkness component are fed into the formula for mMASI to generate the automated MASI (aMASI) score. The mMASI

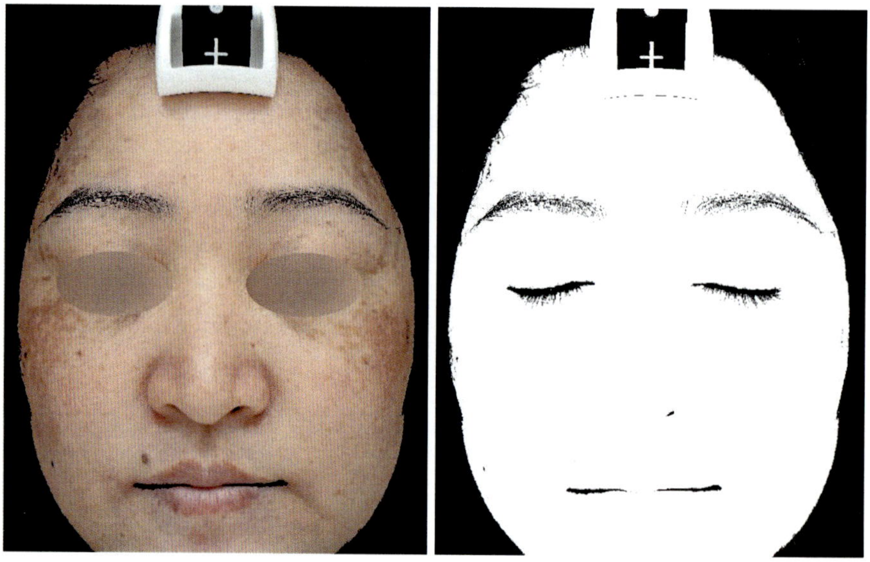

Fig. 8.2 Non-skin set, as defined by *blackened areas*, is excluded from calculation in aMASI

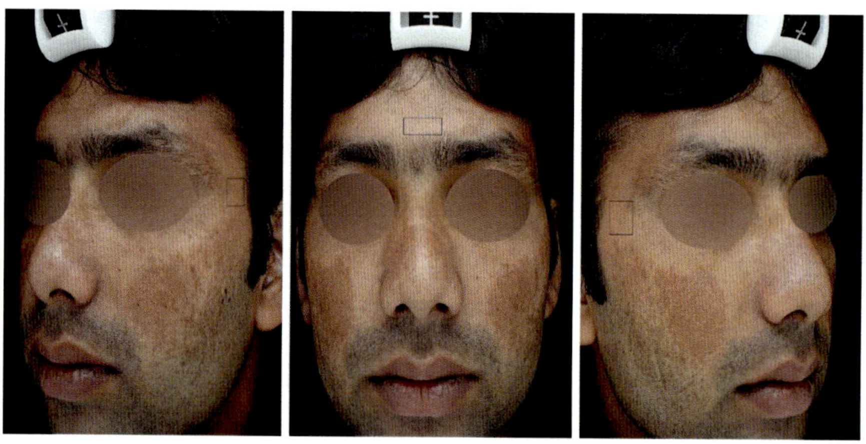

Fig. 8.3 Frontal and two side views at 45° required for aMASI. The aMASI score for this patient calculated through the developed algorithm is 8.6

score was used in the calculation as homogeneity is no longer an important component as the computer algorithm accurately identifies all affected areas on the face regardless of their size and includes them in the final calculation.

The proposed aMASI system seems easy to use as all it requires is a set of three digital photographs (one frontal and two side views) to be taken consistently under the same lighting. The set of three photographs are then fed into the computer algorithm and an aMASI score will be generated within 1 min. As all the assessment and

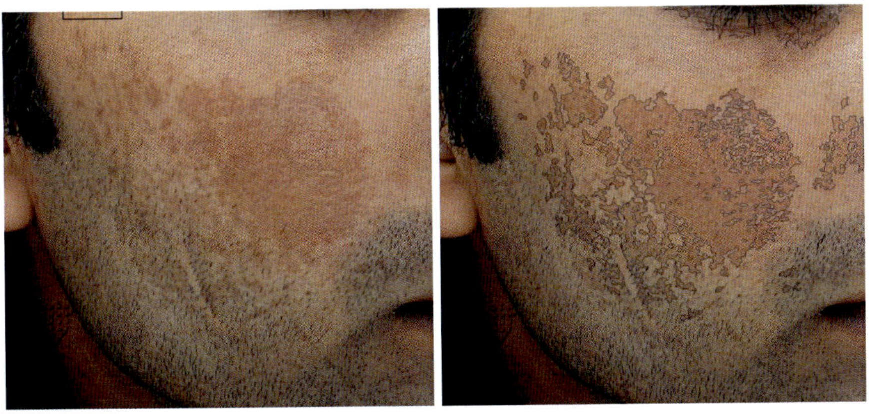

Fig. 8.4 Auto identification of affected areas by computer algorithm

calculations are done automatically, no training is required and the system totally removes all possibility of inter-observer variability as there is no main-in-the-loop for the whole process. The system also totally removes the limitations of banding as all indices used in the calculation (area and darkness) are continuous variables, and these provide a better resolution on the improvement/worsening of melasma.

Despite the obvious advantages, there are several notable weaknesses in this newly developed algorithm. The major weakness would be that the algorithm could not differentiate melasma from other skin hyperpigmentation like Hori's nevus, solar lentigo, nevus, etc. as the algorithm can only differentiate normal skin from abnormally pigmented skin. In addition, for consistent result, the photographs must be taken under the same lighting conditions and at fixed angles. Lastly, while the algorithm has tested and validated patients of skin type 3 and above, it has not been tested in patients with fairer skin types with melasma. Future studies assessing the automated MASI over time in different cohorts of patients should be performed to determine the sensitivity, validity and consistency of this algorithm.

8.6 Conclusion

A good, reproducible, standardized way of scoring melasma severity and response to treatment accurately is important so that efficacy of various treatment modalities can better be compared in meta-analyses. These scoring systems must be inexpensive, with minimal or no inter-assessor variability and more importantly, applicable and adopted worldwide. The scoring of melasma has evolved, over the years, to be closer to the ideal system. The MASI and mMASI are still the gold-standard in melasma scoring systems and should be used routinely in all therapeutic trials for melasma. The automated mMASI (aMASI) system via computer image analysis holds much promise but remains to be validated for consistency and applicability on worldwide basis.

References

1. Griffiths CE, Finkel LJ, Ditre CM, Hamilton TA, Ellis CN, Voorhees JJ. Topical tretinoin (retinoic acid) improves melasma: a vehicle-controlled, clinical trial. Br J Dermatol. 1993;129: 415–21.
2. Taylor SC, Torok H, Jones T, Lowe N, Rich P, Tschen E, et al. Efficacy and safety of a new triple-combination agent for the treatment of facial melasma. Cutis. 2003;72:67–72.
3. Kimbrough-Green CK, Griffiths CE, Finkel LJ, Hamilton TA, Bulengo-Ransby SM, Ellis CN, et al. Topical retinoic acid for melasma in black patients: a vehicle-controlled clinical trial. Arch Dermatol. 1994;130:727–33.
4. Pandya AG, Hynan LS, Bhore R, Riley FC, Guevara IL, Grimes P, et al. Reliability assessment and validation of the Melasma Area and Severity Index (MASI) and a new modified MASI scoring method. J Am Acad Dermatol. 2011;64:78–83.
5. Tay EY, Gan EY, Tan VW, Lin Z, Liang Y, Lin F, Wee S, Thng TG. Pilot study of an automated method to determine Melasma Area and Severity Index. Br J Dermatol. 2015;172(6):1535–40.
6. Liang Y, Lin Z, Gu J, Ser W, Thng TG. Melasma image segmentation using extreme learning machine. In: Cao J, Mao K, Cambria E, Man Z, Toh KA, editors. Proceedings of ELM-2014 Volume 2. Switzerland: Springer International Publishing; 2015. p. 369–77.
7. Khan R, Hanbury A, Stöttinger AB. Colour based skin classification. Pattern Recog Lett. 2012;33:157–63.

Chapter 9
Differential Diagnosis of Melasma in Brown Skin

Evangeline B. Handog and Maria Juliet Enriquez-Macarayo

9.1 Postinflammatory Hyperpigmentation (PIH)

Postinflammatory hyperpigmentation (Fig. 9.1) presents as asymptomatic hyperpigmented macules and patches ranging in color from either tan to dark brown (epidermal melanin) or gray–blue to gray–brown (dermal melanin) caused by numerous preceding cutaneous insults such as drug and phototoxic reactions, infections, physical injury or trauma, allergic reactions and inflammatory diseases [1].

PIH can occur at any age with no gender preference. Epidermal PIH can result from acne, insect bites, pyodermas, atopic dermatitis, psoriasis and pityriasis rosea. It generally resolves over time, although fading may require months or years in darkly pigmented individuals [2].

On the other hand, dermal PIH has been associated with dermatoses characterized by degeneration of the basal layer of the epidermis and inflammation at the dermal-epidermal junction such as lupus erythematosus and fixed drug eruptions. Resolution is slower and longer than epidermal PIH, and treatment is a challenge.

E.B. Handog (✉)
Department of Dermatology, Asian Hospital and Medical Center,
2205 Civic Drive, Alabang, Muntinlupa City, Philippines, 1780
e-mail: vangee@handog.net

M.J. Enriquez-Macarayo
Department of Dermatology, Angeles University Foundation Medical Center,
Pampanga, Philippines

E.B. Handog, M.J. Enriquez-Macarayo (eds.), *Melasma and Vitiligo in Brown Skin*,
DOI 10.1007/978-81-322-3664-1_9

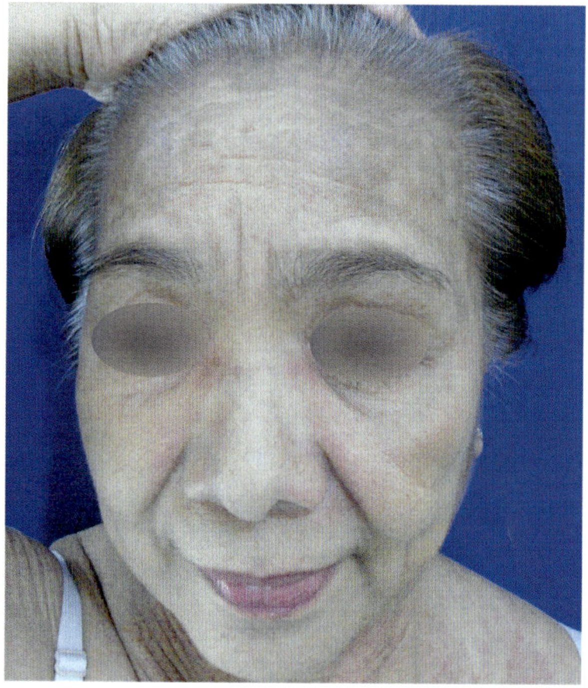

Fig. 9.1 Postinflammatory hyperpigmented patches in an elderly Filipino female with dermatomyositis (Courtesy of the Research Institute for Tropical Medicine, Philippines)

9.2 Exogenous Ochronosis

Exogenous ochronosis is an uncommon disorder characterized by dark brown to black or blue-black hue (Fig. 9.2) caused by the deposition of microscopic, ochre-colored pigment in the dermis [3, 4].

It has been seen as a result of hydroquinone use among dark-skinned individuals. The condition, however, may also develop from the use of antimalarials and products containing resorcinol, phenol, mercury and picric acid [1]. Skin irritation and vigorous friction may be contributory as well. Histopathology is definitive, with the banana-shaped ochronotic fibers in the dermis.

9.3 Acquired Bilateral Nevus of Ota-Like Macules (ABNOM)

Acquired bilateral nevus of ota-like macules are multiple, speckled blue-brown and/or slate-gray macules occurring bilaterally on the malar regions (Fig. 9.3) or less commonly on the forehead, upper eyelids, cheeks and nose. The mucosa is not involved [5]. ABNOM typically affects middle-aged Asians, particularly Chinese

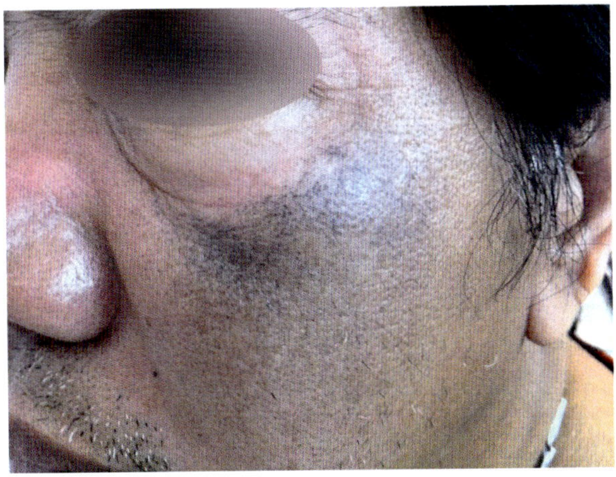

Fig. 9.2 Dark bluish-black pigmentation on the cheeks of a Filipino female after prolonged used of hydroquinone-containing OTC products (Courtesy of the Research Institute for Tropical Medicine, Philippines)

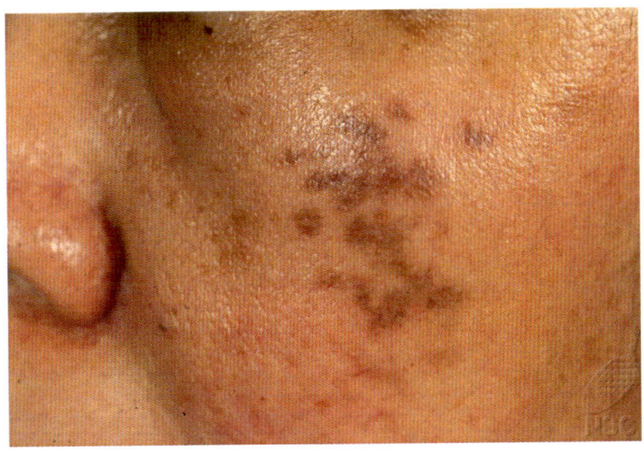

Fig. 9.3 Speckled brown-gray macules on the malar regions in an Asian patient (Courtesy of the National Skin Centre, Singapore)

and Japanese, with age range of 20–70 years [1, 5]. They are thought to increase in thickness with advancing age [6].

9.4 Solar Lentigines

Solar lentigines are characterized by well-circumscribed 1–3 cm pigmented macules on sun-exposed areas [7, 8]. They can occur in children and adults, especially those with skin types I to III.

Children who have xeroderma pigmentosum may develop solar lentigines in the first 6 months of life, after minimal sun exposure. Lesions may vary in color from light yellow to dark brown. The most common sites of predilection are the face (Fig. 9.4), hands, forearms, chest, back and shins.

9.5 Drug-Induced Hyperpigmentation

Hyperpigmentation caused by toxic agents or medications (Fig. 9.5) accounts for 10–20 % of all cases of acquired hyperpigmentation. The most common causes are CNS drugs (e.g, chlorpromazine, amitriptyline), antineoplastic agents (e.g., carmustine, nitrogen mustard, bleomycin, anthracycline, 5-fluorouracil), anti-infectious drugs (e.g., chloroquine, quinacrine, hydroxychloroquine, minocycline, clofazimine, zidovudine), antihypertensive medications (e.g., amiodarone, diltiazem) and hormones (e.g., oral contraceptives) [1, 5].

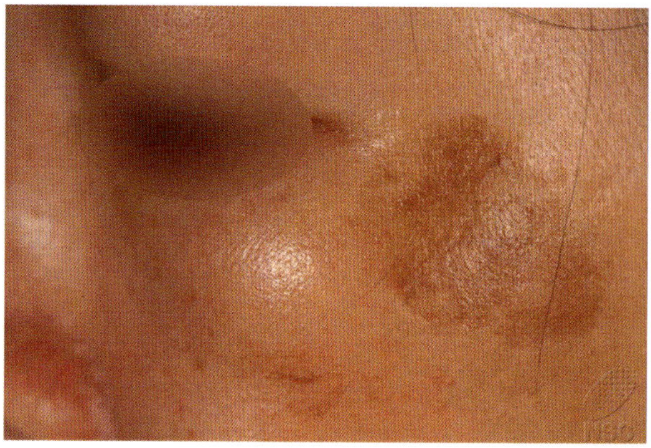

Fig. 9.4 Dark brown patch on the cheekbone area of an Asian patient (Courtesy of the National Skin Centre, Singapore)

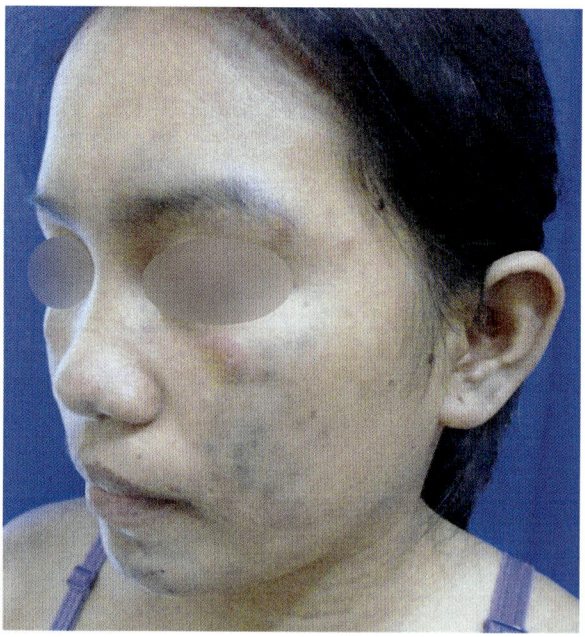

Fig. 9.5 Bluish pigmentation on the face of a Filipino female, developed from intake of minocycline (Courtesy of the Research Institute for Tropical Medicine, Philippines)

9.6 Actinic Lichen Planus

It is a rare variant of cutaneous lichen planus, characterized by the development of lesions on the photodistributed areas (Fig. 9.6a). It is more common in dark-skinned populations, particularly in young adults [9]. Indurated plaques or papules appear on the face, neck and the dorsal surface of hands after exposure to ultraviolet (UV) light [10–12]. Covered areas and mucous membranes are usually spared. In few cases, discrete, confluent papules and hypermelanotic patches, sometimes assuming a melasma-like appearance (Fig. 9.6b), may also be seen. The etiology is unknown.

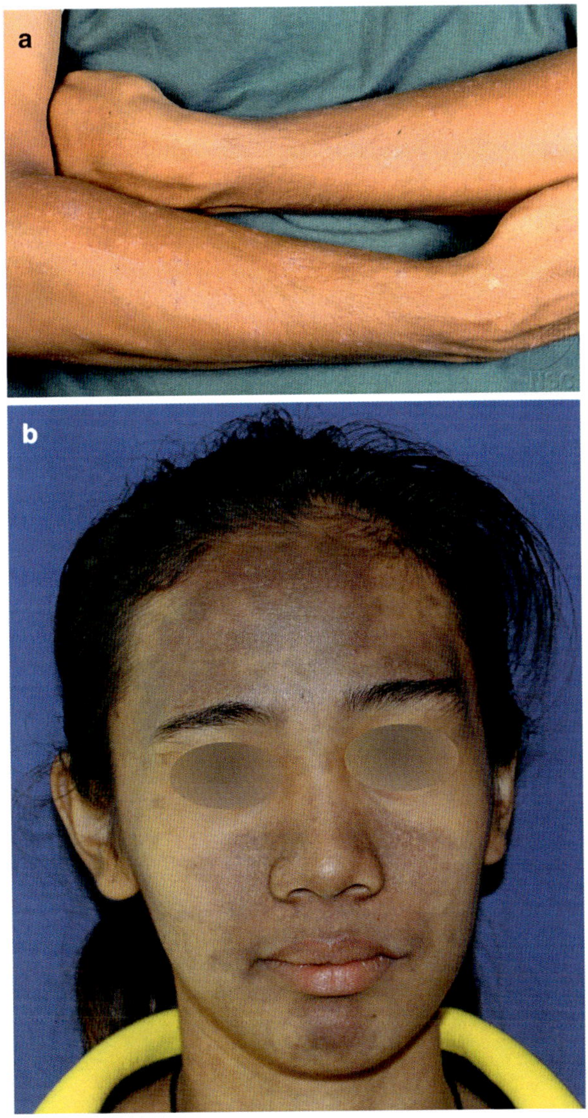

Fig. 9.6 (**a**) Scaly papules on the arms of an Asian male, histopathologically proven as actinic lichen planus (Courtesy of the National Skin Centre, Singapore). (**b**) Hypermelanotic patches on the midface of a young Filipino female, histopathologically proven as lichen planus (Courtesy of the Research Institute for Tropical Medicine, Philippines)

9.7 Erythema Dyschromicum Perstans (Ashy Dermatosis)

Erythema dyschromicum perstans (EDP) is a slowly progressive disease that is more common in children and young adults, particularly those from Latin America with skin phototypes III and IV [5]. It has equal prevalence in both sexes [1]. The common sites of predilection are the neck, proximal upper extremities and trunk [5]. Lesions can follow skin cleavage lines [3]. EDP is characterized by hyperpigmented macules and patches of variable shape and size with an ashen-gray to brown–blue color (Fig. 9.7) [13]. A polymorphic eruption may also be seen, presenting as simultaneous hypo- and hyperpigmented macules [14]. The lesions are usually asymptomatic; however, minimal pruritus can be present. There is a slow progression of the lesions over several years, usually without spontaneous regression.

9.8 Riehl's Melanosis

Also known as female facial melanosis, this condition is more common in middle-aged dark-skinned women, particularly Mexicans and Asians [1]. It is characterized by a rapid onset of a reticular gray-brown to almost black hyperpigmentation on the

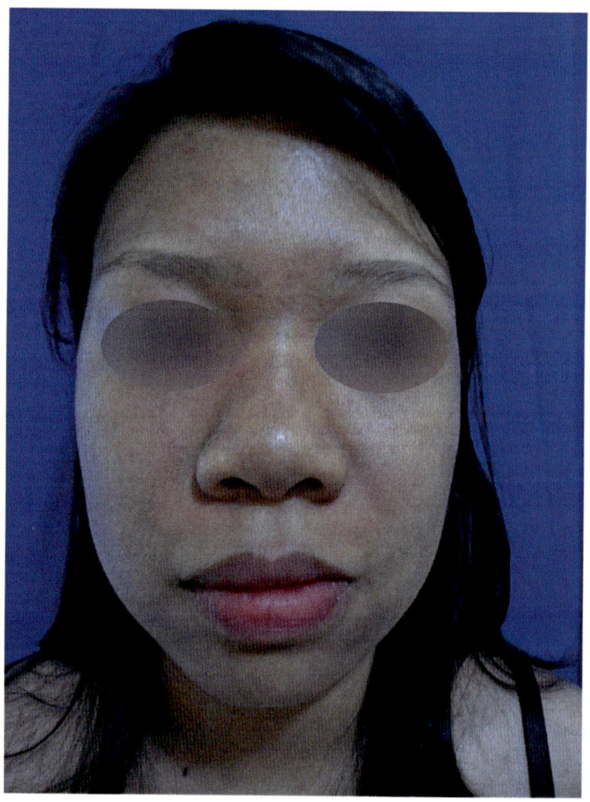

Fig. 9.7 Ashen-brown hyperpigmentation seen on the face of a young Filipino female (Courtesy of The Research Institute for Tropical Medicine, Philippines)

face (particularly on the forehead, zygomatic area and temples) and neck (Fig. 9.8a, b). There is no evidence of any inflammation on the skin [15]. It is induced by repetitive contact with a sensitizer such as fragrances, some pigments and bactericides (carbanilides, ricinoleic acids) used in cosmetics and optical whiteners [16].

9.9 Ephelides

Ephelides or freckles are characterized by small light brown macules appearing on the sun-exposed skin (Fig. 9.9) [1, 8]. It is more common in fair-skinned populations and those with red or blond hair and Celtic ancestry. Onset is usually in early childhood and may or may not disappear later in life.

The table below shows a summary of the differential diagnoses to be considered when dealing with pigmented lesions presenting mostly on the face (Table 9.1).

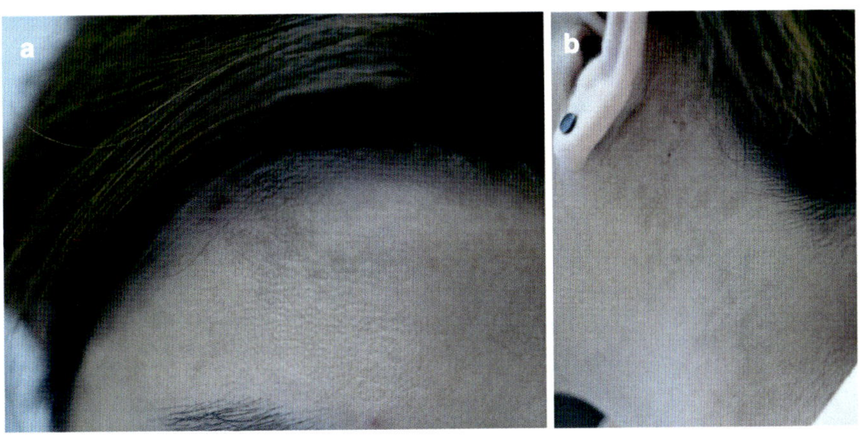

Fig. 9.8 (**a**) Reticulated reddish-brown patch on the forehead and (**b**) neck of a Filipina female (Courtesy of Dr. Johannes F. Dayrit, Philippines)

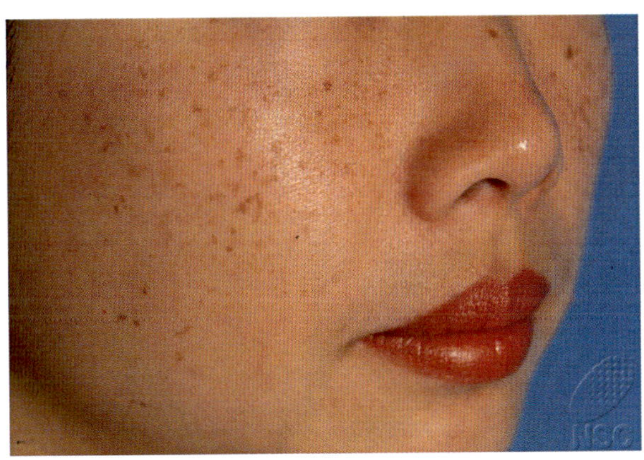

Fig. 9.9 Small brown macules, of different hues, dispersed mostly on the cheeks of an Asian female (Courtesy of the National Skin Centre, Singapore)

Table 9.1 Differential diagnoses summary

Diagnosis	Age/sex	History	Distribution	Color/lesion
Postinflammatory hyperpigmentation	Any age, no gender	History of trauma	Site of previous trauma	Brown/dark gray
Exogenous ochronosis [17, 18]	Rare disease No known age or sex predilection	Prolonged use of hydroquinone (2–5 %) worsened by keratolytic agents and sun exposure	Photodistributed along sites of contact with causative agent Face, neck, back, dorsum of extremities symmetrically distributed	Brown gray or blue black
Aquired bilateral nevus of ota-like macules (ABNOM)/ Hori's nevus	Predominantly among females Mean age is 45.8 years among males and 45.9 among females [19] Median age at onset is 30 years [15]	Become bluer with age among women	Zygomatic area, forehead, temporal area, nasal radix, upper eyelid Zygomatic – most common among women Forehead – most common among men	Brown, blue, slate gray [20]
Solar lentigines	Children and adults	History of sun exposure	Sun-exposed parts	May vary in color
Drug-induced hyperpigmentation	10–20 % of acquired hyperpigmentation; no age or sex predilection	History of drug intake and sun exposure	Sun-exposed areas	Bluish gray
Actinic lichen planus [21]	Mostly younger than 30 years Mean of 14 years No sex predilection	Usually noted in spring or summer Among photosensitive individuals Mainly in tropical areas	Face, dorsal aspect of the hands and outer aspect of the forearms	Atrophic – with hyperpigmentation Dyschromic type – white angular papules and plaques on the neck and dorsa of hands Classic plaque-like – violaceous papules Pigmented type – resembles melasma seen in the face and neck

Erythema dyschromicum perstans [22, 23]	Unrelated to age and sex	Slowly progressive May be pruritic	Symmetric over the trunk, arms, neck and face May occur on any body part except the scalp, palms, soles, mucous membranes	Color may vary from different shades of gray to lead Developing lesions may have raised reddish border
Riehl's hypermelanosis [22]	Not related to age and sex	Develops rapidly Sites previously in contact with allergens, especially cosmetics Associated with positive patch tests to cosmetics or components	Face Highly pronounced on the forehead and temples	Brownish gray
Ephelides [1, 2]	Develop during early childhood then regress with age	Fair-skinned individuals with Celtic ancestry Become more visible at spring and summer, can fade during winter	Face, dorsal aspects of the arms and upper trunk	Light to dark brown

References

1. Lapeere H, Boone B, De Schepper S, Verhaeghe E, Van Gele M, Ongenae K, et al. Hypomelanoses and hypermelanoses. In: Wolff K, Goldsmith L, Katz S, Gilchrest B, Paller A, Leffel D, editors. Fitzpatrick's dermatology in general medicine. 8th ed. New York: McGraw-Hill, Inc; 2012. p. 804–26.
2. Chang M. Disorders of hyperpigmentation. In: Bolognia JL, Jorizzo JL, Schaffer JV, editors. Dermatology. 3rd ed. China: Elsevier Saunders; 2012. p. 1049–50.
3. Kulandaisamy S, Mohan Thappa M, Gupta D. Exogenous ochronosis in melasma: a study from South India. Pigm Int. 2014;1:17–22.
4. Sharma S, Rao R. Exogenous ochronosis masquerading refractory melasma. Our Dermatol Online. 2014;5(4):398–400.
5. Bolognia JL, Schaffer JV, Duncan K, Ko C. Disorders of pigmentation. In: Dermatology essentials. China: Elsevier Inc.; 2014. p. 496–501.
6. Min Park J, Tsao H, Tsao S. Acquired bilateral nevus of Ota-like macules (Hori nevus): etiologic and therapeutic considerations. J Am Acad Dermatol. 2009;61(1):88–92.
7. Grichnik JM, Rhodes AR, Sober AJ. Benign neoplasias and hyperplasias of melanocytes. In: Goldsmith L, Katz S, Gilchrest B, Paller A, Lefell D, editors. Fitzpatricks's dermatology in general medicine. 8th ed. New York: McGraw-Hill, Inc; 2012. p. 1406.
8. Plensdorf S, Martinez J. Common pigmentation disorders. Am Fam Physician. 2009;79(2): 109–16.
9. Verhagen AR, Koten JW. Lichenoid melanodermatitis. A clinicopathological study of fifty-one Kenyan patients with so-called tropical lichen planus. Br J Dermatol. 1979;101(6):651–8.
10. Salman SM, Kibbi AG, Zaynoun S. Actinic lichen planus. A clinicopathologic study of 16 patients. J Am Acad Dermatol. 1989;20(2 Pt 1):226–31.
11. Kim GH, Mikkilineni R. Lichen planus actinicus. Dermatol Online J. 2007;13(1):13. http://escholarship.org/uc/item/98k4v2zx. Accessed: 17 Feb 2016.
12. Meads SB, Kunishige J, Ramos-Caro FA, Hassanein AM. Lichen planus actinicus. Cutis. 2003;72(5):377–81.
13. Bahadir S, Cobanoglu U, Cimsit G, Yayli S, Alpay K. Erythema dyschromicum perstans: response to dapsone therapy. Int J Dermatol. 2004;43(3):220–2.
14. Torrelo A, Zaballos P, Colmenero I, Mediero IG, de Prada I, Zambrano A. Erythema dyschromicum perstans in children: a report of 14 cases. J Eur Acad Dermatol Venereol. 2005;19(4):422–6.
15. Serrano G, Pujol C, Cuadra J, Gallo S, Aliaga A. Riehl's melanosis: pigmented contact dermatitis caused by fragrances. J Am Acad Dermatol. 1989;21:1057–60.
16. Khanna N, Rasool S. Facial melanoses: Indian perspective. Ind J Dermatol Venereol Leprol. 2011;77:552–64.
17. Martins VMR, de Sousa ARD, Portela ND, Tigre CAR, Gonçalves LMS, Filho RJLC. Exogenous ochronosis: case report and literature review. Bras Dermatol. 2012;87(4):633–6.
18. Gandhi V, Verma P, Naik G. Exogenous ochronosis after prolonged use of topical hydroquinone (2%) in a 50-year-old Indian female. Ind J Dermatol. 2012;57(5):394–5.
19. Wang BQ, Shen ZY, Fei Y, Li H, Liu JH, Xu H, et al. A population-based study of acquired bilateral nevus-of-Ota-like macules in Shanghai, China. J Invest Dermatol. 2011;131:358–62.
20. Lee WJ, Lee GY, Won KW, Won CH, Lee MW, Choi JH, Chang SE. Comparison of acquired bilateral nevus of Ota-like macules in men and women. Ind J Dermatol Venereol Leprol. 2014;80(4):313–9.
21. Choi K, Kim H, Kim H, Park Y. A case of actinic lichen planus. Internet J Dermatol. 2009;8(1). http://ispub.com/IJD/8/1/12894. Accessed 17 Feb 2016.
22. Rabinovitz HS, Barnhill RL. Benign melanocytic neoplasms. In: Bologna JL, Jorrizo JL, Schaffer JV, editors. Dermatology. 3rd ed. China: Elsevier Saunders; 2012. p. 1851–83.
23. Convit J, Kerdel-Vegas F, Rodriguez G. Erythema dyschromicum perstans: a hitherto undescribed skin disease. J Invest Dermatol. 1961;36:457–62.

Chapter 10
Melasma and Comorbidities

Ncoza C. Dlova and Levashni Naidoo

10.1 Introduction

The concurrence of multiple diseases or disorders in association with melasma has not been widely reported, and the precise interplay amongst contributory factors that generate this hypermelanization remains the focus of ongoing studies.

Key associated factors identified thus far include endocrine, psychological and emotional disturbance.

10.2 Menstrual Cycle Irregularities

Middle Eastern studies have documented the association of menstrual cycle changes associated with conditions like polycystic ovarian syndrome and insulin resistance, finding them to occur more commonly in patients with melasma [1, 2].

A more recent study from Brazil supported this reporting a greater association with menstrual irregularities and patients diagnosed with melasma. This relationship bordered on significant where a subgroup analysis of females with greater BMI was undertaken [3].

N.C. Dlova, MBChB, FCDerm, PhD (✉) • L. Naidoo
Department of Dermatology, Nelson R Mandela School of Medicine,
University of KwaZulu Natal, Durban, South Africa
e-mail: Dlovan@ukzn.ac.za

E.B. Handog, M.J. Enriquez-Macarayo (eds.), *Melasma and Vitiligo in Brown Skin*,
DOI 10.1007/978-81-322-3664-1_10

10.3 Thyroid Dysfunction

Mild thyroid dysfunction has been found in some studies on females with melasma. The study by Lufti et al. classified melasma patients into two groups: idiopathic versus association with occurrence in pregnancy or subsequent to contraceptive pill use [4]. An association with thyroid abnormalities was found to be higher in the latter group (70 % in the latter versus 39 % in the former group) leading the authors to propose a positive association with thyroid autoimmunity in the setting of pregnancy or contraceptive use.

A more recent study from Iran contrasted the thyroid hormone profile of 70 non-pregnant melasma sufferers with an equal number of age-matched controls [5], with a significantly higher prevalence of thyroid dysfunction in the first group in contrast to the control group, further highlighting the relationship between thyroid autoimmunity and melasma.

Further study regarding this association is necessary before screening policy guidelines for thyroid dysfunction in the setting of melasma can be made [5].

10.4 Hypothalamic and Limbic System Contribution

The hypothalamus acts in the limbic system, and stressors may, therefore, play a part in inciting adrenocorticotrophin- and melanocyte-stimulating hormone release which positively feeds into the melanin pigment production pathway in susceptible individuals [6, 7].

Stress and depression also elevate cortisol levels further augmenting the pathway for melanin production [8]. Patients with melasma have heightened anxiety trait scores and are more frequently on anxiolytics and antidepressants than matched controls [3]. These findings raise our awareness of the importance of our patients' psychological health and its possible impact on pigment alteration.

10.5 Conclusion

Although menstrual irregularities, thyroid dysfunction and higher levels of depression and anxiety have been reported as melasma comorbidities, further studies are still needed to confirm these associations. Validation of the few reports would ensure a future comprehensive and multidisciplinary approach to patients with melasma.

References

1. Mahmood K, Nadeem M, Aman S, Hameed A, Kazmi AH. Role of estrogen, progesterone and prolactin in the etiopathogenesis of melasma in females. J Pak Assoc Dermatol. 2011;21:241–7.
2. Adalatkhan H, Amani F. The correlation between melasma, ovarian cysts and androgenic hormones (a case control study). Res Biol Sci. 2007;2:593–6.

3. Handel AC, Lima PB, Tonolli VM, Mio LDB, Miot HA. Risk factors for facial melasma in women: a case–control study. Br Journ Derm. 2014;171(3):588–94.
4. Lutfi RJ, Fridmanis M, Misiunas AL, Pafume O, Gonzalez EA, Villemur JA, et al. Association of melasma with thyroid autoimmunity and other thyroidal abnormalities and their relationship to the origin of melasma. J Clin Endocrinol Metab. 1985;61:28–31.
5. Rostami Mogaddam M, Iranparvar Alamdari M, Maleki N, Safavi Ardabili N, Abedkouhi S. Evaluation of autoimmune thyroid disease in melasma. J Cosmet Dermatol. 2015;14(2):167–71.
6. Slominski A, Zbytek B, Semak I, Sweatman T, Wortsman J. CRH stimulates POMC activity and corticosterone production in dermal fibroblasts. J Neuroimmunol. 2005;162:97–102.
7. Slominski AT, Botchkarev V, Choudhry M, Fazal N, Fechner K, Furkert J, Krause E, Roloff B, Sayeed M, Wei E. Cutaneous expression of CRH and CRH-R. Is there a 'skin stress response system?'. Ann N Y Acad Sci. 1999;885:287–311.
8. Costin GE, Hearing VJ. Human skin pigmentation: melanocytes modulate skin color in response to stress. FASEB J. 2007;21(4):976–94.

Chapter 11
Melanogenesis and New Signaling Regulators for the Treatment of Melasma

Masakazu Kawaguchi and Tamio Suzuki

11.1 Introduction

Melasma is primarily caused by increased melanin deposition in the epidermis. It often occurs among women with dark complexions and occurs during their reproductive years. Ultraviolet (UV) radiation exposure, hormonal factors, and pregnancy are known risk factors [1, 2].

Melanin is produced by melanocytes and is transferred to surrounding keratinocytes. The most important transcription factor that regulates melanocyte function is the microphthalmia transcription factor (MITF). Genes that encode tyrosinase (TYR), a key enzyme in melanogenesis, tyrosinase-related protein-1 (TRP-1), dopachrome tautomerase (DCT), and PMEL17 are involved in pigmentation disorders and are induced by several factors. MITF plays a fundamental role in the transcriptional regulation of these genes. MITF expression levels are regulated by various transcription factors, including lymphoid enhancer-binding factor 1 (LEF-1)/T-cell factor (TCF), which is a downstream regulator of the Wnt-β-catenin signaling pathway, and cAMP-responsive element-binding protein (CREB). Multiple signaling pathways are involved in the regulation of tyrosinase and MITF, resulting in the stimulation of melanogenesis. The activation of melanocortin-1 receptor (MC1R) by its agonist, α-melanocyte-stimulating hormone (α-MSH), increases cAMP production and leads to the phosphorylation of CREB. Phosphorylated CREB upregulates the transcription of various genes, including MITF. Stem cell factor (SCF, also known as KIT ligand) and its receptor c-KIT link with the Ras-MAP kinase signaling pathway and regulate MITF function *via* MITF phosphorylation [3] (Fig. 11.1).

M. Kawaguchi (✉) • T. Suzuki
Department of Dermatology, Yamagata University Faculty of Medicine,
2-2-2 Iida-Nishi, Yamagata 990-9585, Japan
e-mail: kawaguch@med.id.yamagata-u.ac.jp

E.B. Handog, M.J. Enriquez-Macarayo (eds.), *Melasma and Vitiligo in Brown Skin*,
DOI 10.1007/978-81-322-3664-1_11

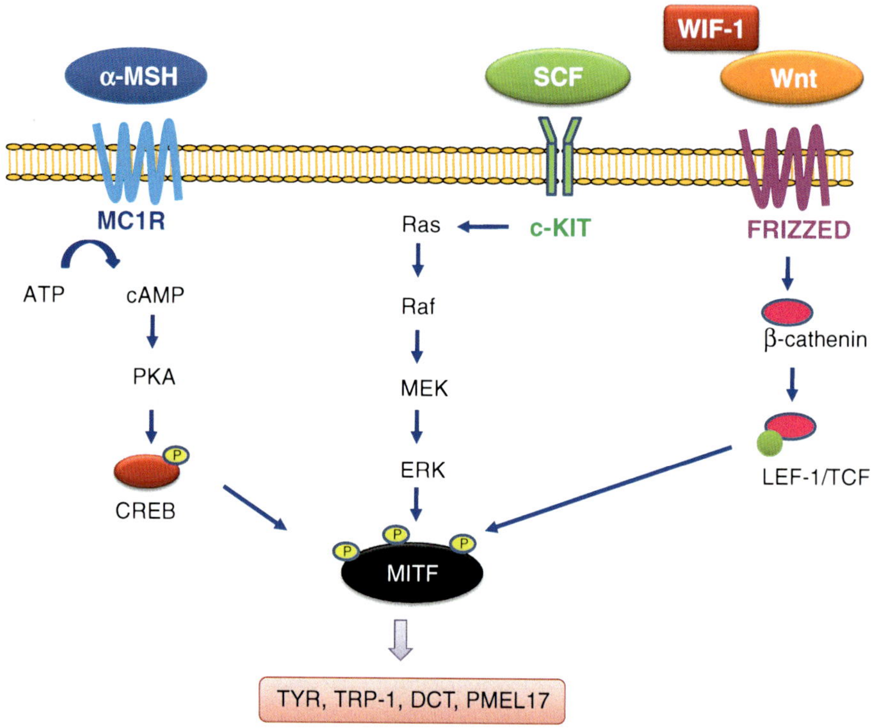

Fig. 11.1 Schematic depiction of melanogenesis in melanocytes. Tyrosinase (TYR), a key enzyme in melanogenesis, tyrosinase-related protein-1 (TRP-1), dopachrome tautomerase (DCT), and PMEL17 are melanogenesis-related proteins involved in pigmentation disorders, and microphthalmia transcription factor (MITF) plays a role in the transcriptional regulation of these factors. MITF expression levels are regulated by various transcription factors, including lymphoid enhancer-binding factor 1 (LEF-1)/T-cell factor (TCF), which is a downstream regulator of the Wnt-β-catenin signaling pathway, and cAMP responsive-element-binding protein (CREB). Melanocortin-1 receptor (MC1R)/α-melanocyte-stimulating hormone (α-MSH) signaling increases cAMP production and leads to the phosphorylation of CREB. Stem cell factor (SCF) and its receptor c-KIT link to the Ras-MAP kinase signaling pathway and regulate MITF function *via* MITF phosphorylation

Recently, novel cellular and molecular mechanisms for skin pigmentation, including melasma, have been identified. These include sex hormonal factors [4], the H19 noncoding RNA [5], microRNAs (miRNA) [6, 7], and Wnt pathway modulators [8–10] (Fig. 11.2).

Sunscreen for protection from sunlight and skin-lightening agents are used to treat melasma. Various well-known agents, such as hydroquinone, arbutin, kojic acid, and ascorbic acid, reduce pigmentation by interfering with several processes involved in melanogenesis 3'-UTR (e.g., the inhibition of melanocyte proliferation, TYR activity and expression, MITF expression, and 5'-UTR melanosome formation). These depigmenting agents have little effect and sometimes have severe side effects. Therefore, it is imperative to identify new agents with better efficacy and fewer side effects.

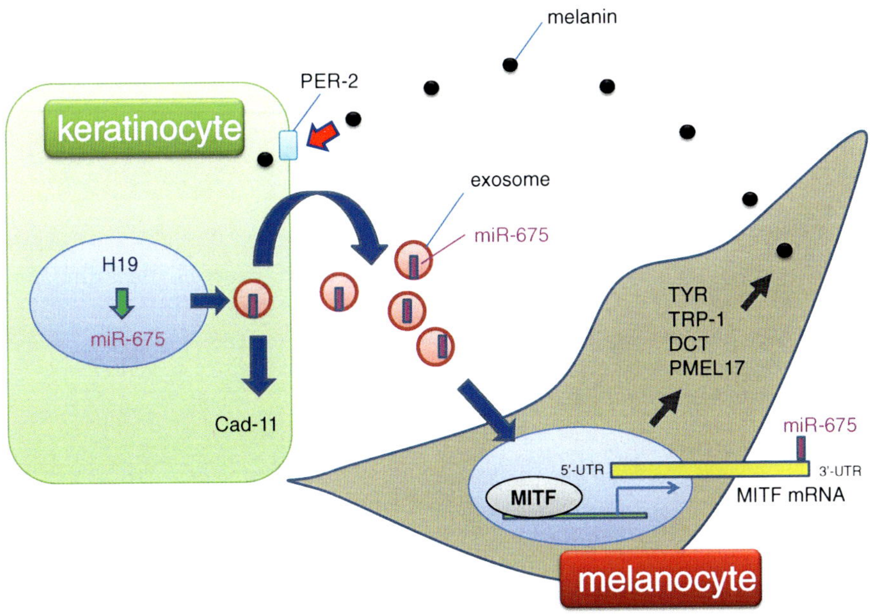

Fig. 11.2 Role of miR-675 in melasma. Downregulation of the H19 noncoding RNA was observed in the hyperpigmented skin of a melasma patient. H19 knockdown reduces miR-675 expression. miR-675 is released from keratinocytes *via* exosomes, a type of extracellular vesicle derived from the endosomal system, and inhibits MITF mRNA expression by targeting its 3′-UTR in melanocytes. Cadherin 11 (Cad-11) is another target of miR-675

The oral antidiabetic drug metformin [11] and omeprazole [12], a gastric proton pump inhibitor, reduce melanin content by decreasing cAMP accumulation and TYR degradation, respectively.

We found that inhibitors of a disintegrin and metalloprotease (ADAM) reduce melanin content by disrupting the processing of the melanosomal protein PMEL17 [13]. PMEL17 (also called gp100 and silver) is a type I transmembrane melanosomal glycoprotein that forms a fibrillar matrix on which melanin is deposited in melanosomes. Proteolytic processing of PMEL17 is required for the formation of functional fibrils during melanogenesis. We demonstrated that ADAM inhibitors disrupt the formation of fibrils and their assembly into sheets in melanosomes *via* the regulation of PMEL17 processing. ADAMs are a family of proteases involved in ectodomain shedding; they play a role in various cellular processes [14, 15]. ADAM17 plays a critical role in the ectodomain shedding of many soluble proteins, including tumor necrosis factor-α (TNF-α), KIT ligand, and its receptor. In humans, *ADAM17* is a candidate gene for the regulation of pigmentation in East Asians [16]. Mutations in *ADAM10* were identified as a cause of reticulate acropigmentation of Kitamura, which is characterized by reticulate, slightly depressed pigmented macules mainly affecting the dorsa of the hands and feet [17]. As ADAMs are involved in multiple signaling pathways that regulate melanogenesis, ADAM proteases could be new potent therapeutic agents for pigmentation disorders.

Identifying the factors involved in the pathogenesis of melasma could facilitate the development of new treatment options for the disorder.

11.2 UV Exposure and Barrier Dysfunction

Based on a transcriptional analysis of melasma skin samples, 279 upregulated genes and 152 downregulated genes have been identified [8]. As expected, the expression levels of melanogenesis-associated factors, such as TYR, TRP-1, DCT, and MITF, are increased in melasma lesions, indicating higher melanogenic activity in lesional skin. As the number of melanocytes is not significantly increased, increased epidermal pigmentation due to increased melanogenesis in lesional melanocytes is expected to be the main physiological mechanism in melasma.

A bioinformatics analysis identified significant modifications of lipid metabolism in melasma. Lipid metabolism genes, such as peroxisome proliferator-activated receptor alpha (*PPARA*), PPAR gamma coactivator 1 alpha (*PPARGC1A*), arachidonate 15-lipoxygenase, type B (*ALOX15B*), and diacylglycerol *O*-acyltransferase 2-like 3 (*DGAT2L3*), were found to be downregulated. It is well known that lipid metabolism of the stratum corneum has an important role in barrier homeostasis. Interestingly, barrier function of melasma lesional skin is damaged compared with perilesional skin [8, 18]; a thinned stratum corneum and delayed barrier recovery rate have been observed for lesional skin.

UV irradiation may play a major role in melasma development based on the location of lesions and the development and/or aggravation of symptoms after sun exposure. Furthermore, chronic UV exposure is known to influence fatty acid metabolism and barrier function of the skin [19]. Free fatty acids and triglycerides in the epidermis of photoaged or acutely UV-irradiated human skin are significantly decreased [20]. The expression levels of genes related to lipid synthesis, including *PPAR*, are also markedly decreased [20]. Ligand activation of PPARs stimulates differentiation, induces lipid accumulation, and accelerates epidermal barrier regeneration in keratinocytes; accordingly, PPAR is an important regulator of lipid metabolism by mediating fatty acids [21]. Therefore, impaired barrier function owing to UV irradiation might be a factor in the pathogenesis of melasma.

11.3 Wnt Signaling

Although the effects of UV exposure are well established, the mechanism of UV-induced pigmentation may not be same for skin pigmentation conditions induced by different causes. In addition, UV irradiation may not be necessary in melasma development. Wnt inhibitory factor 1 (WIF-1) has been identified [9] as a factor involved in melasma pathogenesis that does not exhibit expression changes after UV irradiation. WIF-1 is a secreted antagonist of Wnt signaling; it inhibits the Wnt pathway by binding directly to Wnt ligands and preventing the ligands from binding to cell surface receptors.

The canonical and noncanonical Wnt pathways have important roles in the regulation of melanogenesis. In the canonical pathway, Wnts prevent the degradation of β-catenin, which promotes translocation to the nucleus to stimulate the transcription factor MITF. WIF-1 is reduced in melasma lesions and is expressed in both cultured normal human keratinocytes and fibroblasts, but not in melanocytes. WIF-1 knockdown stimulates TYR expression and melanosome transfer in keratinocyte/melanocyte cocultures. By treatment with recombinant WIF-1 in cocultures, TYR expression is significantly reduced with MITF expression. However, another report has shown that WIF-1 and other Wnt pathway modulators, such as Wnt5a, are upregulated in melasma lesional skin based on a microarray analysis [8]. Currently, decreased expression of WIF-1 is implicated in melasma development via the stimulation of melanogenesis and melanosome transfer through the activation of Wnt signaling.

11.4 Female Sex Hormones

As pregnancy and changes in uterine and ovarian hormones are risk factors for melasma, the female sex hormones estrogen and progesterone have been implicated in the development of hyperpigmentation in melasma [2]. Estrogens stimulate melanogenesis in human melanocytes by inducing the synthesis of melanogenic enzymes, and melanocytes express estrogen receptors [4]. An immunohistochemical analysis has shown that estrogen receptor and progesterone receptor expression levels are increased in affected skin [22, 23].

Recently, based on a microarray analysis, the upregulation of PDZ domain protein kidney 1 (PDZK1) expression was detected in the hyperpigmented skin of melasma patients [4]. PDZK1 is a member of the sodium–hydrogen exchanger regulatory factor (NHERF) family. NHERFs have PDZ domains, which mediate protein–protein interactions and have been shown to bind ion transporters. Estrogen increases MITF and TYR expression via PDZK1 in melanocytes. Knockdown of PDZK1 reduces estrogen-induced TYR expression. PDZK1 overexpression increases estrogen-stimulated TYR expression with ER-α and ER-β expression. PDZK1 also upregulates the expression of several ion transporters such as sodium–hydrogen exchanger (NHE), cystic fibrosis transmembrane conductance regulator (CFTR), and SLC26A3. These transporters are upregulated by estrogen, and specific inhibitors of transporter proteins inhibit the estrogen-induced expression of TYR. Interestingly, PDZK1 upregulation stimulates melanosome transfer to keratinocytes, irrespective of protease-activated receptor-2 (PER-2) expression, which is involved in melanosome transfer. PDZK1 has emerged as an important factor in the development of hyperpigmentation in melasma and is particularly associated with estrogen.

11.5 MicroRNAs and Their Targets

miRNAs have been identified as novel factors in melasma pathogenesis. Downregulation of the expression of the H19 noncoding RNA has been detected in the hyperpigmented skin of a melasma patient, but not in UV-exposed hyperpigmented skin in a microarray analysis [5]. Noncoding RNAs have important roles in the epigenetic regulation of genes. In an examination of the mechanism of H19 downregulation in melasma, one miRNA was identified as its target in melanogenesis [6]. miRNAs are small, 20–24 nucleotide, endogenously expressed noncoding RNAs. They anneal to the 3′-untranslated region (UTR) of mRNAs in a sequence-specific fashion and either block translation or promote transcript degradation, thus playing a major role in the posttranscriptional regulation of gene expression [24].

H19 knockdown reduces miR-675 expression levels in keratinocytes, but not in melanocytes or fibroblasts. In addition, miR-675 overexpression decreases the expression of TYR and TRP-1, whereas its inhibitor increases their expression in keratinocytes and melanocytes in a cocultured system. As the expression levels of miR-675 are correlated with those of H19 in keratinocytes, but not in melanocytes, miR-675 is thought to be released from keratinocytes. Exosomes, which are extracellular vesicles derived from the endosomal system, are secreted from living cells into the extracellular environment. Exosomes can arise from different cell types, including tumor cells but also from normal cells, and contain various cellular proteins, including MHC molecules and adhesion molecules, as well as miRNAs. As the transfer of exosome-derived miRNAs to receipt cells is suggested as a means of cell–cell communication, miR-675 could be released from keratinocytes *via* exosomes and regulate melanogenesis in melanocytes. A microarray analysis has revealed that MITF is a target of miR-675, which inhibits MITF mRNA expression by targeting its 3′-UTR.

Cadherin 11 (Cad-11) is another target of miR-675 [7]. miR-675 similarly inhibits Cad-11 expression by targeting its 3′-UTR. Increased Cad-11 expression is also observed in the hyperpigmented skin of melasma patients, suggesting a role of Cad-11 in melasma. Cad-11 regulates dermal fibroblast migration and β-catenin levels, both of which are important in the development of tissue fibrosis [25]. Although Cad-11 expression is not detectable in melanocytes, Cad-11 in fibroblasts or keratinocytes stimulates melanogenesis, increasing the expression of β-catenin and Wnt, and induces melanocyte migration.

In vivo miR-675 overexpression in mouse skin using a transfection reagent reduces the expression of melanogenesis-related genes [6]. As exosome-derived miRNAs have been shown to be resistant to RNase treatment, miR-675 could be a potent therapeutic target for melasma.

11.6 Conclusion

In this review, we summarize the current understanding of the mechanisms of melasma development. Novel mediators for melasma such as the H19 noncoding RNA, WIF-1, microRNAs, and PDZK1 have recently been identified using large-scale expression profiles. In addition, Cad-11 appears to be an important mediator of melasma, and inhibition of its function is a potential therapeutic approach for the treatment of melasma.

Understanding the pathogenesis of melasma could enable the development of new treatment options for the disorder.

References

1. Ortonne JP, Arellano I, Berneburg M, Cestari T, Chan H, Grimes P, et al. A global survey of the role of ultraviolet radiation and hormonal influences in the development of melasma. J Eur Acad Dermatol Venereol. 2009;23:1254–62.
2. Lee AY. Recent progress in melasma pathogenesis. Pigment Cell Melanoma Res. 2015;28(6): 648–60.
3. Yamaguchi Y, Hearing VJ. Physiological factors that regulate skin pigmentation. Biofactors. 2009;35:193–9.
4. Kim NH, Cheong KA, Lee TR, Lee AY. PDZK1 upregulation in estrogen-related hyperpigmentation in melasma. J Invest Dermatol. 2012;132:2622–31.
5. Kim NH, Lee CH, Lee AY. H19 RNA downregulation stimulated melanogenesis in melasma. Pigment Cell Melanoma Res. 2009;23:84–92.
6. Kim NH, Choi SH, Kim CH, Lee CH, Lee TR, Lee AY. Reduced MiR-675 in exosome in H19 RNA-related melanogenesis via MITF as a direct target. J Invest Dermatol. 2014;134: 1075–82.
7. Kim NH, Choi SH, Lee TR, Lee CH, Lee AY. Cadherin 11, a miR-675 target, induces N-cadherin expression and epithelial-mesenchymal transition in melasma. J Invest Dermatol. 2014;134:2967–76.
8. Kang HY, Suzuki I, Lee DJ, Ha J, Reiniche P, Aubert J, et al. Transcriptional profiling shows altered expression of wnt pathway- and lipid metabolism-related genes as well as melanogenesis-related genes in melasma. J Invest Dermatol. 2011;131:1692–700.
9. Kim JY, Lee TR, Lee AY. Reduced WIF-1 expression stimulates skin hyperpigmentation in patients with melasma. J Invest Dermatol. 2013;133:191–200.
10. Park TJ, Kim M, Kim H, Park SY, Park KC, Ortonne JP, et al. Wnt inhibitory factor (WIF)-1 promotes melanogenesis in normal human melanocytes. Pigment Cell Melanoma Res. 2014;27:72–81.
11. Lehraiki A, Abbe P, Cerezo M, Rouaud F, Regazzetti C, Chignon-Sicard B, et al. Inhibition of melanogenesis by the antidiabetic metformin. J Invest Dermatol. 2014;134:2589–97.
12. Matsui MS, Petris MJ, Niki Y, Karaman-Jurukovska N, Muizzuddin N, Ichihashi M, et al. Omeprazole, a gastric proton pump inhibitor, inhibits melanogenesis by blocking ATP7A trafficking. J Invest Dermatol. 2015;135:834–41.
13. Kawaguchi M, Hozumi Y, Suzuki T. ADAM protease inhibitors reduce melanogenesis by regulating PMEL17 processing in human melanocytes. J Dermatol Sci. 2015;78:133–42.
14. Schlöndorff J, Blobel CP. Metalloprotease-disintegrins: modular proteins capable of promoting cell-cell interactions and triggering signals by protein-ectodomain shedding. J Cell Sci. 1999;112:3603–17.
15. Edwards DR, Handsley MM, Pennington CJ. The ADAM metalloproteinases. Mol Aspects Med. 2008;29:258–89.
16. McEvoy B, Beleza S, Shriver MD. The genetic architecture of normal variation in human pigmentation: an evolutionary perspective and model. Hum Mol Genet. 2006;15 Spec No 2: R176-81.
17. Kono M, Sugiura K, Suganuma M, Hayashi M, Takama H, Suzuki T, et al. Whole-exome sequencing identifies ADAM10 mutations as a cause of reticulate acropigmentation of Kitamura, a clinical entity distinct from Dowling-Degos disease. Hum Mol Genet. 2013;22: 3524–33.

18. Lee DJ, Lee J, Ha J, Park KC, Ortonne JP, Kang HY. Defective barrier function in melasma skin. J Eur Acad Dermatol Venereol. 2012;26:1533–7.
19. Merle C, Laugel C, Baillet-Guffroy A. Effect of UVA or UVB irradiation on cutaneous lipids in films or in solution. Photochem Photobiol. 2010;86:553–62.
20. Kim EJ, Jin XJ, Kim YK, Oh IK, Kim JE, Park CH, et al. UV decreases the synthesis of free fatty acids and triglycerides in the epidermis of human skin in vivo, contributing to development of skin photoaging. J Dermatol Sci. 2010;57:19–26.
21. Schmuth M, Moosbrugger-Martinz V, Blunder S, Dubrac S. Role of PPAR, LXR, and PXR in epidermal homeostasis and inflammation. Biochim Biophys Acta. 1841;2014:463–73.
22. Jang YH, Lee JY, Kang HY, Lee ES, Kim YC. Oestrogen and progesterone receptor expression in melasma: an immunohistochemical analysis. J Eur Acad Dermatol Venereol. 2010;24:1312–6.
23. Tamega Ade A, Miot HA, Moço NP, Silva MG, Marques ME, Miot LD. Gene and protein expression of oestrogen-β and progesterone receptors in facial melasma and adjacent healthy skin in women. Int J Cosmet Sci. 2015;37:222–8.
24. Chekulaeva M, Filipowicz W. Mechanisms of miRNA-mediated post-transcriptional regulation in animal cells. Curr Opin Cell Biol. 2009;21:452–60.
25. Agarwal SK. Integrins and cadherins as therapeutic targets in fibrosis. Front Pharmacol. 2014;5:131.

Chapter 12
Topical Agents in Melasma

Ma. Flordeliz Abad-Casintahan and Hester Gail Lim

12.1 Introduction

Melasma is often difficult to treat, and the condition may be refractory. Principles of therapy include protection from ultraviolet (UV) light, inhibition of melanocyte activity and melanin synthesis, and the disruption and removal of melanin granules [1]. Due to the multiple treatment modalities available, the choice of treatment must take into account the type of melasma (whether epidermal, dermal, or mixed), the skin complexion of the patient, previous treatments, patient expectations, as well as compliance [2].

Topical therapy remains the standard of melasma treatment. It aims to retard the proliferation of melanocytes, inhibit melanosome formation, and enhance melanosome degradation [3]. The epitome of a depigmenting agent should provide powerful, quick, yet selective lightening on hyperactive melanocytes. Resultant elimination of unwanted pigment must be lasting, with no undesirable side effects. Despite the numerous topical therapeutic options in the market, the ideal depigmenting agent has yet to be found. Depigmenting agents can target melanin production at the level of transcription and tyrosinase glycosylation, during the synthesis of melanin as well as the uptake and distribution of melanosomes into recipient keratinocytes, and during tyrosinase degradation and turnover of pigmented keratinocytes. Simply put, depigmenting agents target melanin synthesis before, during, and after the process [4]. Topical agents are especially efficacious in the epidermal type of melasma [5].

This chapter will cover the different types of topical therapy, administered as monotherapy or in combination with different agents. While monotherapy for melasma has been in use the longest, the current trend is toward combination therapy, which has shown greater efficacy.

M.F. Abad-Casintahan (✉) • H.G. Lim, MD
Department of Dermatology, Jose R. Reyes Memorial Medical Center,
Rizal Avenue Extension, Sta. Cruz, Manila, Philippines
e-mail: lizkcmd@yahoo.com; hes.gail@gmail.com

E.B. Handog, M.J. Enriquez-Macarayo (eds.), *Melasma and Vitiligo in Brown Skin*,
DOI 10.1007/978-81-322-3664-1_12

12.2 Monotherapy

12.2.1 Hydroquinone (HQ)

Hydroquinone is the most extensively studied medication in the management of melasma, although most recent studies have hydroquinone in combination with other substances. A dihydric phenol, HQ is an aromatic organic compound with a primary function of hindering melanin production by inhibiting the tyrosinase enzyme [6, 7]. As monotherapy, HQ in itself is effective and used at concentrations ranging from 2 to 5 % [8]. After prolonged use, however, it can cause permanent depigmentation. Other adverse effects include irritant dermatitis, ochronosis, and postinflammatory pigmentation [9].

HQ is often the standard therapy to which other treatment regimens are compared. While it is the gold standard in depigmentation, issues of safety have arisen with this product, thus, it has been banned in several countries. With the risk of exogenous ochronosis and permanent depigmentation following long-term use, it has been banned by the European Committee, with formulations withdrawn from cosmetics in these countries [10]. This has spurred research for its use with other agents and for other equally potent, but safer depigmenting agents.

12.2.2 Azelaic Acid

A dicarboxylic acid derived from *Pityrosporum* mold, azelaic acid is a reversible inhibitor of tyrosinase activity. While it does not affect normal melanocytes, it is antiproliferative and cytotoxic to abnormal melanocytes [3]. This is especially advantageous to patients who only wish to lighten the sites affected with melasma, but not their baseline skin color. In a study by Balina and Graupe, 20 % azelaic acid was found to be comparable with 4 % HQ [11]. In a Thai population comparing 2 % HQ with 20 % azelaic acid, the latter was found to be more efficacious; however this population had a greater incidence of adverse effects which include pruritus, transient erythema, scaling, and, occasionally, sensitization [12].

12.2.3 Kojic Acid

A 7-pyrone compound, produced from fermentation of *Aspergillus* and *Penicillium* [10], kojic acid is a fungal metabolic product that inhibits the catecholate activity of tyrosinase. In addition, kojic acid functions as a potent antioxidant. For the management of hyperpigmentation, a concentration of 1–4 % is often used. While it is more chemically stable than HQ, it is less effective than HQ in its lightening property [13]. The Kojyl-APPA 5-[(3-aminopropyl)phosphinooxy]-2-(hydroxymethyl)-4H-pyran-4-one) synthesized by Kim et al. showed increased skin penetration and pigment lightening efficacy in melanoma and normal human melanocytes [14]. Adverse effects include sensitization, contact dermatitis, and erythema [15, 16].

12.2.4 Vitamin C

Vitamin C chelates copper ions necessary in the enzymatic steps for melanin production. In addition, it can convert melanin from its usual jet-black color to light tan. Vitamin C, however, is very easily oxidized in an aqueous solution. In a study by Espinal-Perez and colleagues, 5 % L-ascorbic acid was found to be equal in efficacy to 4 % HQ [17]. More stable derivatives, such as magnesium 5 % L-ascorbyl-2-phosphate in a 10 % cream compound, have also been found effective in the management of melasma [18]. Iontophoresis has also been used to increase cutaneous penetration of vitamin C [19].

12.2.5 Retinoids

Retinoids have been found to be moderately effective in the management of melasma. It promotes rapid loss of pigment through its effect in increasing epidermopoiesis, thereby decreasing keratinocyte contact time with melanocytes [20]. They also function by decreasing melanosome transfer and inhibiting tyrosinase transcription [21]. Adverse effects include erythema and peeling on application sites. Postinflammatory hyperpigmentation (PIH) should also be considered as a potential adverse effect.

Tretinoin concentrations used for melasma range from 0.05 to 0.1 %. Studies in a predominantly white population [22] have proven moderate effectivity.

Topical isotretinoin studied among Thai patients showed no statistically significant difference in MASI and colorimetry in the 0.05 % isotretinoin group versus a placebo group [23].

Adapalene is a second-generation retinoid. In an RCT of 30 Indian female patients diagnosed with melasma, efficacy and safety of adapalene 0.1 % was compared to that of tretinoin 0.05 %. Melasma area severity index (MASI) scores were recorded at baseline, 2 weeks, 6 weeks, 10 weeks, and 14 weeks. Results showed equal efficacy between the two agents: 37 % reduction in MASI score in tretinoin compared to 41 % reduction in adapalene group, with no statistical difference. There was a greater incidence of adverse effects in the tretinoin group [24].

12.2.6 Tranexamic Acid (TA)

Tranexamic acid is a trans-4(aminomethyl) cyclohexane carboxylic acid, which has been used in medical practice as a fibrinolytic agent. It has shown promise in the management of melasma through inhibition of melanin production. TA binds to plasmin and plasminogen leading to a decrease in the amount of free arachidonic acid. Prostaglandin production is then decreased and so is the melanocyte tyrosinase activity [6].

The injectable and oral forms have been noted to lighten melasma in patients. However, results have been conflicting. In a split-face trial by Kanechorn et al., there appeared to be no significant difference with topical tranexamic acid versus placebo, with a greater incidence of adverse effects in the tranexamic acid group [25]. Banihashemi et al. studied 5 % tranexamic in a liposomal form, a vehicle which may prolong the action of the substance, as well as improve its moisturizing effect. In this form, TA was comparable to HQ [26]. In another randomized, double-blind split-face trial, Ebrahimi et al. compared a topical solution of 3 % tranexamic acid to 0.01 % dexamethasone-3 % hydroquinone combination. Effects were comparable [27]. Velasquez et al. discussed the use of TA intradermally, with favorable results [28]. Due to the paucity of literature, more studies are needed to evaluate this substance for use in melasma.

12.2.7 Arbutin

Arbutin is a β-glycosylated form of HQ present in bearberry extracts [10]. It exists in two forms, α-arbutin and deoxyarbutin, both of which are inhibitors of tyrosinase and melanosome maturation. The synthetic deoxyarbutin, however, is more potent. Arbutin functions through reversible inhibition of melanosomal tyrosinase activity rather than suppression of expression and synthesis of tyrosinase. It shows less melanocyte cytotoxicity than HQ. While higher concentrations appear more efficacious, they may also cause paradoxical hyperpigmentation. In comparison to HQ, where the skin lightening effect is very difficult to sustain, deoxyarbutin-induced skin lightening was maintained without the use of maintenance therapy [29].

12.2.8 Vitamin E

In an in vitro study by Funasaka et al., alpha-tocopheryl ferulate dissolved in lecithin inhibited melanization without significantly inhibiting cell growth, via inhibition of tyrosinase. Added to this is the antioxidant effect of both α-tocopherol and α-tocopheryl through the inhibition of biological reactions induced by reactive oxygen species [30]. Topical vitamin E has been shown to be effective for wrinkles and other signs of photoaging. In porcine skin, vitamin E combination with ascorbic acid works synergistically, providing fourfold protection against UV-induced erythema [31, 32].

12.2.9 Niacinamide

The amide form of vitamin B3, niacinamide, reversibly inhibits melanosome transfer from melanocyte to keratinocyte by 35–68 % [33]. It also decreases collagen oxidation products and improves aging-induced yellowing or sallowness. It has no activity against tyrosinase [4].

12.2.10 Novel Therapeutic Agents

Rucinol serum, a derivative of resorcinol, functions via tyrosinase inhibition [6, 34]. A split-face trial comparing 4-*n*-butylresorcinol 0.1 % cream to placebo showed the former to be more effective [35].

Oligopeptides are a new class of tyrosinase inhibitors. In a study by Ubeid et al., octapeptides P16-18 were more effective than HQ, with minimal toxicity toward major human skin cell types [35]. A split-face, randomized pilot study in cases of recalcitrant melasma was performed, revealing efficacy with no apparent irritation to the skin [36].

Lincomycin and linoleic acid are substances that inhibit melanogenesis by increasing the degradation of tyrosinase and increasing stratum corneum turnover. Lee et al. found that the combination of lincomycin and linoleic acid with 0.05 % betamethasone valerate was found to be more effective than placebo, and the lincomycin group alone [37].

12.3 Combination Topical Therapies

The literature shows multiple variants of the triple combination cream: Kligman's formula (5 % HQ, 0.1 % tretinoin, and 0.1 % dexamethasone), modified Kligman's formula (4 % HQ, 0.05 % tretinoin, and 1 % hydrocortisone acetate), and Pathak (2 % HQ and 0.05–0.1 % tretinoin) and Westerhof's formula (4.7 % N-acetylcysteine, 2 % HQ, and 0.1 % triamcinolone acetonide) [6]. The addition of tretinoin to hydroquinone prevents the oxidation of HQ, ameliorates the side effects of topical steroids, and increases pigment elimination through desquamation. This combination strongly inhibits the production of melanin without the destruction of melanocytes [1].

To date, one of the most effective and widely studied is the triple combination cream utilizing 4 % HQ, 0.05 % tretinoin, and 0.01 % fluocinolone acetonide [38]. In a systematic review of randomized controlled trials (Cochrane), this triple combination was more effective than HQ monotherapy or other individual constituent therapies [39]. The fluocinolone-based triple creams are considered safe up to 24 weeks, with a very low risk of skin atrophy [40, 41]. In an open label study by Grimes et al., the aforementioned triple combination cream improved moderate to severe melasma at 12 weeks. Once patients had improved, they were shifted to maintenance therapy at twice weekly dosing. However, this dosing led to a relapse, prompting resumption of daily therapy [41]. Of significance is that the use of a fluorinated steroid (fluocinolone acetonide) in this triple combination is contributory to its safety, in contrast to the non-fluorinated steroids (dexamethasone, hydrocortisone, mometasone).

Chan et al. compared the efficacy of a fixed triple combination cream (4 % HQ, 0.01 % triamcinolone, and 0.05 % tretinoin) with 4 % HQ for melasma. This triple combination cream was more effective than 4 % HQ monotherapy in an Asian population, despite the high incidence of retinoid dermatitis in this group. Though erythema was a frequently noted adverse reaction, none were severe enough to prompt discontinuation of the study. Even with a corticosteroid containing agent, patients had no reports of skin atrophy at the conclusion of the study [40]. Adverse effects include erythema, peeling, dryness, and irritation. Topical therapy with triple combination cream appears to be the most effective treatment regimen [38].

Hydroquinone 4 % and hyaluronic acid 0.01 % combination was found to be less irritating than HQ alone. The addition of glycolic acid 10 % was found to accelerate desquamation and pigment dispersion, thereby accelerating skin lightening [7]. Unfortunately, many patients found this formula highly irritating. Javaheri et al. suggested the use of glycolic acid 10 % lotion and 2 % HQ [42].

12.4 Maintenance

Melasma is easily triggered by UV exposure and thus tends to be recurrent. Significant in the maintenance phase of melasma management is the diligent daily use of topical sunscreens, in addition to avoidance of UV exposure (by natural or artificial light). Vazquez and Sanchez found that HQ therapy was more effective when sunscreen was added to the treatment regimen. Though most studies include sunscreens in both control and treatment groups, the authors feel that Vazquez and Sanchez's findings can be extrapolated to infer that all other whitening agents are more effective when sunscreen is added [43]. It must be noted, however, that the use of a broad spectrum sunscreen, while important in the management and maintenance therapy of melasma, cannot in itself prevent relapse [44], and thus, maintenance topical regimens are required. The appropriate therapy should be dependent on the patient's compliance and the severity of melasma at initial consult [41, 45].

There are limited studies on the ideal tapering regimen. In a randomized, blinded, controlled study, Arellano et al. compared a tapering regimen (thrice weekly for the first months, then twice weekly for the second month, and then once weekly for the fourth month) versus a twice weekly regimen. Both groups were comparable; however, the twice weekly application postponed relapse for a greater period of time in severe melasma, while the tapering regimen was more effective for patients with moderate melasma [45].

12.5 Conclusion

The management of melasma is no mean task. Topical therapies remain the gold standard in management, with hydroquinone being the most popular and extensively studied agent. In recent years, however, studies have shifted away from hydroquinone monotherapy to search for substances equal in efficacy but superior in safety. Monotherapies such as azelaic acid, retinoids, kojic acid, and other novel agents have found much support in recent years, especially in this era of hydroquinone-free cosmeceuticals. Despite this surge of interest in novel therapies for melasma, the literature considers triple combination cream as the most effective topical therapy for melasma to date. Lastly, of paramount importance is the religious use of broad spectrum sunscreens—success in the treatment of melasma is dependent on rigorous photoprotection as an adjunct to treatment.

References

1. Gupta AK, Nouri K, Taylor S. The treatment of melasma: a review of clinical trials. J Am Acad Dermatol. 2006;55(6):1048–65.
2. Prignano F, Ortonne JP, Buggiani G, Lotti T. Therapeutical approaches in melasma. Dermatol Clin. 2007;25(3):337–42.
3. Rigopoulos D, Gregorious S, Katsamabas A. Hyperpigmentation and melasma. J Cosm Dermatol. 2007;6:195–202.
4. Briganti S, Camera E, Picardo M. Chemical and instrumental approaches to treat hyperpigmentation. Pigment Cell Res. 2003;16(2):101–10.
5. Bandyopadhyay D. Topical treatment of melasma. Ind J Dermatol. 2009;54(4):303–9.
6. Sarkar R, Pooja A, Garg VK, Sonthalia S, Gokhale N. Melasma update. Ind Dermatol Online J. 2014;5(4):426–35.
7. Ibrahim Z, Gheida S, Maghraby G, Farag Z. Evaluation of the efficacy and safety of combinations of hydroquinone, glycolic acid, and hyaluronic acid in the treatment of melasma. J Cosmet Dermatol. 2015;14(2):113–23.
8. Tirado-Sanchez A, Santamaria-Roman A, Ponce Olivera RM. Efficacy of dioic acid compared with hydroquinone in the treatment of melasma. Int J Dermatol. 2009;48:893–5.
9. Marta R, Berneburg M, Arellano I, Picaro M. Treatment of melasma. J Am Acad Dermatol. 2006;54(5):S272–81.
10. Ebanks JP, Wickett RR, Boissy RE. Mechanisms regulating skin pigmentation: the rise and fall of complexion and coloration. Int J Mol Sci. 2009;10(9):4066–87.
11. Balina LM, Graupe K. The treatment of melasma. 20% azelaic acid versus 4% hydroquinone. Int J Dermatol. 1991;30(12):893–5.
12. Sivyathorn A, Verallo-Rowell V, Graupe K. 20% Azelaic acid cream in the topical treatment of melasma: a double-blind comparison with 2% hydroquinone. Eur J Dermatol. 1995;5:680–4.
13. Lim JT. Treatment of melasma using Kojic acid in a gel containing hydroquinone and glycolic acid. Dermatol Surg. 1999;25:282–4.
14. Kim DH, Hwang JS, Baek HS, Lee BG, Chang I, Kang H, et al. Development of 5-[(3-aminopropyl)phosphinooxy]-2-(hydroxymethyl)-4H-pyran-4-one as a novel whitening agent. Chem Pharm Bull (Tokyo). 2003;51(2):113–6.
15. Nakagawa M, Kawai K, Kawai K. Contact allergy to kojic acid in skin care products. Cont Derm. 1995;32:9–13.
16. Badresia B, Draelos ZD. Insight into skin lightening cosmeceuticals for women of color. J Drugs Dermatol. 2007;6:32–9.
17. Espinal-Perez LE, Moncada B, Castanedo-Cazarez JP. A double-blind randomized trial of 5% ascorbic acid vs. 4% hydroquinone in melasma. Int J Dermatol. 2004;43:604–7.
18. Kameyama K, Sakai C, Kondoh C, Yonemoto K, Shigeo N, Tagawa M, et al. Inhibitory effect of magnesium L-ascorbyl-2-phosphate (VC-PMG) on melanogenesis in vitro and in vivo. J Am Acad Dermatol. 1996;34(1):29–33.
19. Huh CH, Seo KI, Park JY, Lim JG, Eun HC, Park KC. A double blind randomized trial of 5% ascorbic acid vs 4% hydroquinone in melasma. Int J Dermatol. 2004;43(8):604–7.
20. Ortonne JP. Retinoid therapy of pigmented disorders. Dermatol Ther. 2006;10:280–8.
21. Sehgal V, Verma P, Srivstava G, Aggarwal AK, Verma S. Melasma: treatment strategy. J Cosm Laser Ther. 2011;13:265–79.

22. Kimbrough-Green CK, Griffiths CE, Finkel LJ, Hamilton TA, Bulengo-Ransby SM, Ellis CN, et al. Topical retinoic acid for melasma in black patients. Arch Dermatol. 1994;130:727–33.
23. Leenutaphong V, Nettakul A, Rttanasuwon P. Topical isotretinoin for melasma in Thai patients: a vehicle-controlled clinical trial. J Med Assoc Thai. 1999;82:868–74.
24. Dogra S, Kanwar AJ, Parasad D. Adapalene in the treatment of melasma: a preliminary report. J Dermatol. 2002;29:539–40.
25. Kanechorn NA, Niumphradit N, Manosroi A, Nakakes A. Topical 5% tranexamic acid for the treatment of melasma in Asians: a double-blind randomized controlled clinical trial. J Cosm Laser Ther. 2012;14:150–4.
26. Banihashemi MD, Zabolinejad N, Jaafari M, Salehi M, Jabari A. Comparison of therapeutic effects of liposomal tranexamic acid and conventional hydroquinone on melasma. J Cosm Dermatol. 2015;14:1–4.
27. Ebrahimi B, Naeini F. Topical tranexamic acid as a promising treatment for melasma. J Res Med Sci. 2014;19(8):753–7.
28. Velasquez S, Bince B, Casintahan MF. Localized intradermal injection of Tranexamic Acid in the treatment of melasma: a randomized placebo-controlled double blind split-face study. Unpublished. JRRMMC Res Archives. Manila.
29. Boissy RE, Visscher M, deLong MA. Deoxyarbutin: a novel reversible tyrosinase inhibitor with effective in vivo skin lightening potency. Exp Dermatol. 2005;14:601–8.
30. Funasaka Y, Komoto MIchihashi M. Depigmenting effect of alpha-tocopheryl ferulate on normal human skin. Pigm Cell Res. 2000;13:170–4.
31. Burke KE. Interaction of vitamins C and E as better cosmeceuticals. Dermatol Ther. 2007;20:314–21.
32. Lin J, Selim A, Shea C, Grichnik J, Omar M, Monteiro-Riviere N, et al. UV photoprotection by combination topical antioxidants vitamin C and E. J Am Acad Dermatol. 2003;48:866–74.
33. Hakozaki T, Minwalla L, Zhuang J, Chhoa M, Matsubara A, Miyamoto K, et al. The effect of niacinamide on reducing cutaneous pigmentation and suppression of melanosome transfer. Br J Dermatol. 2002;147:20–31.
34. Huh SY, Shin JW, Na JI, Huh CH, Youn SW, Park KC. Efficacy and safety of liposome-encapsulated 4-n-butylresorcinol 0.1% cream for the treatment of melasma: a randomized controlled split-face trial. J Dermatol. 2010;37:311–5.
35. Ubeid A, Zhao L, Wang Y, Hantash BM. Short-sequence oligopeptides with inhibitory activity against mushroom and human tyrosinase. J Inves Dermatol. 2009;12(9):2242–9.
36. Hantash B, Jimenez F. A split-face, double-blind, randomized placebo-controlled pilot evaluation of a novel oligopeptide for the treatment of recalcitrant melasma. J Drugs Dermatol. 2009;8:732–5.
37. Lee MH, Kim HJ, Ha DJ. Therapeutic effect of topical application of linoleic acid and lincomycin in combination with betamethasone valerate in melasma patients. J Kor Med Sci. 2002;17:518–23.
38. Sheth V, Pandya A. Melasma: a comprehensive update Part II. J Am Acad Dermatol. 2011;65(4):699–714.
39. Jutley G, Rajaratnam R, Halpern J, Salim A, Emmett C, et al. Systematic review of randomized controlled trials on interventions for melasma: an abridged Cochrane review. J Am Acad Dermatol. 2014;70(2):369–73.
40. Chan R, Park KC, Lee MH, Lee ES, Chang SE, Leow YH, et al. Randomized controlled trial of the efficacy and safety of fixed triple combination (fluocinolone acetonide 0.01%, hydroquinone 4%, tretinoin 0.05%) compared with hydroquinone 4% cream in Asian patients with moderate to severe melasma. Br J Dermatol. 2008;159:697–703.
41. Grimes P, Bhawan J, Guevara I, Colon L, Johnson L, Gottschalk R, et al. Continuous therapy followed by a maintenance therapy regimen with a triple combination cream for melasma. J Am Acad Dermatol. 2010;62(6):962–7.
42. Javaheri SM, Handa S, Kaur I, Kumar B. Safety and efficacy of glycolic acid facial peel in Indian women with melasma. Int J Dermatol. 2001;40:354–7.

43. Vazquez M, Sanchez JL. The efficacy of a broad-spectrum sunscreen in the treatment of melasma. Cutis. 1983;32(1):92–6.
44. Rivas S, Pandya AG. Treatment of melasma with topical agents, peels and lasers: an evidence-based review. Am J Clin Dermatol. 2013;14:359–76.
45. Arellano I, Cestari T, Ocampo-Candiani J, Azulay-Abulafia L, Neto P, Hexsel D, et al. Preventing melasma recurrence: prescribing a maintenance regimen with an effective triple combination cream based on long-standing clinical severity. J Eur Acad Dermatol Venereol. 2012;26:611–8.

Chapter 13
Botanicals in Melasma

Evangeline B. Handog, Maria Juliet Enriquez-Macarayo, and Ricky Hipolito

13.1 Introduction

Greater understanding of the pathogenesis of melasma has given way to more pharmacologic agents especially those of botanical origin. While the role of tyrosinase is well known, many new pathways have been elucidated with molecular research; transcription and posttranslational modification of tyrosinase and other melanogenic enzymes have now been found to be targets of treatment [1].

With free radicals and peroxides inducing melanin formation, molecules with free radical scavenging and antioxidant properties were found to have therapeutic value in melasma. As the understanding of melasma pathophysiology deepens, coupled with clinical research, molecules of botanical origin with less adverse effects than existing therapies are emerging and finding their way into the mainstream treatment regimens.

Even with many currently existing treatments, melasma remains a management challenge. The condition has a tendency to relapse which contributes to patient dissatisfaction. Moreover, the gold standard, hydroquinone has been documented to cause ochronosis with prolonged use. Other available treatments include topical retinoids, azelaic acid, and kojic acid. Peeling agents with benefit in melasma include

E.B. Handog (✉)
Department of Dermatology, Asian Hospital and Medical Center,
2205 Civic Drive, Alabang, Muntinlupa City, Philippines 1780
e-mail: vangee@handog.net

M.J.Enriquez-Macarayo
Department of Dermatology, Angeles University Foundation Medical Center,
Pampanga, Philippines

R. Hipolito
Department of Dermatology, Research Institute for Tropical Medicine, Filinvest Corporate
City, Alabang, Muntinlupa City, Philippines

E.B. Handog, M.J. Enriquez-Macarayo (eds.), *Melasma and Vitiligo in Brown Skin*,
DOI 10.1007/978-81-322-3664-1_13

glycolic, trichloroacetic, salicylic, and lactic acid. All of the above agents either have harmful side effects on prolonged use or does not prevent relapse of melasma [2].

Fisk et al in their review article published in 2014 showed that botanical agents are becoming popular alternative therapies for hyperpigmentation [3]. These agents are more effective in superficial forms of hyperpigmentation and as such should be considered for integration into standard regimens. However, the review also showed that further clinical studies integrating botanicals with accepted treatments are needed.

The following botanicals that will be discussed are well studied, supported by in vitro and clinical research. These are already incorporated into cosmeceuticals available in the market.

13.2 Tyrosinase Inhibitors

Aloe vera, *rumex occidentalis*, bearberry (Figs. 13.1, 13.2, and 13.3, respectively) are some of the botanicals inhibiting tyrosinase.

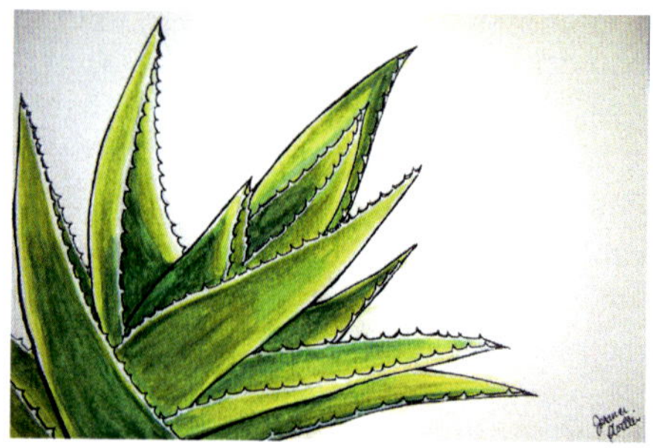

Fig. 13.1 Aloe vera

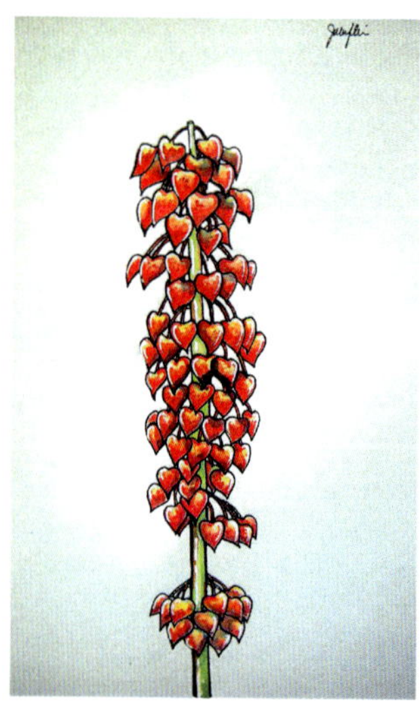

Fig. 13.2 *Rumex occidentalis*

13.2.1 Aloe Vera

Aloe vera is a succulent perennial herb (Fig. 13.1) which is probably native to North Africa but now found in the tropics and warmer areas of the world, including Asia. Viscous, transparent liquid can readily be extracted from the pea green fresh leaves. Some uses described in traditional medicine include minor wounds and burns [4].

Aloesin is a pigment-inhibiting substance derived from aloe vera extract. The study by Choi et al showed that aloesin prevents UV-induced pigment development in the skin of healthy volunteers. The results demonstrated that pigmentation suppression of aloesin was significantly greater than control but less than arbutin. However, aloesin used together with arbutin afforded more pigment suppression than arbutin alone. This study supports the current use of aloesin in nonprescription cosmeceutical formulations [5].

13.2.2 **Rumex Occidentalis**

Rumex occidentalis is a perennial herb (Fig. 13.2) found in North America, Asia, and Europe. It is a small, leafy plant with narrow leaves [6]. *Rumex occidentalis* is a traditional remedy, used as a mild laxative, digestive aid, and liver cleanser. Topical preparations can relieve insect stings [7].

A randomized double-blind study by Mendoza et al showed that *Rumex occidentalis* 3 % extract in cream formulation has lightening efficacy equivalent to hydroquinone 4 %. This study was conducted in 45 Filipino women who were randomized to receive placebo, hydroquinone 4 %, and *Rumex occidentalis* 3 % cream [8].

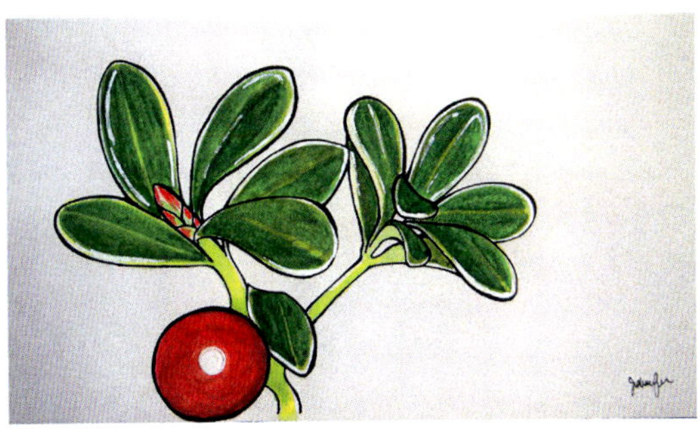

Fig. 13.3 Bearberry

13.2.3 Bearberry

Bearberry is an evergreen shrub (Fig. 13.3) that usually grows less than 6 inches tall. The leaves are alternately on the branches and the flowers are white to pink and bear round. Bearberry is native to Labrador, Alaska, Virginia, Illinois, Nebraska and New Mexico [9].

Arbutin, a tyrosinase inhibitor which comes from bearberry, is a glycosylated form of hydroquinone [10]. It is considered a safer alternative to hydroquinone for long term and regular use due to its comparable efficacy and less side effects [10–12].

13.3 Antioxidants/Free Radical Scavengers/Photoprotective Agents

Under this category are the following botanicals: orchids, proanthocyanidin from grape seed extract, procyanidin from maritime pine bark, coffeeberry, green tree extracts from *Camellia sinensis*, licorice (*Glycyrrhiza glabra*), mulberry (*Morus alba*), soy, and umbelliferone from carrots (Figs. 13.4, 13.5, 13.6, 13.7, 13.8, 13.9, 13.10, 13.11, and 13.12, respectively).

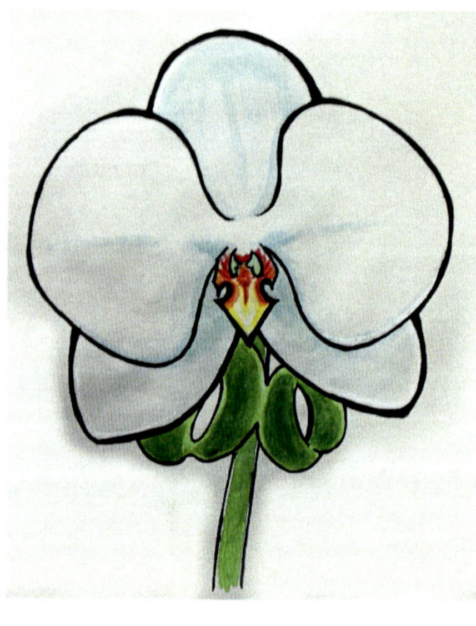

Fig. 13.4 Orchid

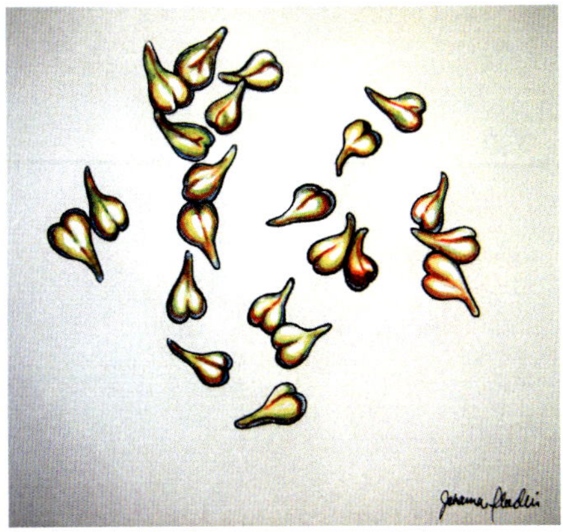

Fig. 13.5 Grape seed

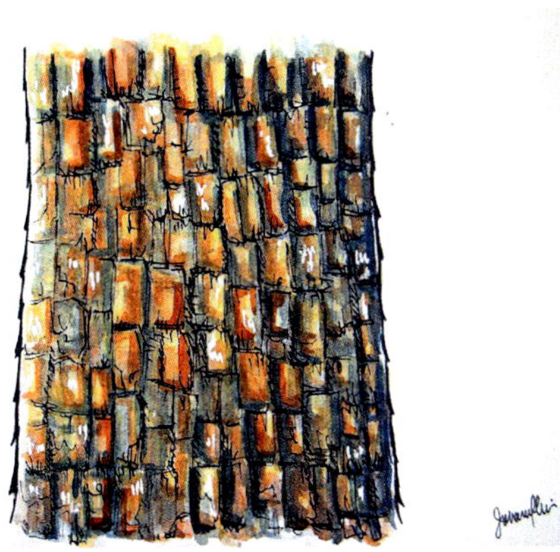

Fig. 13.6 Maritime pine bark

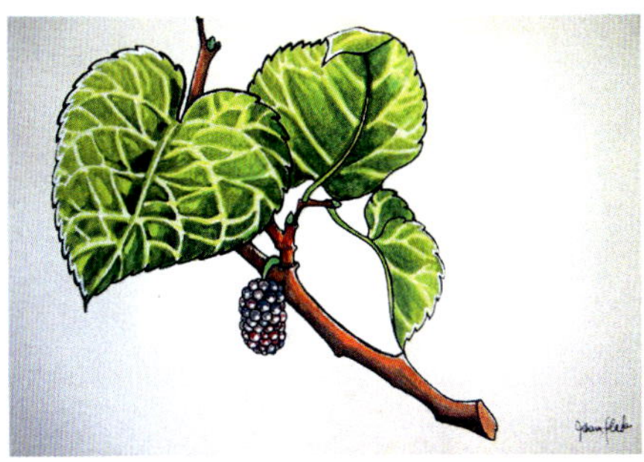

Fig. 13.7 Coffeeberry

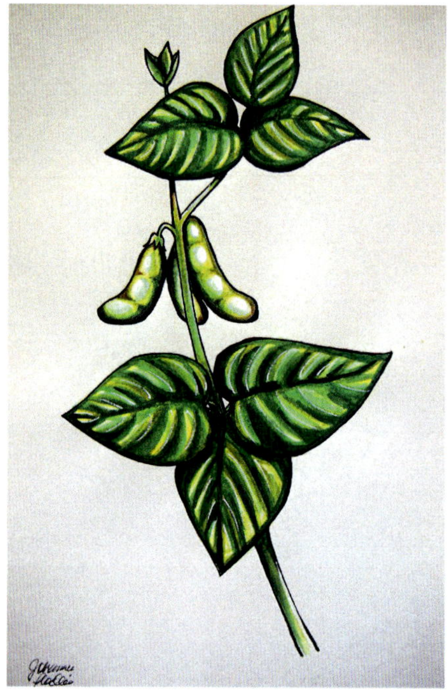

Fig. 13.8 *Camellia sinensis*

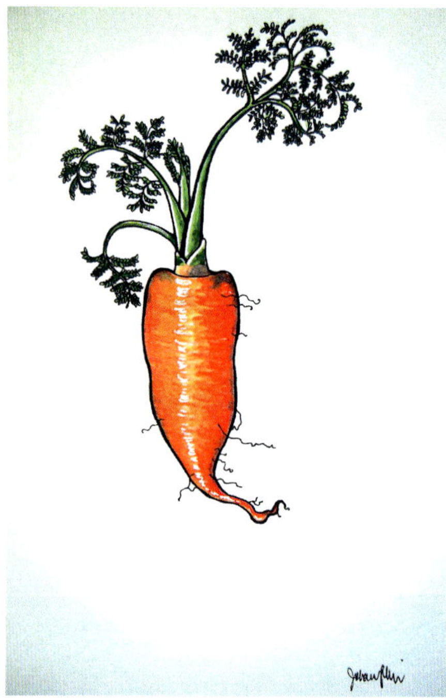

Fig. 13.9 *Glycyrrhiza glabra*

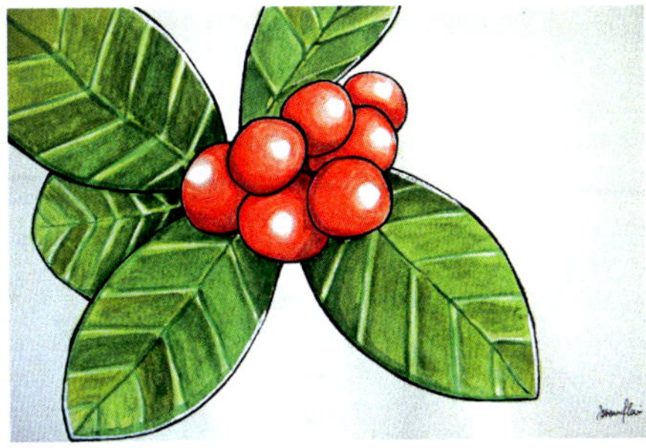

Fig. 13.10 *Morus alba*

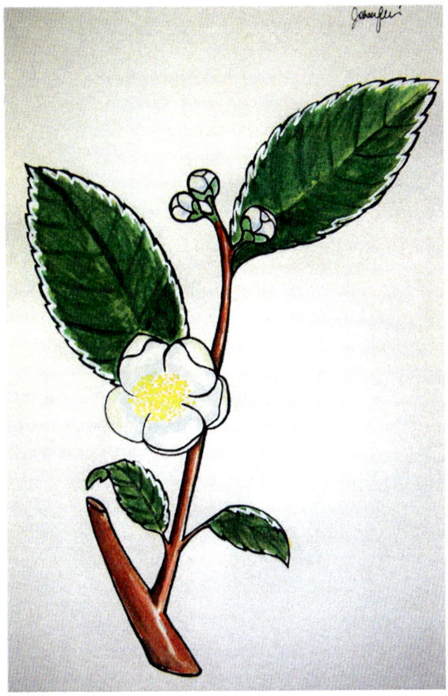

Fig. 13.11 Soybean

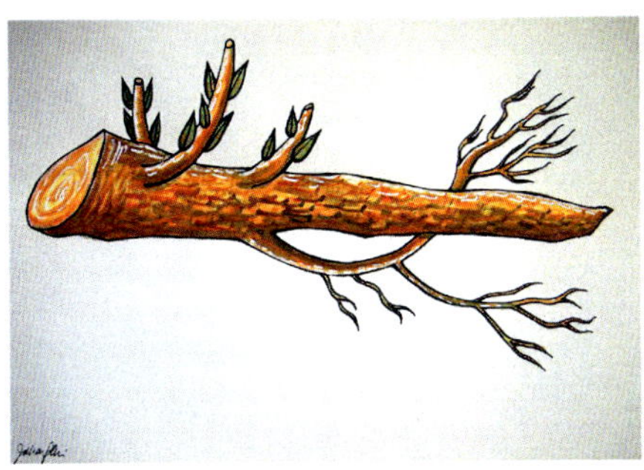

Fig. 13.12 *Daucus carota sativus*

13.3.1 *Orchids*

Orchids are perennial herbs widely distributed mostly in tropical and subtropical forests. While there is much variability in the specialized structures of the Orchidaceae family, the flowers are characteristic, having three petals and three petallike sepals, with a conspicuous central sepal forming a lip (labellum) (Fig. 13.4) [13].

Tadakoro et al conducted a split face study comparing orchid extract cream and vitamin C 3 % cream. Results obtained using the melanin index, clinical evaluation, and skin color tone scale were equivalent for orchid extract and vitamin C at the end of the study [14].

13.3.2 *Flavonoids*

Flavonoids are a group of naturally occurring substances in fruits, vegetables, plant parts, tea and wine. Diversity in their basic phenolic structure is the basis for their grouping and variations in physiologic activities [15, 16]. The main groups of flavonoids are flavones, flavanones, catechins, and anthocyanins [16]. While flavones and anthocyanins are found in berries and grapes, flavanones are sourced from citrus peels and fruits, and catechins are derived from red wine and tea. Several mechanisms have been found in vitro, such as nitric oxide inhibition, leukocyte immobilization, and arachidonic acid metabolism inhibition [16]. Their pigment inhibitory action rests on the antioxidant activity, tyrosinase inhibition and DOPA oxidation [2].

13.3.2.1 Grape Seed Extract

Grapes are climbing shrubs native to different parts of the world, especially in the tropical, subtropical and some temperate regions. The principal genera are *Cissus, Parthenocissus, Ampelopsis and Vitis* [17]. Proanthocyanidin is an antioxidant extracted from grape seeds (Fig. 13.5) [17].

Yamakoshi et al found that intake of the powder form containing 81.0 % proanthocyanidin (Gravinol™) has a beneficial effect on melasma. Eleven patients completed an open-label study for 12 months. Outcomes documented, using colorimetry and melanin index, showed significant improvement in terms of lightening and decrease in lesion size [18].

13.3.2.2 Procyanidin

Procyanidins present in apples, maritime pine bark (Fig. 13.6), cinnamon, aronia fruit, cocoa beans, and grape seeds and skin are flavonoids with high antioxidant properties in vitro [19]. They have been shown to modulate the arachidonic acid pathway, inhibit gene transcription and protein expression of inflammatory mediators, and hence have anti-inflammatory effects [20]. *Pinus pinaster* (French maritime pine), growing in low-lying coastal plains, is found in France, Spain and Portugal [21].

Handog et al conducted a randomized, double-blind, single-center trial to determine the lightening efficacy of tablets containing 24 mg of procyanidin, 6 mg of β-carotene, 60 mg of ascorbic acid, and 15 IU of D-α-tocopherol acetate. After 8 weeks, it was shown that the melanin content decreased significantly among the treatment patients ($p<0.0001$). MASI also decreased for both the treatment and placebo groups ($p<0.001$) with a greater decline noted among the treatment group ($p<0.0001$) [22].

13.3.3 Pycnogenol

Pycnogenol is a dietary supplement with many purported uses. Despite the insufficient evidence for benefit in any chronic condition [23], it remains available in over the counter formulations. Pycnogenol has been reported to have antioxidant and anti-inflammatory properties [24]. Its oral formulation at 50–200 mg per day has been used for a variety of conditions such as chronic venous insufficiency, diabetes, hypertension and retinopathy [24].

For melasma, the recommended dose was 75 mg/day [24]. Ni et al gave 30 women 75 mg of pycnogenol daily. At the end of the thirty-day study, they noted an average decrease in melasma area of 25.86 ± 20.39 mm ($p<0.001$). They also noted an average decrease in pigmentary intensity of 0.47 ± 0.51 unit ($p<0.001$) [25]. Twenty-nine patients with melasma were given 100 mg of daily pycnogenol by Campos et al. Two months of treatment yielded 26–50 % improvement by blind observation verified by digital photography [26]. In another study assessing the preventive action of pycnogenol to IPL-induced melasma-like pigmentation, Campos et al gave 100 mg of daily pycnogenol to 25 patients after three sessions of IPL. None developed melasma-like pigmentation in the treatment arm, while two developed pigmentation in the control group [27].

13.3.4 Coffeeberry

Coffea arabica is one of the two main species of coffee cultivated today, which accounts for 75–80 % of the world's production [28]. It grows best in subtropical and equatorial regions. Coffeeberry extract (Fig. 13.7) is naturally rich in polyphenol antioxidants, specifically cholorogenic acid, condensed proanthocyanidins, quinic acid, and ferrulic acid [29].

McDaniel in 2010 enrolled 30 females with moderate photoaging to determine the beneficial effects of coffee berry extract 1 % for photoaging, including pigmentation. His 6-week protocol included 20 full face and 10 split face participants. The full face participants applied the active product, while split face participants applied the active product on one side of the face and the vehicle on the opposite side. Blinded evaluations were done by dermatologists. Full face participants showed 27 % improvement in global assessment, 16 % for fine lines and wrinkles, 18 % for roughness and dryness, and 25 % for pigment. In the split-face study, notably greater improvement was noted on the active product than vehicle [29].

13.3.5 Green Tea Extracts

Green tea extracts come from *Camellia sinensis* (Fig. 13.8), cultivated in China for the past 3000 years. Polyphenolic compounds from green tea extracts act as anti-inflammatory, antioxidant, and anticarcinogenic. Its antioxidant and in vitro tyrosinase inhibition that may be responsible for its lightening effect [30].

No et al showed that green tea extracts inhibited mushroom tyrosinase in vitro [31].

13.3.6 Licorice

Glycyrrhiza glabra (Fig. 13.9), commonly known as licorice, is a perennial herb belonging to the pea and bean family, native to Eurasia, Northern Africa, and Western Asia. It grows about 1 meter tall with leaflets arranged in pairs along a central axis and light-blue to violet flowers held in loose conical spires [32]. Licorice extract has several pigment inhibitory mechanisms to wit, melanin dispersal, melanin biosynthesis inhibition, and cyclooxygenase inhibition [2].

Glabridin, a polyphenolic flavonoid serving as the main component of the extract, has been shown to prevent UVB-induced hyperpigmentation. It also has anti-inflammatory activity by inhibition of superoxide anion and cyclooxygenase [33]. Liquiritin, another component, has been reported to affect melanin dispersability and epidermal removal [34].

Alobaidi et al conducted a randomized double-blind study among 100 volunteer female patients with melasma. The 28-day study revealed a 93 % improvement of melasma in the group treated with *Glycyrrhiza glabra* 2.5 % cream, while only 4 % improvement was shown among the placebo group. The difference in proportion of improved patients was statistically significant (*p* value: 0.001) [35].

13.3.7 Mulberry

Morus alba (Fig. 13.10), also known as white mulberry, is native to China but is now found in most of the USA [36]. White mulberry is a perennial shrub or tree that can grow as high as 15 meters. The leaves are alternate and ovate, while flowers maybe staminate or pistillate. Fruits can be white, black or purple.

Lee et al measured the tyrosinase and superoxide inhibition of mulberry extract in vitro. Eighty-five percent of methanol extract of dried mulberry leaves was utilized for the experiment. Mushroom and mammalian tyrosinase assays were used to determine tyrosinase inhibition and Oyanagui method for superoxide suppression. In the mushroom tyrosinase assay, inhibition was expressed as IC50, the concentration of sample that inhibits 50% of tyrosinase activity. Strong inhibitory activity for tyrosinase was shown with IC50 of 0.29 ug/ml. Mammalian tyrosinase was suppressed to 50% at a concentration of 68.3 ug/ml. Superoxide inhibition was 8.3% at100 ug/mL. Mulberry extract's tyrosinase inhibition was 4.5 times more potent than kojic acid in mushroom assay with similar results in the mammalian assay [37].

13.3.8 Soy

Soybean is an annual legume of the Fabaceae family (Fig. 13.11), cultivated mainly for its vegetable protein and processed into food and industrial products. Its origin is believed to be from a wild plant in East Asia. It is now grown in most parts of the world, with the largest producers being the USA, Brazil, and China. It is an erect branching plant, which can grow to more than 2 meters. Flowers can be white or a shade of purple. Edible seeds contained in pods can be yellow, green, brown, black or bicolored [38]. Major components of soy reported to be responsible for its pigment inhibitory activity are the protease inhibitors and isoflavones. Protease inhibitors decrease PAR-2 activation, inhibiting melanosome transfer [39]. Isoflavones decrease melanogenesis by inhibiting DOPA oxidase activity [40].

Female patients with Fitzpatrick phototype I–III were enrolled in the study of Wallo et al, evaluating the benefits of soy-containing moisturizer for photoaging. This parallel, randomized, double-blind, vehicle-controlled study lasted for 12 weeks. It was shown that soy moisturizer was significantly better than vehicle (P value <0.05) as to mottled pigmentation, blotchiness, dullness, fine lines, overall texture, overall skin tone, and overall appearance [41].

13.3.9 Umbelliferone

Umbelliferone (UMB) or 7-hydroxycoumarin is a photoprotectant, antioxidant and anti-inflammatory phenolic compound. It is a product of plants belonging to the Apiaceae (Umbelliferae) family including domesticated carrot and coriander [42]. Domesticated carrot (*Daucus carota sativus*) (Fig. 13.12) was developed in the Netherlands in the seventeenth century [43].

13.4 Summary of Studies (Tables 13.1 and 13.2)

Table 13.1 Tyrosinase inhibitors

Component/plant source/ preparation	Study
Aloesin/aloe vera extract/ topical	P: 15 I: Randomized comparative trial of volunteer subjects divided into four groups (control, aloesin, arbutin, and aloesin plus arbutin) Patients were exposed to 210 mJ of UV radiation. Pigment development was determined among the volunteers for 15 days O: Pigmentation suppression was 34 % for aloesin 43.5 % for arbutin, and 63.3 % for combined treatment compared with the control ($N = 15$ p value < 0.05) Choi et al [5]
Rumex occidentalis/3 % *Rumex occidentalis* cream	P: 45 I: Randomized, double-blind, placebo-controlled clinical trial O: Mean decline in MASI and Mexameter values from baseline to week 8 similar for both 4 % hydroquinone and 3 % *Rumex occidentalis* Mendoza et al [8]
Rumex occidentalis with glycolic acid	P: 27 I: Single group, open-label clinical trial O: There was a significant difference between baseline and 12 weeks, baseline and 24 weeks in L*, C*, and h* values. There was a clinically significant response rate Sabancilar et al [44]

Legend: *P* population, *I* intervention, *O* outcome

Table 13.2 Antioxidants/others

Component/plant source/preparation	Depigmenting activity	Study
Orchid extract/topical cream	Antioxidant	P:48 I: Split face study, either side applied with cosmetic formulation with plant including orchid extracts or 3 % vitamin C derivative O: Using melanin index, clinical evaluation, skin color tone scale, and questionnaire, improvement noted to be equivalent for orchid rich extracts and vitamin C derivative Tadokoro et al [14]
Proanthocyanidin/grape seed extract/powder form soluble in water containing 81.0 % proanthocyanidin (Gravinol™) [12]	Antioxidant	P: 12 patients, 12-month study I: Open design, single group of Japanese women with melasma O: Using colorimetry, slight improvement was noted in 5 patients at 3 months ($p<0.05$), 10 patients at 6 months ($p<0.01$) and further improvement on 6 patients at 12 months ($p<0.01$) Melanin index significantly decreased at 6 and 12 months. Size of the lesions also decreased Yamakoshi et al [18]
Procyanidin/bark of *Pinus pinaster* (French maritime pine)/tablets containing procyanidin (24 mg), β-carotene (6 mg), ascorbic acid (60 mg), and D-α-tocopherol acetate (15 IU)	Antioxidant free radical scavenger	P: 56 I: Randomized, double-blind, single-center trial on Filipino subjects. Assessment for outcomes done at baseline and week 8 O: Melanin content decreased significantly among the treatment patients ($p<0.0001$). MASI decreased for treatment and placebo groups ($p<0.001$) but greater among the treatment group ($p<0.0001$) Handog et al [22]

(continued)

Table 13.2 (continued)

Component/plant source/preparation	Depigmenting activity	Study
Pycnogenol/bark of *Pinus pinaster* (French maritime pine)/25, 50, 100 mg tablet	Antioxidant free radical scavenger	P: 30 I: Single group of women with melasma given 75 mg of pycnogenol daily for 30 days O: Average decrease in melasma area was 25.86 ± 20.39 mm (2) ($p < 0.001$) and the average decrease in pigmentary intensity was 0.47 ± 0.51 unit ($p < 0.001$) Ni et al [25] P: 29 I: Single group of patients with melasma given 100 mg of daily pycnogenol O: Blinded observers noted 26–50 % improvement on 48.14 % of patients at 2 months of treatment; results confirmed using standardized digital photography. Campos and Pitassi [26] P: 50 I: Observer blind clinical trial post three sessions of IPL. Pycnogenol 100 mg was given for 3 months post IPL to the treatment group O: Two developed melasma-like pigmentation in the control group and none in the treatment group Campos and Pitassi [27]
Flavonoid/rutin succinate bioflavonoid	Free radical scavenger Photoprotective	I: In vitro investigation of the free radical scavenging activity and photoprotection O: Free radical inhibition was 36.7 %. Chemical structure of rutin succinate supports its photoprotection potential against UVA Velasco et al [45]

Soy/total soy lotion	Inhibits protease receptor-2 leading to decreased phagocytosis of melanosomes by keratinocytes [40, 46]	P: 27, Caucasian females, ages 30–70, Fitzpatrick skin type I–III mild to moderate bilateral photodamage I: 12-week, half-face, double-blind benchmark-controlled clinical study O: Significant improvement in soy treated part on solar lentigenes, mottled hyperpigmentation, fine wrinkling, surface roughness, sallowness and overall damage from week 4 to the end of the study. The improvement was significant (p value: 0.00005) Wu et al [46]
Soy-containing active moisturizer (Aveeno Positively Radiant Daily moisturizer, Johnson and Johnson CCI, Skillman, NJ)		P: 63, female subjects aged 30–61 of Fitzpatrick skin type I to III I: Parallel, randomized, double-blind, vehicle-controlled study O: At the end of 12 weeks, active soy moisturizer was significantly better than control (P value <0.05). Improvements were noted in mottled pigmentation, blotchiness, dullness, fine lines, overall texture, overall skin tone, and overall appearance Wallo et al [41]
UVA/UVB SPF15 moisturizer with nondenatured whole soy extract		P: Women of color with pigmentary problems I: Double-blind, placebo-controlled O: Statistically significant improvement in mottled hyperpigmentation, clarity, texture, and overall appearance compared to placebo noted as early as 2 weeks Finkey [47]
Triterpene, saponins, and flavonoids (Alobaidi)/*Glycyrrhiza glabra* (Licorice)/*G. glabra* 2.5 % extract cream	Inhibits tyrosinase ROS scavenger Melanin dispersibility Epidermal removal	P: 93 females with melasma I: Double-blind placebo-controlled study for 28 days O: Improvement in melasma was 93 % in the treatment and 4 % in the placebo group (p value: 0.007) Zhu and Gao [34]

(continued)

Table 13.2 (continued)

Component/plant source/preparation	Depigmenting activity	Study
Polyphenol antioxidants (specifically, cholorogenic acid, condensed proanthocyanidins, quinic acid, and ferrulic acid)/coffee berry extract/CBE 1 % cream, CBE 0.1 % cleanser	Antioxidant/free radical scavenger	P: 27 (17 = full face protocol, 10 = split face protocol) females with moderate photoaging I: 6-week study; full face subjects applied the active product on the whole face; split face participants applied active product on a side of the face and vehicle on the opposite side O: Blinded evaluations were done by dermatologists. Improvements noted among the full face participants: global improvement (27 %), fine lines and wrinkles (16 %), roughness and dryness (18 %), and pigment (25 %). In the split-face study, notably greater improvement was noted on the active product than vehicle McDaniel [29]
Mulberroside F/mulberry/85 % methanol extract of dried *Morus alba* leaves	Tyrosinase inhibition/inhibition of melanin formation/superoxide scavenging	I: In vitro study; extract was added in mushroom tyrosinase assay, mammalian tyrosinase assay. Superoxide scavenging activity was determined using Oyanagui method O: Extract was shown to have 4.5 times more potent activity than kojic acid on tyrosinase activity on mushroom assay with similar results being noted on mammalian assay Lee et al. [37]

Legend: *P* population, *I* intervention, *O* outcome

13.5 Newer Depigmenting Agents of Botanical Source (Table 13.3)

The list is growing and promising and includes the following:

Table 13.3 Other botanical agents and their sources

Botanical	Source(S)
Artocarpanone	*Artocarpus heterophyllus*, an Indonesian tree
4-n-butylresorcinol or rucinol	May have plant sources
Ursolic acid	Apple peels, holy basil
Anthraquinones	Rhubarb
Cinnamic acid	Various plant sources
Macelignan	*Myristica fragrans*, an evergreen tree
Gallic acid	Gallnuts, grapes, tea, hops, and oak bark
Glycine	Meat, fish, dairy products, legumes
Isopanduratin A and 4-hydroxypanduratin A	*Kaempferia pandurata* Roxb, common name: Chinese ginger
Kurarinol, kuraridinol, and trifolirhizin	*Sophora flavescens*, common names: Ku Shen Gen/bitter root/yellow sophora root
Selina dien-8-one	Atractylodis Rhizoma Alba, Atractylodes rhizome
Taxifolin	Onions, French maritime bark, milk thistle, and tamarind seeds
Deoxyarbutin and its second-generation derivatives	Synthesized by removing the hydroxyl groups from the glucose side chain of arbutin
Hydroperoxytraxastane-type triterpene	*Arnica montana*, common name: leopard's bane
Piceatannol	Grapes, passion fruit, white tea, and Japanese knotweed

13.6 Conclusion

Melasma may be a pigmentary disorder quite elusive to treatment, but continuous efforts are being placed in the discovery of depigmenting agents, with botanicals considered as a safer source.

Grateful acknowledgment to Dr. Johanna O. Flordelis for providing all the artistic original illustrations.

References

1. Ebanks JP, Wickett RR, Boissy RE. Mechanisms regulating skin pigmentation: the rise and fall of complexion coloration. Int J Mol Sci. 2009;10:4066–87.
2. Sarkar R, Chugh S, Garg VK. Newer and upcoming therapies for melasma. Ind J Dermatol Venereol Leprol. 2012;78(4):417–28.
3. Fisk WA, Agbai O, Lev-Tov HA, Sivamani RK. The use of botanically derived agents for hyperpigmentation: a systematic review. J Am Acad Dermatol. 2014;70:352–65.
4. Aloe vera gel. WHO monographs on selected medicinal plants. 1999;1. http://apps.who.int/medicinedocs/en/d/Js2200e/6.html. Accessed Jan 31 2016.
5. Choi S, Park YI, Lee SK, Kim JE, Chung MH. Aloesin inhibits hyperpigmentation induced by UV radiation. Clin Exp Dermatol. 2002;27:513–5.
6. Calflora: information on California plants for education, research and conservation, with data contributed by public and private institutions and individuals, including the Consortium of California Herbaria. The Calflora Database organization, Berkeley. 2016. http://www.calflora.org/. Accessed 16 Jan 2016.
7. Elias J, Ketcham K. Chinese medicine for maximum immunity: understanding the five elemental types for health and well-being. New York: Three Rivers Press, Random House, Inc; 1998. p. 271–2.
8. Mendoza CG, Singzon IA, Handog EB. A randomized, double-blind, placebo-controlled clinical trial on the efficacy and safety of 3% Rumex occidentalis cream versus 4% hydroquinone cream in the treatment of melasma among Filipinos. Int J Dermatol. 2014;53:1412–6.
9. Bearberry. United States Department of Agriculture Plant Fact Sheet. http://plants.usda.gov/factsheet/pdf/fs_aruv.pdf. Accessed 31 Jan 2016.
10. Maeda K, Fukuda M. Arbutin: mechanism of its depigmenting action in human melanocyte culture. J Pharmacol Exp Ther. 1996;276:765–9.
11. Draelos ZD. Skin lightening preparations and the hydroquinone controversy. Dermatol Ther. 2007;20(5):308–13.
12. Boissy RE, Visscher M, DeLong MA. DeoxyArbutin: a novel reversible tyrosinase inhibitor with effective *in vivo* skin lightening potency. Exp Dermatol. 2005;14:601–8.
13. Orchid. The Columbia Encyclopedia. 6th ed. 2015. http://www.encyclopedia.com/doc/1E1-orchid.html. Accessed 17 Jan 2016.
14. Tadokoro T, Bonté F, Archambault JC, Cauchard JH, Neveu M, Ozawa K, et al. Whitening efficacy of plant extracts including orchid extracts on Japanese female skin with melasma and lentigo senilis. J Dermatol. 2010;37(6):522–30.
15. Nijveldt RJ, van Nood E, van Hoorn DEC, Boelens PG, van Norren K, van Leeuwen PAM. Flavonoids: a review of probable mechanisms of action and potential applications. Am J Clin Nutr. 2001;74:418–25.
16. Ververidis F, Trantas E, Douglas C, Vollmer G, Kretzschmar G, Panopoulos N. Biotechnology of flavonoids and other phenylpropanoid-derived natural products. Part I: chemical diversity, impacts on plant biology and human health. Biotechnol J. 2007;2(10):1214–34.

17. Grape. The Columbia Encyclopedia. 6th ed. 2015. http://www.encyclopedia.com/doc/1E1-grape.html. Accessed 17 Jan 2016.
18. Yamakoshi J, Sano A, Tokutake S, Saito M, Kikuchi M, Kubota M, et al. Oral intake of proanthocyanidin-rich extract from grape seeds improves chloasma. Phytother Res. 2004;18(11):895–9.
19. Yang J, Xiao YY. Grape phytochemicals and associated health benefits. Crit Rev Food Sci Nutr. 2013;53(11):1202–25.
20. Martinez-Micaelo N, González-Abuín N, Ardèvol A, Pinent M, Blay MT. Procyanidins and inflammation: molecular targets and health implications. Biofactors. 2012;38(4):257–65.
21. Farjon A. Pinus pinaster. The IUCN Red List of Threatened Species 2013: e.T42390A2977079. http://dx.doi.org/10.2305/IUCN.UK.2013-1.RLTS.T42390A2977079.en. Accessed 31 Jan 2016.
22. Handog EB, Galang MD, de Leon-Godinez MA, Chan GP. A randomized, double-blind, placebo-controlled trial of oral procyanidin with vitamins A, C, E for melasma among Filipino women. Int J Dermatol. 2009;48:896–901.
23. Schoonees A, Visser J, Musekiwa A, Volmink J. Pycnogenol® (extract of French maritime pine bark) for the treatment of chronic disorders. Cochrane Database Syst Rev. 2012;4. Art. No.: CD008294. doi:10.1002/14651858.CD008294.pub4. Accessed 17 Jan 2016.
24. Oliff, HS. Scientific and clinical monograph for the proprietary botanical ingredient pycnogenol. Am Botanical Council. 2010:2. http://abc.herbalgram.org/site/DocServer/Pycnog_FullMono120809_LOW.pdf?docID=1741. Accessed 17 Jan 2016.
25. Ni Z, Mu Y, Gulati O. Treatment of melasma with Pycnogenol. Phytother Res. 2002;16(6):567–71.
26. Campos V, Pitassi L. Oral administration of pycnogenol associated with sunscreen improve clinical symptoms of melasma. J Am Acad Dermatol. 2014;70S1(5):AB19.
27. Campos V, Pitassi L. A comparative study of the efficacy of pycnogenol to prevent the intense pulsed light induced melasma-like hyperpigmentation after treatment. J Am Acad Dermatol. 2014;70S1(5):AB198.
28. Agriculture. Arabica and Robusta Coffee Plant. Coffee Research institute. Coffee research.org. http://www.coffeeresearch.org/agriculture/coffeeplant.htm. Accessed 31 Jan 2016.
29. McDaniel DH. Clinical safety and efficacy in photoaged skin with coffeeberry extract, a natural antioxidant. Cosmet Dermatol. 2009;22:610–6.
30. Camellia sinensis (L.) Kuntze, Purdue University, Center for new crops and plant products. 1996. https://hort.purdue.edu/newcrop/duke_energy/Camellia_sinensis.html. Accessed 21 Jan 2016.
31. No JK, Soung DY, Kim YJ, Shim KH, Jun YS, Rhee SH, et al. Inhibition of tyrosinase by green tea components. Life Sci. 1999;65:PL241–6.
32. Glycyrrhiza glabra (liquorice). Kew, Royal Botanical Gardens. http://www.kew.org/science-conservation/plants-fungi/glycyrrhiza-glabra-liquorice. Accessed 23 Jan 2016.
33. Yokota T, Nishio H, Kubota Y, Mizoguchi M. The inhibitory effect of glabridin from licorice extracts on melanogenesis and inflammation. Pigment Cell Res. 1998;11:355–61.
34. Zhu W, Gao J. The use of botanical extracts as topical skin-lightening agents for the improvement of skin pigmentation disorders. J Invest Dermatol Symp Proc. 2008;13:20–4.
35. Alobaidi AH, Hamad EH, Alsamarai AM, Kudair KA. Evaluation of *Glycyrrhiza glabra* cream as treatment for melasma. INTECH. 2015. http://cdn.intechopen.com/pdfs-wm/47519.pdf. Accessed 23 Jan 2016.
36. Stone, KR. Morus alba. In: Fire Effects Information System. U.S. Department of Agriculture, Forest Service, Rocky Mountain Research Station, Fire Sciences Laboratory (Producer). 2009. http://www.fs.fed.us/database/feis/accessed 24 Jan 2016.
37. Lee SH, Choi SY, Kim H, Hwang JS, Lee BG, Gao JJ, et al. Mulberroside F isolated from the leaves of Morus alba inhibits melanin biosynthesis. Biol Pharm Bull. 2002;25:1045–8.
38. Soybean plant. Encyclopedia Britannica, School and Library Subscribers. http://www.britannica.com/plant/soybean#_comments. Accessed 31 Jan 2016.
39. Thornfeldt C. Cosmeceuticals containing herbs: fact, fiction, and future. Dermatol Surg. 2005;31:873–80.

40. Leyden J, Wallo W. The mechanism of action and clinical benefits of soy for the treatment of hyperpigmentation. Int J Dermatol. 2011;50:470–7.
41. Wallo W, Nebus J, Leyden JJ. Efficacy of a soy moisturizer in photoaging: a double-blind, vehicle-controlled, 12-week study. J Drugs Dermatol. 2007;6(9):917–22.
42. Sarkar R, Arora P, Garg KV. Cosmeceuticals for hyperpigmentation: what is available? J Cutan Aesthet Surg. 2013;6(1):4–11.
43. Shapiro L. Dauscus carota subsp sativus. Encyclopedia Life. 2012. http://eol.org/pages/1278046/overview. Accessed 31 Jan 2016.
44. Sabancilar E, Aydin F, Bek Y, Ozden MG, Ozcan M, Senturk N, et al. Treatment of melasma with a depigmentation cream determined with colorimetry. J Cosmet Laser Ther. 2011;13(5):255–9.
45. Velasco MV, Baby AR, Pedriali-Moraes CA, Dario MF, Villa RT, et al. Antioxidant activity and photoprotection of rutin succinate bioflavonoid. J Am Acad Dermatol. 2013;68S1(4):AB188.
46. Wu J, Kollias N, Liu JC, Leiden J. Total soy to diminish wrinkles and hyperpigmentation in photoaged population. J Am Acad Dermatol. 2004;50S(3):26.
47. Finkey MB, Herndon J, Stephens T, Appa Y. Soy moisturizer spf 15 improves dyschromia. J Am Acad Dermatol. 2005;52S(3):170.

Chapter 14
Oral Lightening Agents

Evangeline B. Handog and Maria Juliet Enriquez-Macarayo

14.1 Introduction

Uneven skin color especially among female patients with melasma always illustrates a lot of concern and anxiety. For several decades now, having a fair face and an even skin tone have not only been symbols of prominence but also of preeminence and advantage. In India, attitudes towards skin color have developed over two centuries and reflect consideration of class and background [1].

Systemic skin whitening agents are very rapidly attaining popularity. Commercialism has gone far hence has become a multimillion dollar business. Women who believe that being fair has more advantages and can afford to buy them will not have second thoughts even if there is not much evidence in its efficacy.

14.2 Tranexamic Acid (TA)

Known to be a hemostatic agent, tranexamic acid (trans-4-aminomethyl cyclohexane carboxylic acid) (Fig. 14.1) is a synthetic derivative of the amino acid lysine. Foremost, it is being used especially in surgery, because of its antifibrolytic action [2]. As early as 1979, Nijor's first study and report paved the way for more researches especially on its action on melasma [3]. Being a synthetic lysine analogue that reversibly blocks lysine binding sites on plasminogen molecules, TA's efficacy lies in its being an inhibitory plasminogen activator (PA) of plasmin.

E.B. Handog (✉)
Department of Dermatology, Asian Hospital and Medical Center,
2205 Civic Drive, Alabang, Muntinlupa City, Philippines 1780
e-mail: vangee@handog.net

M.J. Enriquez-Macarayo
Department of Dermatology, Angeles University Foundation Medical Center,
Pampanga, Philippines

E.B. Handog, M.J. Enriquez-Macarayo (eds.), *Melasma and Vitiligo in Brown Skin*,
DOI 10.1007/978-81-322-3664-1_14

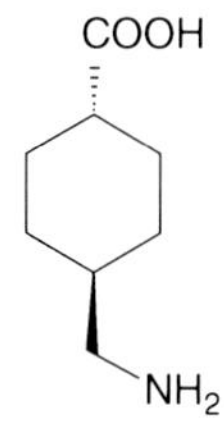

Fig. 14.1 Tranexamic acid (trans-4-amonimethyl cyclohexane carboxylic acid)

Keratinocytes produce PA. Epidermal basal cells contain plasminogen molecules. Plasmin plays a role in the release of basic fibroblast growth factor, which is a potent growth factor for melanocytes [4]. Wu et al reported that TA in animal models has been shown to prevent ultraviolet light-induced pigmentation by preventing the binding of plasminogen to keratinocytes that resulted in a decrease in the tyrosinase activity of melanocytes [5]. He further stated that research by Zhang et al showed that TA is able to inhibit melanogenesis by interfering with the catalytic reaction of tyrosinase. Sarkar et al showed that TA is able to decrease α-melanocyte-stimulating hormone that stimulates melanin synthesis [6].

Karn et al evaluated the efficacy of TA as an adjunct to topical hydroquinone and sunscreen for melasma in 260 subjects [7]. In this randomized controlled trial done for 3 months, Group A received TA at a dose of 250 mg twice daily in addition to topical treatment, and Group B received topical treatment alone. Results indicated that there was a statistically significant decrease in the mean Melasma Assessment Severity Index (MASI) from baseline to 8 and 12 weeks among group A patients (11.08 ± 2.91 vs. 8.95 ± 2.08 at week 8 and vs. 7.84 ± 2.44 at week 12; $p < 0.05$ for both). Among group B patients, the decrease in mean score was significant at 8 weeks and insignificant at 12 weeks follow-up (11.60 ± 3.40 vs. 9.9 ± 2.61 at 8 weeks and vs. 9.26 ± 3 at 12 weeks; $p < 0.05$ for former but $p > 0.05$ for later). TA was found effective for the treatment of melasma at a low dose of 250 mg twice a day for at least 3 months.

Because of its antihemorrhagic property, it is not safe to use it for a long duration. Unwanted side effects can include venous thromboembolism, myocardial infarction, cerebrovascular accidents and pulmonary embolism.

14.3 Pycnogenol/Procyanidin

Pycnogenol is derived from the extract of the French maritime pine bark, *Pinus pinaster* (Fig. 14.2). It contains 65–75 % procyanidin as its main ingredient. It also contains other phenolic compounds such as catechin, epicatechin, caffeic acid and ferulic acid [8]. It was found to be more potent than vitamins C and E in vitro, in its anti-inflammatory and antioxidant properties [9]. It has been demonstrated to protect against UV-induced erythema through mechanisms that inhibit the expression of nuclear factor (NF-kB) [8].

Ni et al in an open-label trial of 30 Chinese women with melasma taking oral Pycnogenol 25 mg thrice daily for 30 days demonstrated an 80 % response rate with no significant side effects observed [9]. Handog et al, in a randomized,

Fig. 14.2 French maritime pine bark

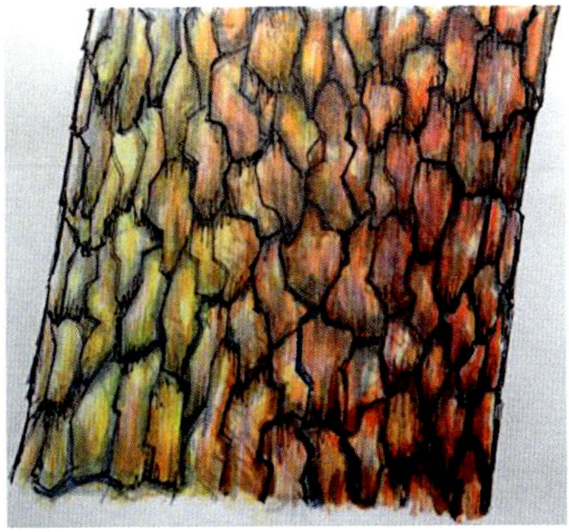

double-blind, placebo-controlled trial, reported that a fixed combination of oral procyanidin plus vitamins A, C, E given to 60 Filipino women with bilateral epidermal melasma resulted in a significant decrease in the degree of pigmentation in both malar regions (left: 165.85 ± 70.909; right: 161.33 ± 61.824, $p < 0.0001$). MASI scores showed similar significant improvements (left: 2.4862 ± 1.67816; right: 1.8889 ± 1.67110, $p < 0.001$). Procyanidin + vitamins A, C, E proved to be safe and well tolerated, with minimal adverse events. The combination contained 24 mg of procyanidin and was taken twice daily for 8 weeks. No serious adverse reaction was reported in the study [10].

14.4 Polypodium leucotomos (PL)

Polypodium leucotomos is a tropical species of fern (Fig. 14.3) that contains polyphenols, which are potent inhibitors of reactive oxygen species with anti-inflammatory, antioxidant, and photoprotective properties. PL inhibits matrix metalloproteinase-1-photoinduced membrane damage and reduces psoralen/UVA-induced phototoxicity [11].

Martin et al demonstrated the clinical efficacy of *P. leucotomos* for the treatment of melasma. Female subjects aged 18–50 years with epidermal melasma ($N = 21$) were randomized to receive oral *P. leucotomos* or placebo twice daily for 12 weeks. Each subject applied SPF45 sunscreen daily. Efficacy measures included changes in the Melasma Quality of Life Scale, MASI and clinical evaluation by the study investigator. Plain and UV-lamp photographs obtained at baseline and weeks 4, 8, and 12 were evaluated by an independent, blinded investigator. At 12 weeks, patients treated with *P. leucotomos* had significantly decreased mean MASI scores (5.7–3.3; $p < 0.05$), whereas the placebo group did not (4.7–5.7; $p = \text{NS}$). Photographic assessment revealed that mild and marked improvement was achieved by 43 and 17 % of *P. leucotomos*-treated patients, respectively, versus 14 and 0 % of placebo-treated patients. Similarly, patient self-assessments revealed 50 and 13 % of patients achieved mild and marked improvement, respectively, versus 17 and 0 % for placebo-treated patients. Seventeen percent of

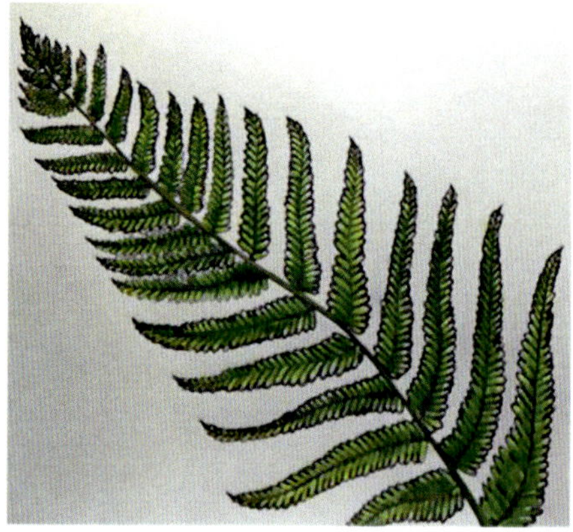

Fig. 14.3 *Polypodium leucotomos*

placebo-treated patients reported worsened melasma severity versus none of *P. leucotomos*-treated patients [12].

A review by Nestor et al quoted a randomized, placebo-controlled trial, which evaluated oral PL in 21 females (18–50 years) with epidermal melasma. PL was given twice daily (dose not stated) for a duration of 12 weeks in addition to daily use of sunscreen. Outcome measures included change in the Melasma Quality of Life Scale, MASI score, clinical evaluation by the study investigator and photographic evaluation by an independent, blinded investigator. At the end of the study, subjects who received PL had significantly decreased mean MASI scores which was not observed in the placebo group. All other parameters improved [13].

14.5 Glutathione (GSH)

Glutathione is a ubiquitous compound containing a biologically active sulfhydryl (SH) group found in our bodies. It is a tripeptide composed of glutamate, L-cysteine and glycine (Fig. 14.4), that has been recognized to be the master antioxidant. As a skin lightening agent, several mechanisms were proposed. These include: (1) a shift in the production of pheomelanin over eumelanin, (2) the effects of glutathione on tyrosinase, and (3) the quenching of ROS and free radicals that influence tyrosinase activation [14, 15].

The first published study on glutathione as an oral whitening agent was by Arjinpathana et al in 2012. It was a randomized, double-blind, placebo-controlled trial involving 60 medical students, where 250 mg capsules were taken twice daily on an empty stomach for 4 weeks. Changes in melanin indices and digital photographs comparing baseline and after treatment were significant. Limitations of the study, however, were: plasma glutathione levels were not measured, limited study period of only 4 weeks, and no follow-up on the participants to determine when the skin melanin indices return to their baseline value [16].

Handog et al did an open-label, single-arm pilot study enrolling 34 patients, 30 of whom completed the study. Subjects were healthy women (aged 22–42) having

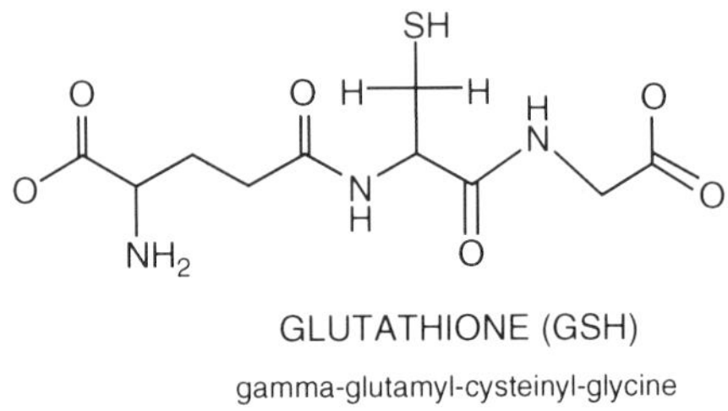

Fig. 14.4 Glutathione (GSH), gamma-glutamyl-cysteinyl-glycine

Fitzpatrick skin types IV or V. Subjects received 500 mg of GSH in the form of lozenges and were instructed to melt in their mouth (or side of buccal cavity) every morning for eight weeks. Mucosal delivery avoids the first pass metabolism and hence the dosage is uniform. Complete blood count and liver profile tests were done before and after the study. Melanin indices were determined every 2 weeks. Mexameter reading from both the sun exposed (mid sternum) and sun protected areas (extensor right wrist) were recorded. Global assessment scores were obtained at the end of the study. Statistical analysis revealed significant lowering of the melanin indices as early as 2 weeks, in both areas. Ninety percent of the subjects noted moderate degree of skin lightening while 3 % had mild change [17].

14.6 Conclusion

Systemic lightening agents may be useful as adjuvant management for patients seeking to have fairer complexion. More studies are needed to evaluate GSH's efficacy when used for a long time.

Grateful acknowledgment to Dr. Johanna O. Flordelis for providing all the artistic original illustrations.

References

1. Malathi M, Thappa DM. Systemic skin whitening/lightening agents: what is the evidence? Ind J Dermatol Venereol Leprol. 2013;79:842–6.
2. Dunn CJ, Goa KL. Tranexamic acid: a review of its use in surgery and other indications. Drugs. 1999;57:1005–32.
3. Nijor T. Treatment of melasma with tranexamic acid. Clin Res. 1979;13:3129–31.
4. Tse TW, Hui E. Tranexamic acid: an important adjuvant in the treatment of melasma. Aesthetic Plas Surg. 2012;36:964–70.
5. Wu S, Shi H, Wu H, Yan S, Guo J, Sun Y, et al. Treatment of melasma with oral administration of tranexamic acid. Aesthetic Plas Surg. 2012;36:964–70.
6. Sarkar R, Chugh S, Garg VK. Newer and upcoming therapies for melasma. Ind J Dermatol Venereol Leprol. 2012;78:417–28.

7. Karn D, Kc S, Amatya A, Razouria EA, Timalsina M. Oral tranexamic acid for the treatment of melasma. Kathmandu Univ Med J. 2012;10(4):40–3.
8. Konda S, Geria AN, Halder RM. New horizons in treating disorders of hyperpigmentation in skin of color. Semin Cutan Med Surg. 2012;31:133–9.
9. Ni Z, Mu Y, Gulati O. Treatment of melasma with Pycnogenol. Phytother Res. 2002;16(6):567–71.
10. Handog EB, Galang DA, de Leon Godinez MA, Chan GP. A Randomized, double-blind, placebo-controlled trial of oral procyanidin with vitamins A, C, E for melasma among Filipino women. Int J Dermatol. 2009;48:896–901.
11. Philips N, Smith J, Keller T, Gonzalez S. Predominant effects of *Polypodium leucotomos* on membrane integrity, lipid peroxidation, and expression of elastin and matrix-metalloproteinase-1 in ultraviolet radiation exposed fibroblasts, and keratinocytes. J Dermatol Sci. 2003;32:1–9.
12. Martin lK, Caperton C, Woolery-lloyd H, et al. A randomized double-blind placebo controlled study evaluating the effectiveness and tolerability of oral *Polypodium leucotomos* in patients with melasma. Presented at: American Academy of Dermatology Annual Meeting. San Diego; 2012.
13. Nestor M, Bucay V, Callender V, Cohen J, Sadick N, Wadorf H. Polypodium leucotomos as an adjunct treatment of pigmentary disorders. J Clin Aesthetic Dermatol. 2014;7:13–7.
14. Villarama CD, Maibach HI. Glutathione as a depigmenting agent: an overview. Int J Cosmet Sci. 2005;27:147–53.
15. Ebanks JP, Wickett RR, Boissy RE. Mechanisms regulating skin pigmentation: the rise and fall of complexion coloration. Int J Mol Sci. 2009;10:4006–87.
16. Arjinpathana N, Asawanonda P. Glutathione as an oral whitening agent: a randomized, double-blind, placebo-controlled study. J Dermatolog Treat. 2012;23:97–102.
17. Handog EB, Datuin MSL, Singzon IA. An open-label, single-arm trial of the safety and efficacy of a novel preparation of glutathione as a skin-lightening agent in Filipino women. Int J Dermatol. 2016;55:153–7.

Chapter 15
Chemical Peeling for Melasma

Rosalina E. Nadela

15.1 Introduction

Melasma is characterized by increased melanin in the skin. This increased epidermal pigmentation, as evidenced from histological studies of lesional skin, is the hallmark of melasma and must be the main target for melasma treatment [1]. With this in mind, the use of chemical peeling, as an ancillary procedure in the treatment of this disorder is a warranted option. The basic mechanism of action of the chemical peel is to remove the unwanted epidermal melanin by creating a controlled injury to the skin. This entails special consideration in brown to dark brown skin, as the risk of post-inflammatory hyperpigmentation (PIH) and the exacerbation of the existing melasma is high.

15.2 Chemical Peels for Use in Brown Skin

Chemical peeling is a mainstay in a dermatologists' workbox due to its simple technique, inexpensive cost, and relatively low rate of adverse effects. The application of a caustic agent causes a penetration to a specific skin depth depending on the type of agent selected. The net effect of a superficial peel is to increase epidermal cell turnover, stimulate collagen production, and generate a more rejuvenated even skin color. Specifically for melasma, a peel removes unwelcome melanin.

R.E. Nadela, MD
MEDderm Asia Clinic and Laser Surgicentre,
35 Wilson St. Greenhills, San Juan 1500, Philippines
e-mail: rona.nadela@gmail.com

E.B. Handog, M.J. Enriquez-Macarayo (eds.), *Melasma and Vitiligo in Brown Skin*,
DOI 10.1007/978-81-322-3664-1_15

15.2.1 Alpha Hydroxy Acids (AHA)

15.2.1.1 Glycolic Acid Peels (GAP)

Fast Facts

- Sugar cane derivative.
- Anti-inflammatory, keratolytic, and antioxidant effect.
- Serial peels for 3–5 min once every 2 weeks (Fig.15.1).
- Mild desquamation.
- Uneven penetration into the skin.
- Neutralization with sodium bicarbonate solution is needed.
- Adverse events are slight discomfort, burning, erythema, and pigmentary changes.

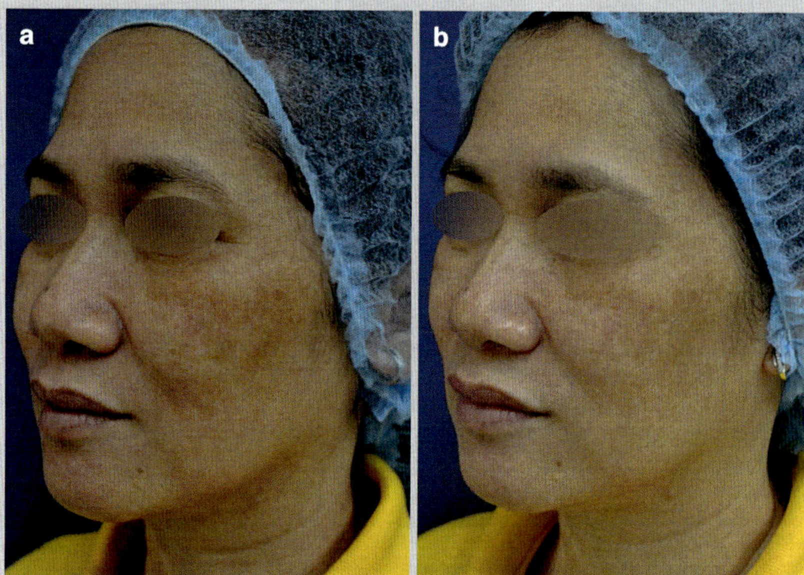

Fig. 15.1 (**a**) Before 70 % glycolic acid peels (**b**) after 4 biweekly sessions of 70 % glycolic acid peels

Glycolic acid, a derivative of sugar cane, is the most widely used alpha hydroxy acid. It has the smallest molecular weight of the AHAs and thus is able to penetrate the skin easily. Often used in concentrations of 20–70 %, its absorption into the skin is dependent on its pH, concentration, and length of application time on the skin. It should be used in lower concentrations initially, gradually increasing the concentration in subsequent sessions with an interval of 2 weeks between treatments. Peel neutralization is particularly important and should immediately follow the timed application of the peel. The longer the duration on the skin, the deeper the depth of the peel. Application of the GAP is associated with a mild stinging and/or a burning sensation. To counter this discomfort, the author prefers to use an ice cube wiped over the face followed by a peel neutralizer significantly alleviating any distress that the patient might be experiencing. Advising the patient in advance of the discomfort will also help them mentally prepare for this.

The usefulness of GAP for the treatment of melasma has been widely documented. In a study by Erbil et al., 28 women with melasma underwent serial glycolic acid peels (35–50 %, and 70 % every second peel) alone and in combination with topical azelaic acid 20 % cream and adapalene 0.1 % gel over a 20 week period [2]. There was significant decrease in the Melasma Area Severity Index (MASI) scores ($p=0.048$) in the group receiving the chemical peels plus topical treatment but only with GAP of 50 % and higher. However, three patients in the glycolic acid peel group developed a mild degree of PIH with total clearance at the end of the treatment period.

Lim, et al. demonstrated in ten Asian women the efficacy of GAP done every 3 weeks (20–70 %) alone or in combination with 2 % hydroquinone and 10 % glycolic acid cream. After eight peels, the subjects on GAP with combination cream trended towards significant improvement ($p<0.06$) in their melasma with lightening of the condition [3].

Sarkar, et al. found a significant decrease in the MASI scores ($p<0.001$) of 20 Indian patients receiving six serial GAP (30–40 %) combined with a topical modified Kligman's formula (2 % hydroquinone, 0.025 % tretinoin, and 1 % mometasone) as compared to the 20 patients who received the cream alone. The only adverse events observe with GAP were mild burning, erythema, desquamation, and transient hyperpigmentation [4]. A similar result was shown by Chaudhary and Dayal on 20 Indian patients who underwent serial GAP with a topical regimen (2 % hydroquinone, 1 % hydrocortisone, and 0.05 % tretinoin) versus cream alone. After 24 weeks, there was an overall decrease in MASI from baseline in both the groups (p value <0.05). The group receiving the glycolic acid peel with topical regimen showed early and greater improvement than the group which was receiving topical regimen only [5].

15.2.1.2 Lactic Acid Peel (LAP)

Fast Facts

- Sour milk derivative.
- Serial peels done every 2–3 weeks.
- Peel neutralization is needed.
- Adverse effects are uncommon: mild erythema, flaking, and burning sensation rare.

This is often called a "starter peel" because the lactic acid peel is the most gentle of all the chemical peels and usually results in few side effects. The following support its use as an option in brown skin. Lactic acid peels were found to be an effective and safe peeling agent in a study involving 20 Fitzpatrick skin type IV patients with melasma. Lactic acid peels (92 %, pH 3.5) were applied on the face once every 3 weeks. A maximum of six sessions resulted in marked improvement as seen in the MASI scores (56 % decrease) [6].

Sharquie compared the use of LAP (92 %, pH 3.5) on the left side of the face and Jessner's solution on the right side of the face on 30 Fitzpatrick skin type IV patients with melasma. Peeling was done once every 3 weeks for 2–5 sessions. There was significant improvement in MASI scores from baseline in both groups without any side effects noted. LAPs were shown to be as effective as Jessner's solution [7].

Further, Magalhães also reported the successful use of serial sessions of 85 % LAP on 33 melasma patients, predominantly of phototype IV. There was a significant reduction in both MASI (average decrease of 7 points) and melasma quality of life scales. This peel was also found to be safe, with an almost total absence of adverse events. The only events verified were light and transient erythema and edema immediately after the procedure [8]. Singh used LAP 82 % applied every 2 weeks for 12 weeks on 20 patients Fitzpatrick skin type IV–V with melasma. The decrease in MASI score was statistically significant ($p < 0.05$) at 12 weeks and all follow-ups. There was 35.7 % of total improvement at final visit (24 weeks) with a burning sensation noted as the only side effect of treatment [9].

15.2.2 Beta Hydroxy Acids (BHA)

15.2.2.1 Salicylic Acid Peels (SAP)

Fast Facts
- Beta hydroxy acid from willow bark.
- Anti-inflammatory and antimicrobial effects.
- Lipophilic nature with a comedolytic effect.
- White precipitate represents crystallization of the acid (pseudofrost).
- Adverse events are a stinging sensation on application, erythema, dryness, excessive crusting and desquamation, and salicylism.

Salicylic acid is beta hydroxy acid which can be used in low concentrations of 1–2 % in over the counter acne products or in higher concentration of 20–30 % to produce a superficial chemical peel.

Its efficacy as a peeling agent has been demonstrated in darker skin patients treated with a series of 20–30 % SAP for acne vulgaris, post-inflammatory hyperpigmentation, and melasma [10]. Bari likewise documented its use in Fitzpatrick skin type IV and V patients, treated with a series of eight weekly sessions of 30 % SAP. There was a 35–63 % improvement ($p < 0.05$) in all facial dermatoses treated such as melasma, acne vulgaris, and post-inflammatory hyperpigmentations without significant side effects [11]. In a comparison of 30 % SAP and Jessner's solution for epidermal melasma, it was shown that both were equally effective peeling agents with only mild adverse effects in sixty Asian patients predominantly skin type V with melasma [12]. Sarkar has documented the use of three consecutive 20 % and

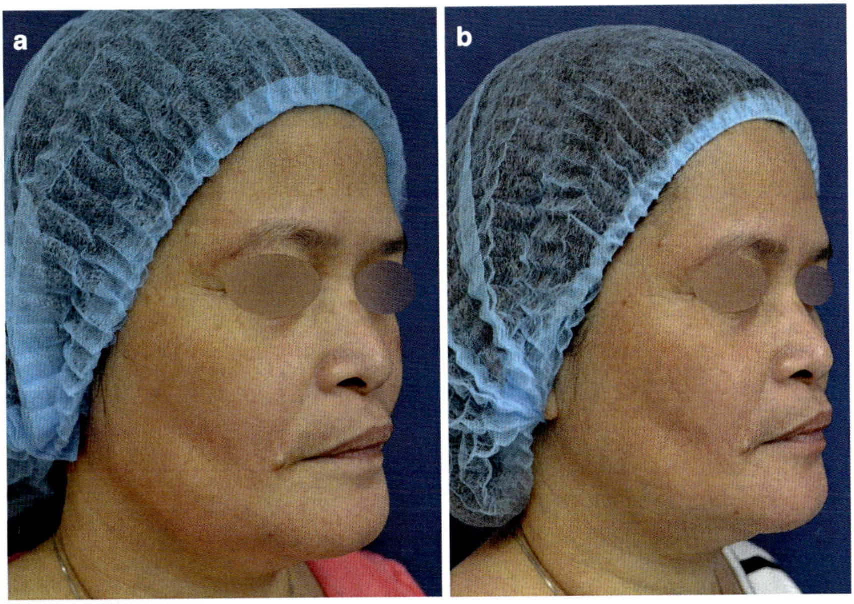

Fig. 15.2 (**a**) Before salicylic acid 20 % peels (**b**) after 4 biweekly sessions of salicylic acid 20 % peels

30 % salicylic acid peels done weekly followed by the 2 % hydroquinone/0.025 % tretinoin cream in between peels in 20 Indian patients. This led to a significant decrease in MASI scores ($p < 0.05$) [13].

In the treatment of melasma, the author recommends a series of SAP done once every 2 weeks using a 20–30 % concentration (Fig. 15.2). As a precautionary measure, start with a 20 % SAP, left on the skin for 3 min to test the patient's reaction to the solution. Frequently a stinging or burning sensation is experienced during the peel, followed by skin dryness lasting for a few days. The discomfort lasts only for 1–2 min and can be eased with the use of a handheld fan and application of ice post peel. There is also more visible peeling as compared to a GAP.

15.2.3 *Trichloroacetic Acid Peels (TCA)*

Fast Facts

- Colorless crystalline solid.
- Formulated using weight-in-volume method (TCA 10 % solution is 10 g TCA + water to make a 100 ml solution).
- Uniform application.
- Endpoint is frosting which indicates protein denaturation (Fig. 15.3a).
- No need to neutralize.
- Adverse events are a moderate to severe burning sensation, erythema, post-peel cracking (Fig. 15.3b), PIH, scarring.

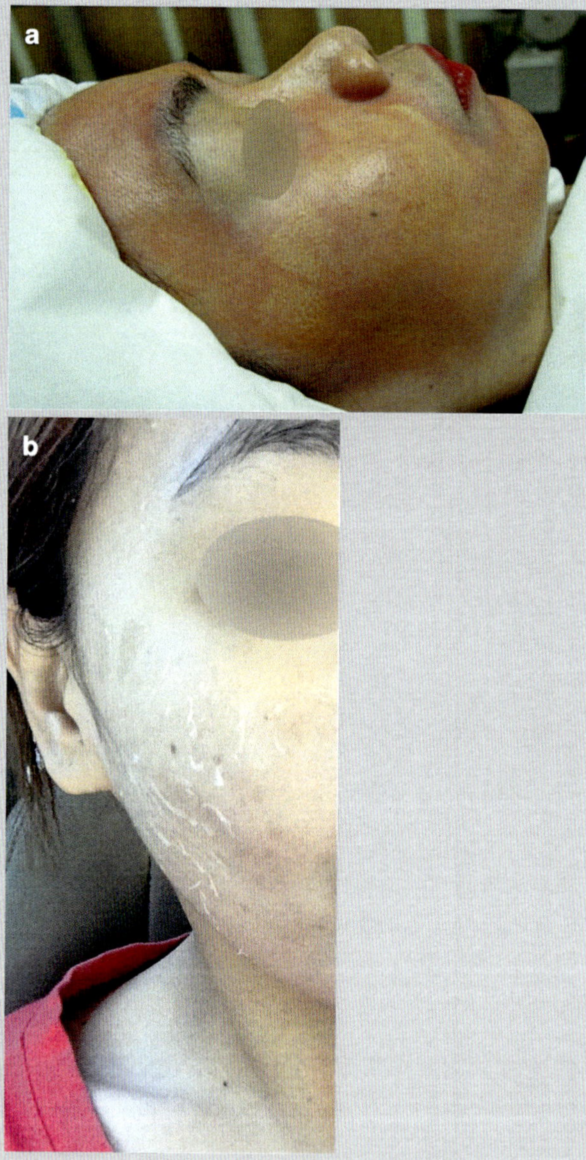

Fig. 15.3 (**a**) Immediately after a TCA 30 % peel with frosting and erythema (**b**) post-peel cracking

Considered the gold standard of chemical peels, TCA is well researched, stable, and easy to prepare and has no systemic toxicity. It is considered the most versatile of the peeling agents and can be used alone or in combination with glycolic acid or

Jessner's solution to produce a medium-depth peel. TCA is a coat-dependent peel, and the operator has to carefully observe the skin for the frost which may be seen as only a wisp in brown skin patients. At times, erythema is seen, but frosting is not observed. Thus relying on the number of coats is more important than waiting for the frost. It is best to wait for a coat to sufficiently dry and observe for the color changes on the skin before applying another coat. The more coats, the deeper the peel; consequently, multiple coats of a 15 % TCA can mimic the results of one to two coats of 35 % TCA [14, 15]. Thus, it is prudent to use only TCA 10–30 % in the management of melasma in brown-skinned patients and start off with 1–3 coats. Using a lower concentration of TCA will likewise decrease the likelihood that the peel will cause uneven penetration into skin, so-called hot spots. A major complaint by most patients is the initial experience of heat that develops into a moderate to severe burning sensation, lasting for a couple of minutes. The use of a handheld battery-operated fan and the application of cold wet compresses alleviate the discomfort. Soliman, et al. reported that 20 % TCA plus 5 % ascorbic acid cream was superior to TCA alone in 30 women with Fitzpatrick skin type III-IV. There was a significant decrease in MASI score for this group ($p<0.001$) as compared to TCA alone [16]. Some studies have compared the efficacy of TCA to GAP with insignificant differences between the two agents.

Kumari compared the efficacy of 20–30 % GAP to 10–20 % TCA in 40 Indian women with melasma. Gradually increasing peel concentrations were applied once every 15 days for a total of six treatments for both groups. There was a significant reduction in MASI scores from baseline but no difference between the two groups. Moderate to severe burning and post-peel cracking was reported in the TCA group but not in the GAP group [17]. Similar findings were reported by Puri who compared a 15 % TCA peel versus a 35 % glycolic acid peel for the treatment of melasma in 30 Indian patients. After six sessions spaced 3 weeks apart, the decrease in MASI score from baseline in both the groups was found to be statistically significant ($p=0.269$). However, there was no difference between the two regimens in terms of efficacy. The adverse effects of burning, erythema, and hyperpigmentation were more common in the TCA group rather than in the GAP group [18].

For the author, the burning discomfort and the downtime associated with the TCA peel are the major drawbacks to this modality. The deeper penetration and injury to the skin means that there is more visible peeling and a higher risk for PIH.

15.2.4 Jessner's Solution

Fast Facts

- Classic – 14 % resorcinol, 14 % lactic acid, and 14 % salicylic acid.
- Modified – 17 % lactic acid, 17 % salicylic acid, and 8 % citric acid.
- Keratolytic.
- Adverse effects are moderate burning sensation, peeling, and PIH.

Jessner's solution, like TCA, is coat dependent. Increasing the number of coats will increase the depth of penetration as well as the skin reaction. For melasma, serial peels done once every 2–3 weeks can be utilized. Modified Jessner's solution proved to be useful as an adjuvant treatment with TCA in the treatment of 20 females, Fitzpatrick skin type III–IV with epidermal melasma (TCA 15 % on 1 side of the face and TCA 15 % + modified Jessner's solution on the contralateral side). Peel sessions were done once every 10 days for eight sessions. There was a decrease in MASI scores for both sides; however, the side with the combination TCA and Jessner's solution showed a higher decrease in MASI scores (54.76 vs. 71.72). As regards the side effects, they were the same on both sides, in the form of erythema, swelling, acne, and folliculitis [19]. The efficacy of Jessner's solution was also described by Sharquie on 30 melasma patients, Fitzpatrick skin type IV who underwent one treatment session every 3 weeks for 2–5 times. There was a significant decrease in MASI scores on both the Jessner's side and lactic acid side without any side effects [20].

15.2.5 Tretinoin Peel

Fast Facts

- On application leaves a yellowish discoloration on the skin.
- No neutralization needed.
- Should be left on the skin for 4–5 h before washing.
- Adverse effects are erythema and peeling.

Tretinoin promotes the rapid loss of pigment through epidermopoiesis, and increased epidermal turnover decreases the contact time between keratinocytes and melanocytes [21]. It has produced good results in melasma clinical trials [22, 23]. Khunger, in a split-face study involving ten Indian women with melasma, compared 1 % tretinoin solution on half face to 70 % GAP on the opposite side. After 12 weekly peels, there was a significant improvement on both sides as assessed by photography and decreased MASI scores ($p < 0.001$). Both peels were well tolerated with minimal side effects [24]. More recently, a study on 63 Asian women with melasma compared the split face use of tretinoin 1 % and GAP 70 % every 2 weeks for four sessions. The efficiency of tretinoin 1 % peelings in decreasing the MASI score was similar to GA 70 %. Patient discomfort was significantly lower with tretinoin 1 % compared to GAP 70 % [25]. Ghersetich, et al., using a modification, i.e., 10 % tretinoin peel mask on 20 melasma patients, has shown that there was significant improvement ($p < 0.05$) after the peels [26].

From the author's experience, the use of a tretinoin peel (Fig. 15.4) is likewise comparable to a higher-strength GAP although more treatment sessions are needed with a tretinoin peel.

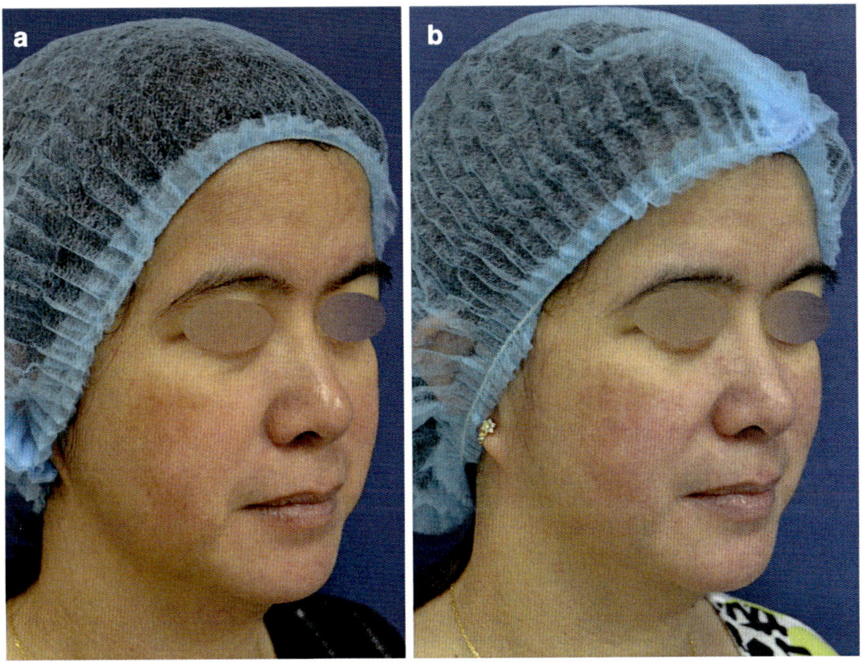

Fig. 15.4 (**a**) Before tretinoin 1 % peel (**b**) after 4 biweekly sessions of tretinoin 1 % peel

15.3 Considerations for an Optimum Result

The management of melasma remains a challenge. It is imperative to devise a therapeutic regimen that will target the disease progression and prevent relapse. Of particular concern is the propensity of brown skin to develop post-inflammatory hyperpigmentation (PIH). The high incidence of PIH in darker skin is attributable to its faulty pathophysiological response to cutaneous injury, owing, in turn, to its increased melanocyte activity [27].

Chemical peels are generally used to treat only the epidermal and mixed forms of melasma, as an attempt to treat the deeper variant often leads to unwanted complications like hypertrophic scarring and permanent depigmentation [1, 28]. The main advantage of chemical peels lies in the fact that they can be tailored for use according to the needs of the patient and can be used synergistically with other in-office procedures and topical creams to achieve synergistic effects [29].

15.3.1 Patient Preparation

15.3.1.1 Assessment and History

A thorough patient evaluation is done on the first consultation. Eliciting a detailed medical history with attention to details (e.g., family history of melasma, use of oral contraceptives, current medications, and sun exposure history) will reveal the underlying causes of pigmentation, as well as factors that may hinder treatment. Evaluate the skin type of the patient, paying attention to a history of post-inflammatory hyperpigmentation and a keloidal tendency. As part of the preparations, it is essential to take good photographs before and during treatment to properly document a patient's response. Consistent serial photos can be acquired if guidelines are maintained such as the same color background, distance of camera from patient, good overhead lighting, as well as angles taken like front, 45°, and 90°. Photographs prove particularly useful to show the patients, as improvement rates vary. General contraindications to peeling include active inflammation or infection of the treatment site, oral isotretinoin intake within the last 6 months, and allergies to any component of the peel solution such as resorcinol or salicylic acid. Start oral antivirals (acyclovir 400 mg BID or valciclovir 500 mg BID) if there is a history of recurrent herpes simplex infection, 2 days before the peel.

15.3.1.2 Priming the Skin

The preparation of the skin prior to the peel procedure is essential to obtain the best results while minimizing the risk of post-peel complications. Two to four weeks prior to the peel, the patient is put on a topical regimen of a daily sunscreen SPF 30–50, an alpha hydroxy acid cream to promote a mild exfoliation, and a depigmenting agent like 2 % hydroquinone or arbutin cream to reduce epidermal melanin.

In dark-skinned patients, the choice of a retinoid cream or a 4 % hydroquinone or higher is not the best option since irritation can occur, leading to more complications. In a study, Garg compared the beneficiary effects of with and without a priming agent (2 % hydroquinone or 0.025 % retinoic acid) before a series of glycolic acid peels in 60 melasma patients. There was an overall decrease in MASI scores from baseline for the three groups, but the results were more significant for the group that used 2 % hydroquinone as a priming agent compared to tretinoin [30]. According to Javaheri, the use of daily sunscreen and a night time 10 % glycolic acid lotion for 2 weeks prior to monthly 50 % glycolic acid peels, improved melasma in 91 % of the Indian patients studied who had melasma [31].

When patients are given a priming routine to follow, the physician will be able to gauge adherence to treatment. If a patient is uncooperative or has an irregular application, then this might affect the overall success of a peel.

15.3.2 Peel Procedure

Obtain an informed consent prior to the peel procedure. Tailor the therapy to the patient. If downtime is a problem because of work, then a series of superficial peels may be the better option. Regardless of the chemical peel solution selected, the physician has to be very familiar with the peel agent, the application procedure, as well as its removal and whether or not neutralization is needed. Prepare all the needed equipment by the bedside prior to the peel. A precise technique is paramount to ensure a satisfactory result. The mode of application affects the evenness of application and the penetration of the peeling agents. Remember to practice the cautious application of the solution, especially around the periorbital area, proper neutralization of agents if needed, and documentation in the chart of the procedure [32].

15.3.3 Post Peel Care

It is best to explain to the patient what to expect after a chemical peel. A printed handout with detailed instructions maybe given so that they patient remembers all the do's and don'ts. A skin care regimen inclusive of a gentle cleanser, sunscreen, and moisturizer, if needed, is prescribed for the patient to take home and use. More importantly, schedule a return visit for a checkup. The necessity for maintenance treatment is likewise emphasized.

15.4 Conclusion

Despite ongoing researches on the pathophysiology of melasma, it remains difficult to treat and is recurrent despite therapy. Chemical peels for the treatment of melasma remain to be a worthwhile adjunct in its management for both the patient and physician. For the author, the glycolic acid peel remains the best option for epidermal melasma in the hands of an experienced physician. Careful consideration must be made to avoid PIH which is common in Asian skin. While promises cannot be made on the outcome, careful selection of the chemical peeling agent, patients, and use of precise technique will ensure a satisfactory result.

References

1. Kang HY. What should be considered in treatment of melasma. Ann Dermatol. 2010; 22(4):373–8.
2. Erbil H, Sezer E, Taştan B, Arca E, Kurumlu Z. The efficacy and safety of serial glycolic acid peels and topical regimen in the treatment of recalcitrant melasma. J Dermatol. 2007;34(1):25–30.
3. Lim JT, Tham SN. Glycolic peels in the treatment of melasma among Asian women. Dermatol Surg. 1997;23(3):177–9.
4. Sarkar R, Kaur C, Bhalla M, Kanwar AJ. The combination of glycolic acid peels with a topical regimen in the treatment of melasma in dark-skinned patients: a comparative study. Dermatol Surg. 2002;28(9):828–32.
5. Chaudhary S, Dayal S. Efficacy of combination of glycolic acid peeling with topical regimen in treatment of melasma. J Drugs Dermatol. 2013;12(10):1149–53.
6. Sharquie KE, Al-Tikreety MM, Al-Mashhadani SA. Lactic acid as a new therapeutic peeling agent in melasma. Dermatol Surg. 2005;31(2):149–54.

7. Sharquie KE, Al-Tikreety MM, Al-Mashhadani SA. Lactic acid chemical peels as a new therapeutic modality in melasma in comparison to Jessner's solution chemical peels. Dermatol Surg. 2006;32(12):1429–36.
8. Magalhães GM, Borges MFB, Oliveira PJV, Neves DR. Lactic acid chemical peel in the treatment of melasma: clinical evaluation and impact on quality of life. Surg Cosmet Dermatol. 2010;2(3):173–9.
9. Singh R, Goyal S, Ahmed OR, Gupta N, Singh S. Effect of 82% lactic acid in treatment of melasma. International Scholarly Research Notices. 2014; Article ID 407142, p. 7.
10. Grimes PE. The safety and efficacy of salicylic acid chemical peels in darker racial-ethnic groups. Dermatol Surg. 1999;25(1):18–22.
11. Bari AU, Iqbal Z, Rahman SB. Superficial chemical peeling with salicylic acid in facial dermatoses. J Coll Physicians Surg Pak. 2007;17(4):187–90.
12. Ejaz A, Raza N, Iftikhar N, Muzzafar F. Comparison of 30% salicylic acid with Jessner's solution for superficial chemical peeling in epidermal melasma. J Coll Physicians Surg Pak. 2008;18(4):205–8.
13. Sarkar R, Puri P. A study to assess the safety and tolerability of salicylic acid peels for melasma in dark skinned patients. JAAD. 2012;6(4 Suppl 1):AB178.
14. Al-Waiz MM, Al-Sharqi AI. Medium-depth chemical peels in the treatment of acne scars in dark skinned individuals. Dermatol Surg. 2002;28:383–7.
15. Monheit GD. Medium-depth chemical peels. Dermatol Clin. 2001;19:413–25.
16. Soliman MM, Ramadan SA, Bassiouny DA, Abdelmalek M. Combined trichloroacetic acid peel and topical ascorbic acid versus trichloroacetic acid peel alone in the treatment of melasma: a comparative study. J Cosmet Dermatol. 2007;6(2):89–94.
17. Kumari R, Thappa DM. Comparative study of trichloroacetic acid versus glycolic acid chemical peels in the treatment of melasma. Indian J Dermatol Venereol Leprol. 2010;76(4):447.
18. Puri N. Comparative study of 15% TCA peel versus 35% glycolic acid peel for the treatment of melasma. Indian Dermatol Online J. 2012;3(2):109–13.
19. Safoury OS, Zaki NM, El Nabarawy EA, Farag EA. A study comparing chemical peeling using modified Jessner's solution and 15% trichloroacetic acid versus 15% trichloroacetic acid in the treatment of melasma. Indian J Dermatol. 2009;54(1):41–5.
20. Sharquie KE, Al-Tikreety MM, Al-Mashhadani SA. Lactic acid chemical peels as a new therapeutic modality in melasma in comparison to Jessner's solution chemical peels. Dermatol Surg. 2006;32(12):1429–36.
21. Bandyopadhyay D. Topical treatment of melasma. Indian J Dermatol. 2009;54(4):303–9.
22. Griffiths CE, Finkel LJ, Ditre CM, Hamilton TA, Ellis CN, Boorhees JJ. Topical tretinoin (retinoid acid) improves melasma: a vehicle-controlled, clinical trial. Br J Dermatol. 1993;129:415–21.
23. Kimbrough-Green CK, Griffiths CE, Finkel LJ, Hamilton TA, Bulengo-Ransby SM, Ellis CN, et al. Topical retinoid acid (tretinoin) for melasma in black patients: a vehicle-controlled clinical trial. Arch Dermatol. 1994;130:727–33.
24. Khunger N, Sarkar R, Jain RK. Tretinoin peels versus glycolic acid peels in the treatment of melasma in dark-skinned patients. Dermatol Surg. 2004;25:270–3.
25. Faghihi G, Shahingohar A, Siadat AH. Comparison between 1% tretinoin peeling versus 70% glycolic acid peeling in the treatment of female patients with melasma. J Drugs Dermatol. 2011;10(12):1439–42.
26. Ghersetich I, Troiano M, Brazzni B, Arunachalam M, Lotti T. Melasma: treatment with 10% tretinoin peeling mask. J Cosmet Dermatol. 2010;9:117–21.
27. Ho SG, Chan HH. The Asian dermatologic patient: review of common pigmentary disorders and cutaneous diseases. Am J Clin Dermatol. 2009;10:153–68.
28. Sarkar R, Bansal S, Garg V. Chemical peels for melasma in dark-skinned patients. J Cutan Aesthet Surg. 2012;5(4):247–53.
29. Sarkar R, Chugh S, Garg VK. Newer and upcoming therapies for melasma. Ind J Dermatol. 2012;78(4):417–28.
30. Garg VK, Sarkar R, Agarwal R. Comparative evaluation of beneficiary effects of priming agents (2% hydroquinone and 0.025% retinoic acid) in the treatment of melasma with glycolic acid peels. Dermatol Surg. 2008;34(8):1032–9.

31. Javaheri SM, Handa S, Kaur I, Kumar B. Safety and efficacy of glycolic acid facial peel in Indian women with melasma. Int J Dermatol. 2001;40(5):354–7.
32. Drake LA, Dinehart SM, Goltz RW, Graham GF, Hordinsky MK, Lewis CW, Pariser DM, Salasche SJ, Skouge JW, Turner ML, et al. Guidelines of care for chemical peeling. Guidelines/Outcomes Committee: American Academy of Dermatology. J Am Acad Dermatol. 1995;33(3):497–503.

Chapter 16
The Role of Lasers and Light Devices for the Treatment of Melasma

Chee Leok Goh

16.1 Introduction

Melasma is a common pigmentary disorder among Asians, Hispanics, and the Mediterraneans. The etiology is multifactorial, and there is no single treatment (topical or procedural) that can completely cure melasma. The first-line treatment of melasma is sun avoidance, sun protection, and elimination of aggravating factors together with topical skin whitening agents. Oral tranexamic acid and chemical peels are generally second-line treatment [1], and lasers and light devices are generally used as second- or third-line treatment after a failed topical treatment. None of these second- and third-line treatments are curative either, and relapse is commonly observed upon cessation of treatment.

Lasers and light devices have a role in the management of melasma. Generally, such devices must be used with caution in skin of color, especially among Asians, as the risk of post-inflammatory hyperpigmentation (PIH) following treatment is high (Fig. 16.1). Melasma may occasionally darken following laser and light treatment and patients should be counseled and advised on such complications. But as a second- or third-line treatment, lasers and light devices can offer patients with melasma, who are recalcitrant to topical treatment, a respite and improvement in the quality of life. Laser and light treatment can be a therapeutic option that will provide benefits to the patients.

C.L. Goh
National Skin Centre, Singapore, YLL School of Medicine, National University of Singapore, 1 Mandalay Road, Singapore 308205, Singapore
e-mail: drgohcl@gmail.com

E.B. Handog, M.J. Enriquez-Macarayo (eds.), *Melasma and Vitiligo in Brown Skin*,
DOI 10.1007/978-81-322-3664-1_16

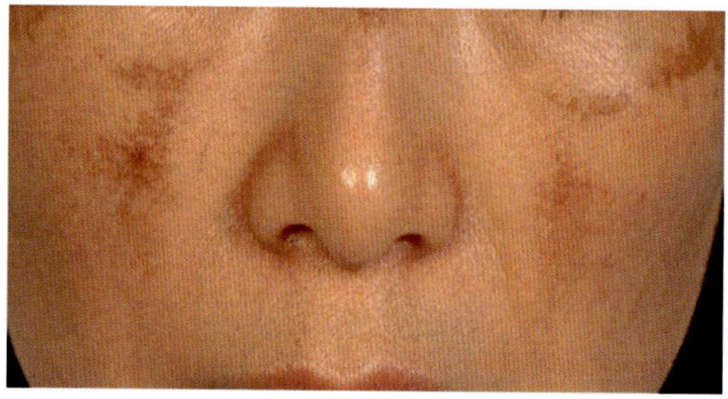

Fig. 16.1 PIH 2 months following QS Nd:YAG 1064-nm laser using convention treatment protocol for treating melasma. This patient was treated with QS Nd:YAG 1064 nm 4 ns pulsed duration and fluence of 8 J/cm^2 (Photograph courtesy of National Skin Centre, Singapore)

16.2 Laser and Light Therapies

16.2.1 The Q-Switched Lasers (Pigment Lasers)

The Q-switched (QS) lasers are lasers with short pulse duration in nanosecond domain. They are suited to treat pigmentary skin disorders because of melanin's short thermal relaxation time and absorption spectrum. These lasers include the QS ruby, alexandrite, and Nd:YAG lasers. The QS lasers are wonderful devices for removing tattoos, nevus of Ota, Hori's nevus, lentigines, and some other pigmentary disorders. Initially, it was thought that adopting the same treatment protocol used to treat other pigmentary skin disorders will also be suitable for melasma [2, 3]. But experience showed that they are not, as severe PIH is common and often no improvement could be achieved.

Taylor reported eight patients with melasma or PIH treated with the QS ruby laser (694 nm, 40 ns pulse duration) at fluences of 15–7.5 J/cm^2. It was shown that regardless of fluence, there was no permanent improvement of their melasma; in some cases, darkening of melasma was even observed. Histologic sections of biopsy specimens taken before and after treatment showed extracellular melanin immediately after the procedure. Several months after the last treatment, epidermal pigmentation was back to baseline levels, and dermal melanophages were focally increased [4].

Given these results, the Q-switched lasers used in conventional treatment parameter for pigmentary skin lesions are not a recommended method to treat melasma.

16.2.2 Ablative Skin Resurfacing (Erbium: Yttrium-Aluminum-Garnet Lasers)

The erbium:YAG laser (Continuum Biomedical, Dublin, CA) emits 2940-nm laser wavelengths. This wavelength is highly absorbed by tissue water as its chromophore and is an effective ablative resurfacing wavelength. Manaloto et al. treated ten patients of Fitzpatrick skin phototypes II–V with refractory melasma using the erbium:YAG laser. Utilizing MASI scores and spectrophotometer for assessment, the authors found that there was improvement immediately after the laser treatment. However, all patients developed PIH after 3–6 weeks follow-up, despite prophylaxis oral steroids for 5 days post procedure [5].

While the PIH improved with serial glycolic acid peels, this side effect appears to outweigh the benefit derived from this ablative procedure.

16.2.3 Combination of Carbon Dioxide and QS Alexandrite Laser

Various combination treatments with ablative laser resurfacing with the QS lasers were tried too, but the problem of post-inflammatory hyperpigmentation remained.

Theoretically, pulsed CO_2 laser wavelength targets water as its chromophore and can be helpful in removing epidermal pigmentation. The QS alexandrite laser emits 755 nm wavelength energy that targets melanin up to the dermis. A study reported the combination of the CO_2 laser ablation followed by the QS alexandrite laser treatment to enhance the penetration of the pigment laser to remove dermal melanin in melasma. Nouri et al. treated eight patients with Fitzpatrick skin phototypes IV–VI with dermal melasma who were pretreated with 14 days of 0.05 % tretinoin cream, 4 % hydroquinone cream, and 1 % hydrocortisone cream twice daily. Four patients were randomized to receive spot treatment with one pass of the CO_2 laser, followed by one pass of the Q-switched alexandrite laser. The other four patients received treatment with one pass of the CO_2 laser alone. Using blinded subjective investigator evaluation as the primary end point, the authors felt that the combination therapy led to better resolution of the treated area with less peripheral hyperpigmentation. However, the sample size was small, as was the area being treated, limiting the generalizability of these results [6].

Niwat et al. reported a split-face study among Thai patients with refractory melasma on the efficacy of the Q-switched alexandrite 755-nm laser (Accolade; Cynosure, Chelmsford, United Kingdom) with or without one pass of the Ultrapulse CO_2 laser (Coherent, Palo Alto, CA). Among the six females with Fitzpatrick skin phototypes II–V with refractory melasma who were treated, there was no statistically significant difference between the two treatment modalities at the end of the study. MASI and melanin index evaluation, however, showed Ultrapulse CO_2 laser + QSAL gave better improvement but more severe PIH. Importantly, three (33 %) patients with Fitzpatrick skin phototypes IV–V had PIH on both sides at 2–4 weeks lasting up to 3 months, and one patient had transient hypopigmentation lasting 6 months. The authors' conclusion was that given the risk of postoperative dyspigmentation, neither modality was safe for routine use for treating melasma in Asians [7].

It is generally felt that combination ablative and pigment lasers are not a recommended treatment for melasma in view of the high risk of PIH among Asians.

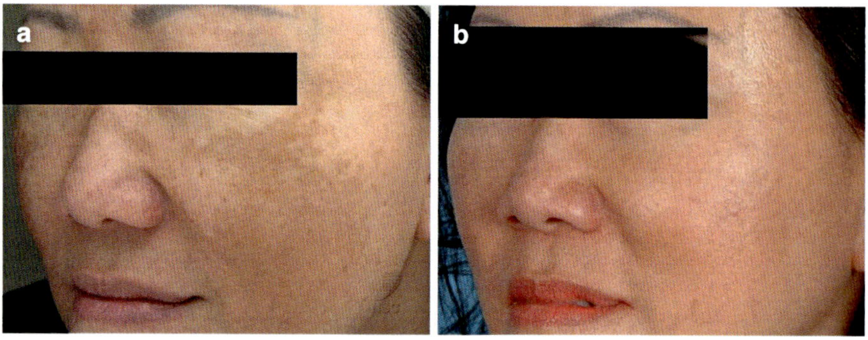

Fig. 16.2 Significant improvement of melasma after three treatments at monthly interval with non-ablative fractional laser. But recurrence appeared 3 months after stopping treatment (Photographs courtesy of National Skin Centre, Singapore)

16.2.4 Fractional Laser Resurfacing

Fractional laser resurfacing is a procedure that uses laser light to create scattered microzones of thermal damage on the skin. It does not cause confluent full-thickness skin wounds, and the in-between normal undamaged skin acts as a reservoir to regenerate the laser damaged skin. This results in more rapid skin repair and recovery [8]. This laser is approved by the Food and Drug Administration (FDA) for the treatment of melasma, periorbital rhytides, pigmented lesions, skin resurfacing, acne scars, and surgical scars [9]. The microthermal zones of injury limit the area of the skin that is damaged with each treatment, which may decrease the risk of PIH.

The transepidermal elimination of debris and tissue through the microthermal treatment zones after injury could serve as an effective method of removing dermal melanophages [10]. Good clinical results may be seen in some patients (Fig. 16.2).

Roshkar evaluated ten patients with Fitzpatrick skin phototypes III–V treated with a fractional laser (Fraxel; Reliant Technologies, Palo Alto, CA) for four to six sessions, 1–2 weeks apart [11]. None of the patients were pretreated with hydroquinone. The authors found that six out of the ten patients had 75–100 % clearing of melasma based on clinical evaluation and 30 % had less than 25 % improvement. The nonresponders were all Hispanic patients. There was a 10 % risk of post-inflammatory hypopigmentation. The risk of delayed PIH and relapse were not assessed (level of evidence, II-iii).

However, the incidence of post-inflammatory pigmentation (Fig. 16.3) following fractional laser resurfacing in Asians is high ranging from 10 to 90 % [12]. It is likely that those with melasma will experience higher risk of PIH. Hence such modality of treatment is not suitable for Asian melasma patients especially those with darker skin type.

Another study looked at the histopathologic effects of fractional laser technology on melasma. The study failed to support the efficaciousness of fractional laser resurfacing for melasma [13]. The authors treated ten patients with epidermal melasma

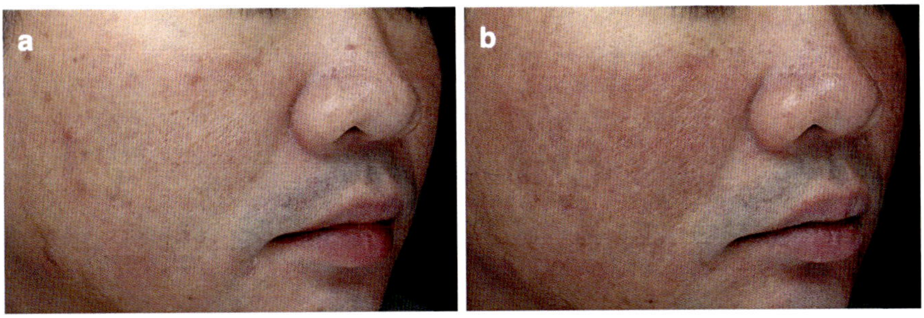

Fig. 16.3 PIH following a single treatment with the non-ablative fractional laser treatment for melasma (Photographs courtesy of National Skin Centre, Singapore)

who had Fitzpatrick skin phototypes III–IV every 2 weeks for four sessions. Biopsy specimens were obtained before treatment and 3 months after the final treatment. Sunscreen use was advocated but depigmenting agents were avoided. After treatment, lesional skin showed a decrease in the number of epidermal melanocytes and fewer enlarged melanocytes on electron microscopy; however, there was no correlation between histologic improvement and investigator-rated improvement.

Several later studies also reported lack of efficaciousness of fractional lasers for melasma. Lee et al. reported 25 melasma patients who received four monthly fractional laser treatments who achieved reduction of mean MASI score from 7.6 to 6.2. There was 60 % improvement at 4 weeks after treatment which deteriorated to 52 % at 24 weeks after treatment. Mean melanin index decreased significantly after the first two sessions, but it relapsed in subsequent follow-ups. The treatment did not alter skin elasticity. Hyperpigmentation was observed in three of 23 subjects (13 %). The authors concluded that fractional laser treatment of melasma led to some clinical improvements, but it was not as efficacious as previously reported. They recommend judicious use of fractional laser for melasma in Asian skin because of its limited efficacy. There is also risk of PIH [14].

Wind et al. treated 29 melasma patients with a split-face study using four to five treatments with non-ablative 1550-nm fractional laser on half the face compared to daily topical triple combination therapy (hydroquinone 5 %, tretinoin 0.05 %, triamcinolone acetonide 0.1 % cream) alone on the other half in a 15-week study. After the last treatment session, patients were asked to apply the triple combination cream twice weekly on both sides of the face during follow-up. Mean patient global assessment and satisfaction were significantly lower at the fractional laser-treated side ($p<0.001$). Physician global assessment, melanin index, and L-value showed a significant worsening of hyperpigmentation at the fractional laser-treated side. At the triple cream-treated side, no significant change was observed. At 6-month follow-up, most patients preferred the triple cream treatment. Side effects of the fractional laser-treated side were erythema, burning sensation, edema, and pain. Nine patients (31 %) developed PIH after two or more laser sessions. The authors concluded that given the high rate of PIH, non-ablative 1550-nm fractional laser at 15 mJ/microbeam is not recommendable in the treatment of melasma. Triple cream treatment remains the gold standard treatment [15].

Subsequently, the same group of authors reported a somewhat similar study in 2011. Twenty female patients with moderate to severe melasma and Fitzpatrick skin phototypes II–V were treated either with non-ablative fractional laser therapy or triple topical therapy (hydroquinone 5 %, tretinoin 0.05 %, and triamcinolone acetonide 0.1 % cream) once daily for 8 weeks in a randomized controlled observer-blinded study. Laser treatment was performed every 2 weeks for a total of four times. Physician global assessment improved ($p < .001$) in both groups at 3 weeks. There was no difference in physician global assessment between the two groups. Mean treatment satisfaction and recommendation were significantly higher in the laser group at 3 weeks ($p < .05$). However, melasma recurred in five patients in both groups after 6 months. Side effects in the laser group were erythema, burning sensation, facial edema, and pain; in the triple topical therapy group, side effects were erythema, burning, and scaling. The authors concluded that non-ablative fractional laser therapy is safe and comparable in efficacy and recurrence rate with the triple topical therapy. It may be a useful alternative treatment option for melasma when topical bleaching is ineffective or not tolerated [16].

Fractional laser appears to show satisfactory results for melasma in Caucasians with lighter skin type but is associated with unacceptable PIH and relapses in Asians with darker skin types. It is at most equivalent to topical triple cream therapy.

16.2.5 Laser Toning with QS Nd:YAG Lasers

A procedure called "laser toning" that uses a low-energy 1064-nm Q-switched Nd:YAG laser was recently introduced for the treatment of melasma, demonstrating good results (Fig. 16.4). The procedure involves using the QS Nd:YAG laser setting at large spot size of 6 mm or 8 mm, with fluence of 2–3 J/cm^2 and 1–2 J/cm^2, respectively, and waving the laser beam on the surface of melasma lesions for 5–10 passes. The procedure is carried out once a week or fortnightly. The proposed mechanism of action of laser toning is subcellular selective photothermolysis of melanosomes and not melanocytes. It is speculated that melanocytes survived but the melanogenic activity downregulated such that they did not produce fully matured melanosomes [17].

There have been numerous reports of "laser toning" using the QS Nd:YAG laser. The initial reports generally concluded that the 1064-nm Q-switched Nd:YAG laser is a safe and effective modality for treating melasma in Asian patients [18–21].

A recent study comparing "laser toning" with hydroquinone and hydroquinone alone confirmed the efficacy of the treatment. Twenty-two Thai patients on split-face randomized study, combination of low-fluence QS Nd:YAG laser + 2 % hydroquinone versus topical treatment only, showed that the laser-treated side achieved 92.5 % improvement in relative lightness index and 75.9 % improvement in mMASI score, against 19.7 % and 24 %, respectively, on the topical HQ alone side ($p < .001$). However, the report indicated that "laser toning" procedure was associated with side effects including mottled hypopigmentation in three patients (14 %) and rebound

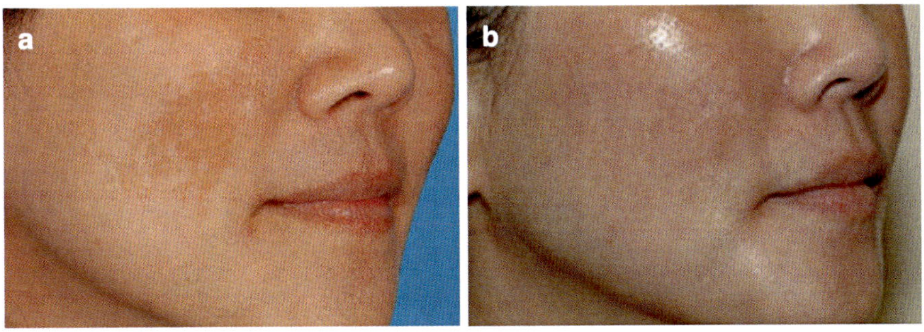

Fig. 16.4 Good improvement of melasma following eight treatments of laser toning with the QS Nd:YAG 1064-nm laser performed every 2 weeks. Fluence was 2.5 J/cm^2, 6 mm spot size, 5 ns pulsed duration. Recurrence appeared 3 months after cessation of treatment (Photographs courtesy of National Skin Centre, Singapore)

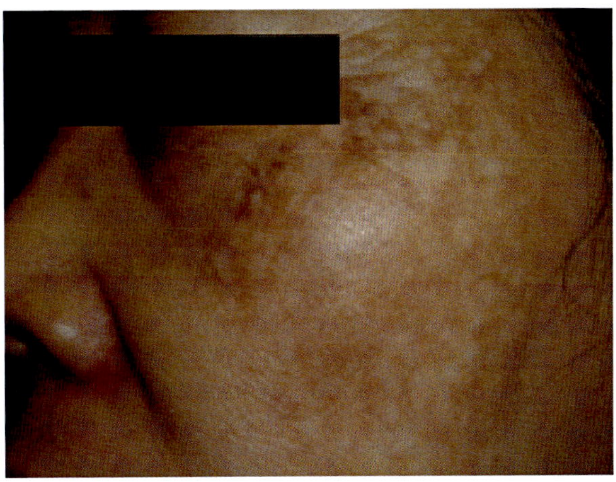

Fig. 16.5 Guttate hypomelanotic macules following too frequent and high-dose laser toning with the QS Nd:YAG 1064-nm laser for melasma (Photograph courtesy of National Skin Centre, Singapore)

hyperpigmentation in four (18 %) at 12-week follow-up. Melasma relapse is the rule upon cessation of treatment. Their conclusions were that QS Nd:YAG laser treatment ("laser toning") for melasma in Asians produced only temporary improvement and had side effects. Common complications were hypopigmentation, melasma recurrence, and rebound hyperpigmentation [22]. Hypomelanosis following "laser toning" with QS Nd:YAG laser is a serious complication (Fig. 16.5). There have been several reports on this difficult to treat complication which may last several years [23–25].

"Laser toning" appears to be a useful adjunct to topical treatment for melasma. But it should be used with caution. The laser physician should use conservative treatment protocol when carrying out "laser toning." Generally, the frequency of "laser toning" should not exceed more often than once fortnightly, and the fluence should be kept low. "Laser toning" should be stopped at the earliest indication of guttate hypomelanotic macules appearing.

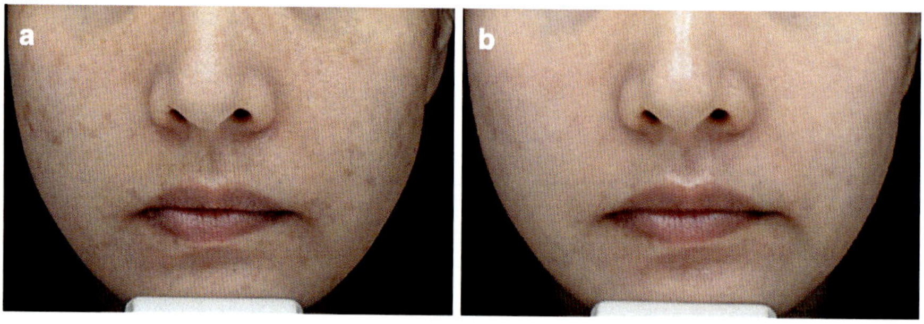

Fig. 16.6 Fairly good response of melasma to six sessions at monthly interval of IPL

16.2.6 Intense Pulsed Light

Intense pulsed light (IPL) is a broadband light source and is not a laser device. The IPL emits light of wavelength stretching from 500 to 1200 nm. This spectrum of wavelength falls within the absorption spectrum of melanin and oxyhemoglobin. Hence, it can be used to treat superficial pigmentary lesions including melasma. "Cutoff" filters can be placed across IPL sources to eliminate unwanted shorter wavelengths to prevent epidermal burn. These filters are especially useful when using IPL on darker skin type.

Several studies have reported improvements of melasma with IPL with minimal side effects. But patients often require multiple treatments (Fig. 16.6).

A report from Taiwan compared IPL treatment with HQ against HQ alone on 33 patients with Fitzpatrick skin phototypes III and IV having mixed melasma. Patients received four monthly sessions of IPL. Using the mexameter, the authors calculated a relative melanin index (defined as the difference between the melanin index of lesional skin and the melanin index of normal skin). In the IPL/HQ group (17 females), 35 % had greater than 50 % improvement compared to the HQ-alone group (16 control) with only 14 % experiencing greater than 50 % improvement. The patients who received IPL treatment had a 39.8 % decrease in the relative melanin index after four treatments (16 weeks), while the control group receiving topical therapy alone had only an 11.6 % decrease. At 24-week posttreatment, the improvement on the IPL-treated side had decreased less to a mean of 24.2 %, suggesting the need for maintenance treatments. Side effects of the IPL included some crusting lasting for 1–2 weeks; transient PIH seen in 12 % was resolved with the use of HQ [26].

In another report from China, 89 Chinese females with predominantly mixed melasma unresponsive to topical therapy and chemical peels were treated with IPL every 3 weeks for four sessions. Patients were instructed to use broad-spectrum sunscreen and avoid bleaching creams. Improvement of melasma was assessed using the MASI score. Pigmentation and erythema were objectively measured with a mexameter. Mean MASI scores dropped significantly, from 15.2 to 5.2 after four sessions and to 4.5 at the 3-month follow-up visit. Epidermal melasma responded better than the mixed type. The melanin index as measured by the mexameter dropped from a mean value of 140.8 to a value of 119; the erythema index dropped significantly as well. The most common side effects included temporary erythema and edema and microcrusting. PIH was observed in three cases [27].

16.2.7 Newer Intense Pulsed Light Treatment Protocol and Devices

16.2.7.1 Low-Fluence and Short-Pulse Intense Pulsed Light

Low-fluence and short-pulse IPL has been reported to be effective and safe in the treatment of melasma. The low-fluence IPL has nanosecond-level pulse duration and allows selective thermolysis of melanosomes with minimal side effects. Twenty Korean adults with melasma were randomly assigned to two groups and treated at fluences of 10 or 13 J/cm^2 of IPL weekly over 6 weeks. Subjects were evaluated at baseline and weekly during the 6 weeks of treatment and at 3 weeks following the final treatment. Melanin and erythema indices were scored using a spectrophotometer. The mMASI score of 20 patients at inclusion was 11.6. Both 10 J and 13 J IPL treatment groups had decreased mMASI scores from 2 weeks onward at statistically significant levels. Both 10 J and 13 J IPL treatment groups showed decreased melanin indices with statistically significant differences from 3 weeks onward. The authors concluded that a low-fluence IPL protocol could provide effective treatment for melasma with minimal side effects in Asian skin [28].

16.2.7.2 Fractionated Intense Pulsed Light Device

A recent report on a prospective, split-face, randomized study of the efficacy and safety of a novel fractionated IPL with microsecond domain to treat melasma in 30 Asian women showed significant improvement of melasma. In this 14-week split-face study, one side of the face received weekly fractionated IPL and the other side biweekly conventional IPL. The non-inferiority of a weekly fractionated IPL regimen to a biweekly conventional IPL regimen was verified by a lower margin of the 95 % confidence interval for the difference in the MASI change from baseline of 2.61 for each side. This value was greater than the previously determined non-inferiority margin of −2.68 ($p < 0.025$). On the fractionated IPL side, the mMASI score decreased continuously, but in the conventional IPL group, the mMASI score rebounded during the treatment course. The authors concluded that fractionated IPL shows moderate efficacy as a melasma treatment and is therefore a good alternative to conventional IPL. Fractionated IPL can also be used as a maintenance treatment for melasma [29].

IPL appears to be moderately effective in the treatment of melasma. It does not clear nor cure the condition. However, because of its safety and a lower percentage of producing PIH, IPL can be considered as an adjunct in the treatment of recalcitrant melasma.

16.2.8 Combination of Laser Toning and IPL

"Laser toning" with Q-switched Nd:YAG 1064-nm laser combined with IPL for the treatment of melasma has been reported to enhance the efficaciousness of the two individual procedures. Skin toning with the QS Nd:YAG laser targets deeper pigment, while IPL targets a wide range of superficial cutaneous structures.

In a study among 20 females with mixed-type melasma on both cheeks, laser toning with the QS Nd:YAG laser was done full face for five sessions at 1-week interval. One side of the face was randomly assigned to receive additional three sessions of IPL treatments at 2-week intervals. At 12 weeks after the last treatment, 18 patients completing the study showed both sides of the face with significant improvement in their mMASI score and melanin indices. A more rapid improvement of mMASI score and melanin indices, however, was observed on the combined side. At the end of treatment, 55 % improvement and 37 % improvement of melanin indices were observed on the combined side and monotherapy side, respectively. The overall patients' satisfaction was in favor of the combined side. Recurrence occurred on both sides but there was still a significant decrease compared to baseline. No serious side effect was noted. The authors concluded that combination of "skin toning" with QS Nd:YAG lasers and IPL results in faster clearance of melasma and is more effective than skin toning with QS Nd:YAG laser alone. However, recurrence is still inevitable [30].

16.2.9 Pulsed Dye and Copper Bromide Lasers

The vascular lasers were used to treat melasma with variable results. There are not enough good scientific reports to confirm the role of vascular laser and copper bromide lasers for the treatment of melasma at present.

The basis for the role of vasculature in melasma was reported by Kim et al. It was shown that melasma lesions have, in addition to increased pigmentation, more elastosis and vascularization than perilesional skin. Chromometer measurements were significantly higher in the melasma lesion than the nonlesional skin. Histology showed that factor VIIIa-related antigen staining showed a significant increase in the number and size of dermal blood vessels in the lesional skin. Added to the significant relationship between the number of vessels and pigmentation, expression of vascular endothelial growth factor (VEGF) was significantly increased in melasma skin [31, 32].

16.2.9.1 Pulsed Dye Laser (PDL)

Pulsed dye laser was reported to improve the topical treatment outcome of melasma and prolong remission period. Passeron et al. carried out a controlled, randomized, single-blind, split-face clinical trial evaluating the effectivity of dual treatment of fixed triple combination cream (TCC) and PDL in the treatment of melasma. Patient satisfaction was significantly greater for the combination treatment. Half of the patients with dark skin type IV developed PIH. PDL in association with a bleaching cream appears beneficial in treating melasma in patients with skin phototypes II and III [33].

Following the same study, Passeron reported that melasma lesion treated with PDL and triple cream showed long remission indicating enhanced effects of PDL on melasma lesions [34].

16.2.9.2 Copper Bromide Laser

The copper bromide laser (Dual Yellow; Norseld) is a laser with a concomitant-output dual-wavelength light source comprising 90 % yellow light at 578 nm targeting vascular lesions and 10 % green light at 511 nm which targets pigmentary lesions. These two light wavelengths can be emitted separately or simultaneously. Recent studies have suggested the potential effectiveness of targeting the vascular component of melasma [33, 34, 35, 37].

In a recent pilot study, ten Korean women with mixed or epidermal melasma were treated with a copper bromide laser emitting both wavelengths simultaneously at 2-week intervals for a total of 8 weeks. MASI scores decreased modestly from an average of 12.3 pretreatment to 9.5 at 1-month posttreatment follow-up. Using a chromometer, the authors noted measurable lightening of lesional skin after treatment, but the effects appeared to wane slightly at 1-month posttreatment follow-up. The same findings were seen when erythema was measured. Clinically, three patients were noted to have recurrence at the 6-month posttreatment follow-up. The histologic examination of lesional skin before and 3 months after treatment showed decreased levels of basal layer melanin (Melan-A) and fewer melanosomes in the epidermis after treatment, suggesting some longer-term benefit. In addition, CD34 staining for blood vessels showed a decrease in the number and size of dermal vessels after treatment. Staining for endothelin 1 and VEGF antigen showed decreased numbers in keratinocytes posttreatment, indicating some effect of the laser on vascularity within treated lesions. It is significant to note that none of the ten patients exhibited scarring or dyspigmentation from treatment. The authors concluded that the copper bromide lasers seem relatively safe and at least moderately effective for melasma in Asian patients (level of evidence, II-iii). Additional studies in other patient populations will help determine the generalizability of these results [35].

A study done in Thailand, however, did not corroborate these positive results. Among 20 melasma patients treated with the copper bromide laser, the mean melanin index (MI) showed no statistically significant improvement compared with baseline measurements at any of the follow-up visits. Though there were significant improvements in clinical evaluation after three treatments ($p=0.00$), this difference was no longer visible after six treatments. There was no improvement as measured by clinical evaluation or MI. The authors concluded that copper bromide laser does not improve melasma in patients with skin phototypes III–V [36].

Ghorbel et al. from France conducted a randomized split-face study comparing copper bromide lasers with the triple cream (a combination of hydroquinone, 5 %;

dexamethasone acetate, 0.1 %; and retinoic acid, 0.1 %). All patients applied the topical cream to their entire face once a day for 4 weeks. A hemiface was then randomly assigned to be treated with the copper bromide laser, while the other side of the face continued to receive daily application of the topical cream for 3 additional months. Four sessions of copper bromide laser were given at weeks 4, 6, 9, and 12. The yellow and green wavelengths were simultaneously produced at a ratio of 9:1. The treatments' effectiveness was assessed using the MASI score for each hemiface. Follow-up visits were conducted at 3 and 6 months. The main evaluation criterion was the patient's MASI score 6 months after the end of treatment. At the end of treatment, the topical cream resulted in a greater decrease in the MASI score compared with the laser treatment ($p = .006$). The MASI score at 6 months was comparable with the score at the beginning of the study in both groups; no significant difference was observed between the two groups. No difference could be found when results were analyzed according to the localization and duration of the melasma ($p > .99$ and $p = .87$, respectively). An increased vascularization was noted on the melasma lesions at baseline compared with perilesional skin. However, no decrease in vascularization was observed on the laser-treated side between the baseline and posttreatment visits. At the final visit, no changes in vascularization were noted between the two sides. Neither scarring nor PIH was noted. The authors concluded that results showed that Kligman's formula combination cream is more effective than the copper bromide laser for treating melasma [37].

It would appear that there is little role for the copper bromide laser in the treatment of melasma since the latter two reports appear to indicate lack of superiority over topical treatment. The role of other vascular lasers remains to be ascertained.

16.3 Level of Evidence for Using Lasers and Light Procedures for Treating Melasma Using the GRADE Working Group Recommendation [38–40]

Levels of evidence for aesthetic procedures

Level of evidence	Quality of evidence and definitions
A: High	Further research is very unlikely to change our confidence in the estimate of effect Several high quality studies with consistent results
B: Moderate	Further research is likely to have an important impact on our confidence in the estimate of effect and may change the estimate One high quality study or several studies with limitations
C: Low	Further research is very likely to have an important impact on our confidence in the estimate of effect and is likely to change the estimate One or more studies with limitations
D: Very low	Any estimate of effect is very uncertain Expert opinion with No direct research experience One or more studies with very severe limitations

GRADE Working Group [38], Guyatt et al. [39]

Reference	Procedures	Quality of evidence (A–D)
[5–7]	Full ablative lasering	D (very low)
[11, 13, 14]	Fractional lasers	B (moderate)
[2–4]	QS Nd:YAG laser	C (low)
[18–22, 28]	QS Nd:YAG laser toning	A (high)
[26, 27, 29]	Intense pulsed light	C (low)
[33, 34]	Pulsed dye laser	C (low)
[37, 38]	Copper bromide laser	C (low)

16.4 Conclusion

Topical treatment together with sun avoidance and protection remains to be the first-line treatment for melasma. Lasers and light devices are reserved as second- or third-line treatments, as they are not curative, do not clear melasma completely, and may be associated with post-inflammatory hyperpigmentation and relapses. They do have a role to play in recalcitrant melasma unresponsive to topical treatment, providing a respite and improvement of quality of life.

IPL appears to be the safest among the laser/light devices. However, it modestly offers only mild to moderate improvement, requires multiple sessions, and necessitates the need of maintenance treatment. Laser toning is the other alternative, but complications including rebound pigmentation and guttate hypomelanosis are serious impediments to watch out for. The QS pigment lasers using standard protocols, fractional lasers, and copper bromide lasers do not appear to be useful for melasma. The role of pulsed dye lasers remains unclear. More studies are needed to ascertain their effectiveness for melasma.

Given their cost and the need for multiple treatments, laser and light therapies should be considered third-line treatments in severe refractory melasma patients who have not responded to topical preparations or chemical peels and who are willing to accept the risks of these procedures.

References

1. Na JI, Choi SY, Yang SH, Choi HR, Kang HY, Park KC. Effect of tranexamic acid on melasma: a clinical trial with histological evaluation. J Eur Acad Dermatol Venereol. 2013;27(8):1035–9.
2. Tse Y, Levine VJ, McClain SA, Ashinoff R. The removal of cutaneous pigmented lesions with the Q-switched ruby laser and the Q-switched neodymium: yttrium-aluminum-garnet laser. A comparative study. J Dermatol Surg Oncol. 1994;20:795–800.
3. Alster TS, Lupton JR. Laser therapy for cutaneous hyperpigmentation and pigmented lesions. Dermatol Ther. 2001;14:46–54.
4. Taylor CR, Anderson RR. Ineffective treatment of refractory melasma and post-inflammatory hyperpigmentation by QS ruby laser. J Dermatol Surg Oncol. 1994;20(9):592–7.
5. Manaloto RMP, Alster T. Erbium: YAG laser resurfacing for refractory melasma. Dermatol Surg. 1999;25:121–3.

6. Nouri K, Bowes L, Chartier T, Romagosa R, Spencer JM. Combination treatment of melasma with pulsed CO2 laser followed by Q-switched Alexandrite laser: a pilot study. Dermatol Surg. 1999;25:494–7.
7. Angsurarangsee S, Polnikorn N. Combined ultrapulse CO2 laser and Q-switched alexandrite laser compared with Q-switched alexandrite laser alone for refractory melasma: Split face design. Dermatol Surg. 2003;29:59–64.
8. Manstein D, Herron GS, Sink RK, Tanner H, Anderson RR. Fractional photothermolysis: a new concept for cutaneous remodeling using microscopic patterns of thermal injury. Lasers Surg Med. 2004;34(5):426–38.
9. Rahman Z, Alam M, Dover JS. Fractional laser treatment for pigmentation and texture improvement. Skin Therapy Lett. 2006;11:7–11.
10. Laubach HJ, Tannous Z, Anderson RR, Manstein D. Skin responses to fractional photothermolysis. Lasers Surg Med. 2006;38(2):142–9.
11. Rokhsar CK, Fitzpatrick RE. The treatment of melasma with fractional photothermolysis: a pilot study. Dermatol Surg. 2005;31:1645–50.
12. Ong MW, Bashir SJ. Fractional laser resurfacing for acne scars: ablative vs non-ablative. Br J Dermatol. 2012;166:1160–9.
13. Goldberg DJ, Berlin AL, Phelps R. Histologic and ultrastructural analysis of melasma after fractional resurfacing. Lasers Surg Med. 2008;40:134–8.
14. Lee HS, Won CH, Lee DH, An JS, Chang HW, Lee JH, et al. Treatment of melasma in Asian skin using a fractional 1,550-nm laser: an open clinical study. Dermatol Surg. 2009;35(10): 1499–504.
15. Wind BS, Kroon MW, Meesters AA, Beek JF, van der Veen JP, Nieuweboer-Krobotová L, et al. Non-ablative 1,550 nm fractional laser therapy versus triple topical therapy for the treatment of melasma: a randomized controlled split-face study. Lasers Surg Med. 2010;42(7): 607–12.
16. Kroon MW, Wind BS, Beek JF, van der Veen JP, Nieuweboer-Krobotová L, Bos JD, Wolkerstorfer A. Nonablative 1550-nm fractional laser therapy versus triple topical therapy for the treatment of melasma: a randomized controlled pilot study. J Am Acad Dermatol. 2011;64(3):516–23.
17. Jang YH, Park JY, Park YJ, Kang HY. Changes in melanin and melanocytes in mottled hypopigmentation after low-fluence 1,064-nm Q-switched Nd:YAG laser treatment for melasma. Ann Derm. 2015;27(3):341.
18. Polnikorn N. Rx of refractory dermal melasma with QS Nd:YAG laser: 2 case reports. J Cosmet Laser Ther. 2008;10:167–73.
19. Cho SB, Kim JS, Kim MJ. Melasma treatment in Korean women using a 1064-nm Q-switched Nd:YAG laser with low pulse energy. Clin Exp Dermatol. 2009;34:e847–50.
20. Jeong SY, Shin JB, Yeo UC, Kim WS, Kim IH. Low-fluence QS Nd:YAG laser for melasma with pre- or post-treatment triple combination cream. Dermatol Surg. 2010;6:909–18.
21. Choi M, Choi JW, Lee SY, Choi SY, Park HJ, Park KC, et al. Low-dose 1064-nm Q-switched Nd:YAG laser for the Rx of melasma. Dermatol Treat. 2010;21:224–8.
22. Wattanakrai P, Mornchan R, Eimpunth S. Low-fluence Q-switched Nd:YAG (1,064 nm) Laser for the treatment of facial melasma in Asians. Dermatol Surg. 2010;36(1):76–87.
23. Shek SY, Yeung CK, Chan HH. A case series of facial depigmentation associated with low fluence Q-switched 1,064 nm Nd:YAG laser for skin rejuvenation and melasma. Lasers Surg Med. 2010;42(8):712–9.
24. Kou S, Yasumura K, Satake T, Maegawa J. Influence of the frequency of laser toning for melasma on occurrence of leukoderma and its early detection by ultraviolet imaging. Lasers Surg Med. 2015;47(2):161–7.
25. Jang YH, Park JY, Park YJ, Kang HY. Changes in melanin and melanocytes in mottled hypopigmentation after low-fluence 1,064-nm Q-switched Nd:YAG laser treatment for melasma. Ann Derm. 2015;27(3):340–2.

26. Wang CC, Hui CY, Sue YM, Wong WR, Hong HS. Intense pulsed light for the treatment of refractory melasma in Asian persons. Dermatol Surg. 2004;30:1196–200.
27. Li YH, Chen ZS, Wei HS, Wu Y, Liu M, Xu YY, et al. Efficiency of and safety of Intense pulsed light in treatment of melasma in Chinese patients. Dermatol Surg. 2008;34:1–9.
28. Bae MI, Park JM, Jeong KH, Lee MH, Shin MK. Effectiveness of low-fluence and short-pulse intense pulsed light in the treatment of melasma: a randomized study. J Cosmet Laser Ther. 2015;17(6):292–5.
29. Jun WJ, Lee SM, Han JS, Lee SH, Chang SY, Haw S, et al. A prospective, split-face, randomized study of the efficacy and safety of a novel fractionated intense pulsed light treatment for melasma in Asians. J Cosmet Laser Ther. 2015;17(5):259–66.
30. Vachiramon V, Sirithanabadeekul P, Sahawatwong S. Low-fluence Q-switched Nd:YAG 1064-nm laser and intense pulsed light for the treatment of melasma. J Eur Acad Dermatol Venereol. 2015;29(7):1339–46.
31. Kim EH, Kim YC, Lee ES, Kang HY. The vascular characteristics of melasma. J Derm Sci. 2007;46:111–6.
32. Passeron T. Melasma pathogenesis and influencing factors: an overview of the latest research. J Eur Acad Dermatol Venereol. 2013;27(S1):5–6.
33. Passeron T, Fontas E, Kang HY, Bahadoran P, Lacour JP, Ortonne JP. Melasma treatment with pulsed-dye laser and triple combination cream: a prospective, randomized, single-blind, split-face study. Arch Dermatol. 2011;147(9):1106–8.
34. Passeron T. Long-lasting effect of vascular targeted therapy of melasma. J Am Acad Dermatol. 2013;69(3):e141–2.
35. Lee HI, Lim YY, Kim BJ, Kim MN, Min HJ, Hwang JH, Song KY. Clinicopathologic efficacy of copper bromide plus/yellow laser (578 nm with 511) for treatment of melasma in Asian patients. Dermatol Surg. 2010;36:885–93.
36. Eimpunth S, Wanitphadeedecha R, Triwongwaranat D, Varothai S, Manuskiatti W. Therapeutic outcome of melasma treatment by dual-wavelength (511 and 578 nm) laser in patients with skin phototypes III-V. Clin Exp Dermatol. 2014;39(3):292–7.
37. Ghorbel HH, Boukari F, Fontas E, Montaudié H, Bahadoran P, Lacour JP, Passeron T. Copper bromide laser vs triple-combination cream for the treatment of melasma: a randomized clinical trial. JAMA Dermatol. 2015;151(7):791–2.
38. GRADE Working Group. Grading quality of evidence and strength of recommendations. BMJ. 2004;328:1490.
39. Guyatt GH, Oxman AD, Vist GE, Kunz R, Falck-Ytter Y, Alonso-Coello P, Schünemann HJ, Grade Working Group. GRADE: an emerging consensus on rating quality of evidence and strength of recommendations. BMJ. 2008;336:924–6.
40. GRADE Working Group. Rating quality of evidence and strength of recommendations: What is "quality of evidence" and why is it important to clinicians? BMJ. 2008;336(7651):995–8.

Chapter 17
Iontophoresis and Mesotherapy in Melasma

Maria Suzanne L. Datuin

17.1 Introduction

Melasma is a chronic, acquired pigmentary disorder that affects individuals worldwide. The mainstays for the treatment of melasma are topical depigmenting agents such as hydroquinone, kojic acid, arbutin, and azelaic acid. Procedural treatments are usually considered as second line options and include chemical peels, intense pulsed light, and various lasers among others, which have yielded mixed success rates [1]. Therefore, there is a continuous search for treatments that are safe, effective, accessible, cost-effective, and capable of providing long-term clearance of the pigment. This chapter discusses the available evidence of two other procedural treatments that have been used for melasma: iontophoresis and mesotherapy.

17.2 Iontophoresis

Iontophoresis is the facilitated movement of both ionic and nonionic molecules across a membrane through the application of an electric potential that enhances the delivery of these molecules. It is based on the principle that like charges repel, while unlike charges attract each other [2]. Iontophoresis applied to the skin is known as transdermal iontophoresis [3].

Under normal conditions, the lipophilic nature of the skin limits the permeation of high molecular weight, hydrophilic, and charged compounds [2]. The main barrier for transdermal delivery of these molecules is the stratum corneum, which is around 10–100 μm thick [3]. Iontophoresis can enhance the absorption of these

M.S.L. Datuin
St. Luke's Medical Center-Global City, Department of Dermatology, Taguig, Philippines
e-mail: suzanne_datuin@yahoo.com

E.B. Handog, M.J. Enriquez-Macarayo (eds.), *Melasma and Vitiligo in Brown Skin*,
DOI 10.1007/978-81-322-3664-1_17

molecules without injuring the skin and occurs by any of three main pathways, namely, intracellular, intercellular, or the appendageal pathways [3, 4].

The advantages of iontophoresis include the noninvasive delivery of ionized and unionized drugs, improvement in the delivery of polar molecules and high-molecular-weight compounds, and controlled and easy termination of drug delivery, all with restoration of the skin barrier without producing severe skin irritation [2]. The treatment time is between 10 and 30 min, as most of the ions pass through the skin at about 8–15 min, and very little passage occurs after 30 min [4].

Historically, iontophoresis has been used in the treatment of several dermatologic indications such as warts, softening of scar tissue, and wound care [2, 5]. Other applications include local delivery of anesthetics (i.e., lidocaine), steroids, retinoids, as well as the temporary relief of acral hyperhidrosis [3, 5].

17.2.1 Vitamin C

Among the studies on iontophoresis for melasma, Vitamin C has been the most utilized molecule. The role of vitamin C in melasma lies in its antioxidant properties, reducing the formation of *o*-quinone and reducing oxidized melanin [6, 7]. Vitamin C (as L-ascorbic acid) is a negatively charged ion in solution and may be transported transdermally for the treatment of melasma [5]. However, it is quickly oxidized and decomposes in an aqueous solution. For this reason, more stable forms of vitamin C have been used which includes magnesium-L-ascorbyl-2-phosphate (MAP) and ascorbyl glucoside [5, 6].

One of the earlier clinical trials on vitamin C iontophoresis for melasma was done in Korea involving 15 patients. Vitamin C was applied under a constant direct current of 0.4–0.8 A for 15 min, and the treatment was performed twice weekly for 6 weeks. Outcome measures were the Melasma Area and Severity Index (MASI) score and light reflectance as measured by a colorimeter, taken at baseline and at the end of the study. Results showed a decrease in the MASI score and light reflectance and significant clinical improvement of the melasma [8].

Subsequent to this trial, a randomized, double-blind, placebo-controlled trial using vitamin C was conducted also in Korea among 29 females with melasma. Vitamin C, as MAP 3.75 % solution, was applied to half of the face, while distilled water was applied to the other half as the control. A direct current of 0.5 mA was used, and the treatment was done for 8 min with the patients treated twice a week for 12 weeks. The objective outcome measures were the MASI score and the change in the luminance value (*L* value), as measured by a colorimeter, and patient self-assessment using a 5-point scale. At the end of the study, clinical photography showed improvement only on the side treated with vitamin C. The *L* values also decreased on the treated side ($p=0.002$), which were not observed on the side of the control ($p=0.142$). However, patients reported an improvement on both sides, which could be attributed to the placebo effect. Side effects were mild and transient and included mild burning sensation and mild sense of electric shock, pruritus, erythema, and dryness of the skin. The authors concluded that vitamin C iontophoresis is a useful modality in treating melasma [6].

17.2.2 Vitamin C Versus Glycolic Acid

Comparative studies have also been done, specifically with glycolic acid peel. An early study evaluated the efficacy of vitamin C iontophoresis and 30 % glycolic acid peel. Thirty-four patients were enrolled in the study. The first group received vitamin C only, the second group received only the peel, and last group received both treatments. Iontophoresis was done weekly for 12 weeks, under a direct current of 0.3 mA/cm^2 for 6 min. The glycolic acid peel, on the other hand, had a contact time of only 2 min. Outcome measures were the modified MASI (mMASI) score and melanin indices measured by a Mexameter. At the end of the study, all groups had lower mMASI scores and Mexameter readings ($p < 0.05$) [9].

More recently, a single-blinded study was done that compared topical nanosome vitamin C to 70 % glycolic acid peel. Fourteen patients with skin types IV and V were enrolled, with each patient receiving the glycolic acid peel on the right side of the face, while 0.5 ml solution containing 10 % ascorbic acid liposome was applied on the left side using iontophoresis at 50 mA for 10 min. Each patient received a total of six treatments. Photographs, MASI scores, and global evaluation were taken at baseline and at the end of the study.

Results showed a statistically significant improvement of both sides, but the side treated with the vitamin C had a greater improvement, with a 43 % decrease in the MASI score (versus 22 % for right side) at end point. Global assessment by the patient, attending physician, and two blinded physicians likewise revealed greater improvement on the vitamin C treated side. The authors concluded that nanosome vitamin C delivered via iontophoresis was safe and effective in the treatment of melasma and was superior to the glycolic acid peel [10].

17.2.3 Vitamin C Versus Multivitamin Mixture

Another Korean study enrolled 20 women in a randomized, split-face, double-blind trial that compared vitamin C to a multivitamin mixture composed of vitamins A, D, E, B1, B2, B5, B6, C, and nicotinamide. Vitamin C alone was applied on one side of the face, while the multivitamin was applied on the other side. Iontophoresis was performed for 6 min, and a sunscreen was applied after. All patients received treatments twice a week for 12 weeks. The outcome measures were the *L* value and the patient self-assessment at baseline, 6 weeks and 12 weeks.

As early as 6 weeks, patients already reported lightening of both sides of the face which was sustained until 12 weeks. At the end of the study, both sides had decreased *L* values and were equally effective in lightening the hyperpigmented patches. There was no statistically significant difference between the two ($p > 0.05$). Side effects for both treatments were burning sensation, erythema, and pruritus with fewer events recorded in the multivitamin treated side [7].

17.2.4 Iontophoresis Home Device

The latest study on vitamin C iontophoresis for melasma involves a novel home device called the full-face iontophoresis mask (FFIM). The FFIM mask was made of biocompatible gels with an adhesive back surface for direct contact with the whole face. The device was connected to 6-V power source with an output of 1.8 μA per cm^2. From a larger study that originally involved 101 patients with both postinflammatory hyperpigmentation (PIH) and melasma, outcomes of 35 patients with melasma who received the FFIM with vitamin C (as ascorbyl glucoside 20 %) and an alpha hydroxy acid-based skin care regimen were reported. A sunscreen was also incorporated into the program. Majority of the patients had skin types III, IV, and V.

After one in-office treatment, the FFIM together with the ascorbyl glucoside preparation was applied by the patients at home. The mask was left on for 1 h, three times a week for 1–2 months, in conjunction with the previously mentioned skin care regimen. Patients were followed up from 1 up to 54 months, with a mean follow-up length of 26 months. The mean improvement in the pigmentation was 73 %, with more than 50 % improvement in 22 out 35 of patients. The authors concluded that the use of the FFIM was able to sufficiently increase the levels of vitamin C to therapeutic levels, which led to favorable clinical outcomes, and the addition of the skin care regimen led to long-term sustained results [5].

17.2.5 Glutathione

Glutathione (GSH) is the most abundant low-molecular-weight thiol in mammalian cells. It is composed of the amino acids L-cysteine, glutamate, and glycine and is involved in many important biological processes such as protection of cells through the metabolism of xenobiotics and carcinogens. Glutathione, at high concentrations, can influence melanogenesis by several proposed mechanisms. These include a shift toward the production of the lighter pigment, pheomelanin over eumelanin; the direct and indirect effects of glutathione on the enzyme tyrosinase; and the quenching of free radicals and reactive oxygen species which increase tyrosinase activity [11].

GSH iontophoresis has been used by the author in an open-label pilot study where 10 Filipino patients with malar melasma, all with skin type IV, received eight weekly treatments. GSH 12 % solution (600 mg/5 ml) 1 ml was applied on the hyperpigmented patches under a direct current. Since GSH is a negatively charged molecule, the cathode was the active electrode used. Iontophoresis was done for 8 min on each side of the face, while the forehead was used as the control. Patients were instructed to use a sunscreen daily and to avoid direct sun exposure.

Clinical photography and mMASI scoring were done at baseline and 1 week after the last treatment session. Melanin indices (Mexameter readings) of both cheeks and the control were taken at baseline, after the fourth treatment and 1 week after the last treatment. A patient global assessment using a 5-point scale was done after the eighth treatment. At the end of the study period, there was a significant decrease in the

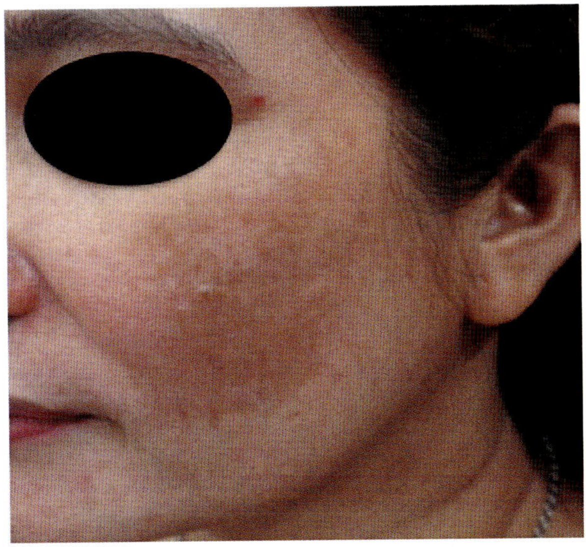

Fig. 17.1 Before treatment

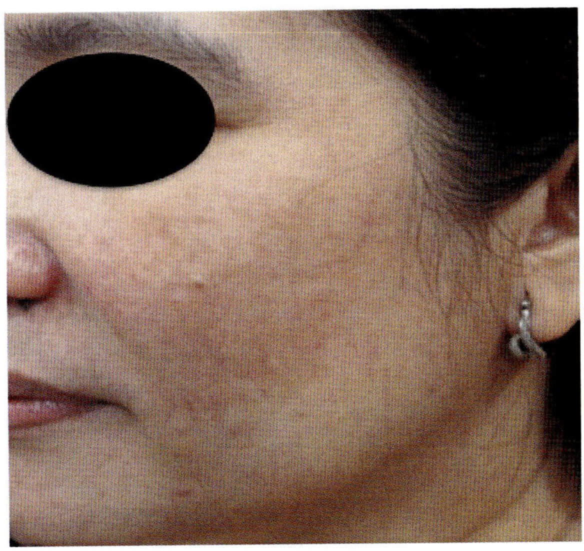

Fig. 17.2 After treatment

mMASI scores ($p=0.0015$), which was evident on clinical photography. There was likewise a decrease in the melanin indices of both cheeks ($p=0.0108$), which was not observed with the control ($p=0.5619$). Six patients graded themselves as having slight to moderate improvement while four graded themselves as having marked to excellent improvement (Figs. 17.1, 17.2, 17.3, and 17.4). Side effects were transient erythema on the treated areas and a sensation of mild electric shock. In conclusion, glutathione solution, when delivered topically via iontophoresis, was considered safe and effective as an adjunctive treatment for melasma.

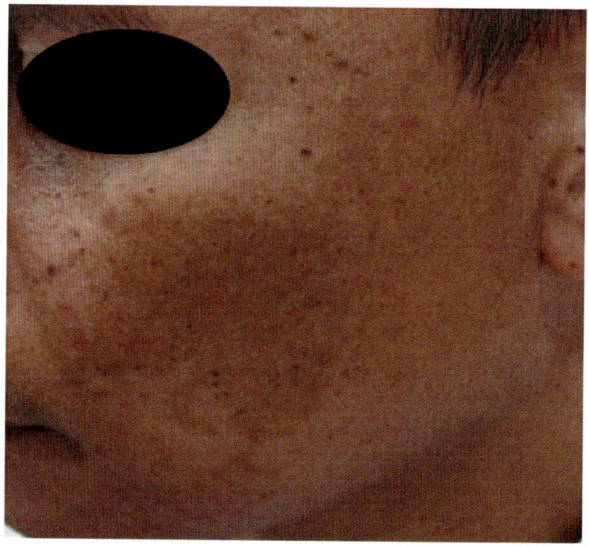

Fig. 17.3 Before treatment

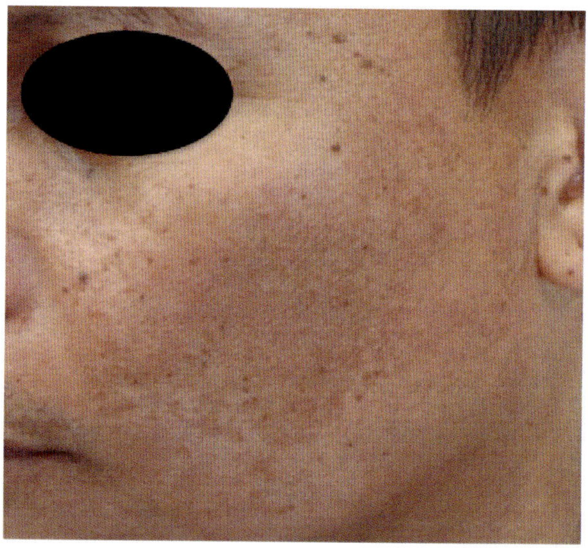

Fig. 17.4 After treatment

17.3 Mesotherapy

Mesotherapy is a technique where drugs or substances are introduced into the dermis or subcutaneous tissue through localized microinjections. All intravenously injectable compounds may be used except for alcoholic and oily solvents [12]. There were two studies found on the use of mesotherapy for melasma, both using tranexamic acid.

17.3.1 Tranexamic Acid

Tranexamic acid (TA), a plasmin inhibitor, is a synthetic analog of the amino acid lysine [12]. TA reversibly blocks lysine-binding sites on plasminogen molecules and prevents plasminogen activator from converting plasminogen to plasmin [13, 14]. Plasmin is a protease that enhances the release of intracellular arachidonic acid and also increases levels of alpha-melanocyte-stimulating hormone (α-MSH). These two molecules are known to increase melanocyte synthesis of melanin [15].

TA inhibits UV-induced plasmin activity by preventing the binding of plasminogen to keratinocytes, which results in a decrease in free arachidonic acid and therefore a decrease in prostaglandins that are known to increase melanocyte tyrosinase activity [12, 15, 16]. Prostaglandins D_2, E_2, and F_2 have been reported to increase melanogenesis [12].

Mesotherapy using TA for melasma among Asians was first done in Korea. Eighty-five females with Fitzpatrick skin types IV to V completed an open-label pilot study, which involved weekly intradermal injections of 0.5 ml of TA (4 mg/ml) directly into the hyperpigmented lesions. Injections were spaced 1 cm apart after topical anesthesia was applied. The study ran for 12 weeks with clinical evaluation and MASI scoring done every 4 weeks. Subjective assessment was done using a patient satisfaction questionnaire at the end of week 12. Results showed a significant decrease in the MASI scores from baseline to 8 and 12 weeks ($p<0.05$ for both). The authors observed that from week 8, there was a decrease in the darkness of the lesions followed by a decrease in the area of the hyperpigmented patches. However, only 8/85 patients (9.4 %) graded their improvement as good (51–75 % lightening), while majority of the patients (65/85, 76.5 %) graded their improvement as fair (26–50 % lightening). None graded their improvement as excellent (>75 % lightening), and 12/85 (14.1 %) graded themselves as poor (<25 % improvement). No significant side effects were noted [12].

A more recent study compared two methods of delivering TA on patients with melasma: through mesotherapy (microinjections) and microneedling. Microneedling is a minimally invasive procedure that involves passing a handheld device studded with numerous microneedles (frequently called a dermaroller) on the skin in order to create hundreds of microchannels where specific molecules or medications can be delivered transdermally. Normally, several passes are done on any given area, and the target medication/product is applied directly on the skin while these microchannels are still open. This facilitates entry into the skin of substances that would normally take longer or be more difficult to be absorbed topically such as proteins that would not otherwise pass through intact skin [15]. Microneedling has other dermatologic applications, most notably for skin rejuvenation and in the treatment of acne scars.

In this randomized open-label trial of 60 patients with Fitzpatrick skin types IV and V, half of the group (arm 1) received microinjections of TA (4 mg/ml) using a 4 mm meso needle into lesional skin. The other half (arm 2) underwent microneedling using a roller studded with fine needles 1.5 mm in length and 0.25 mm in diameter. After the skin was sufficiently wounded using the microneedles after four to five passes, the TA solution was directly applied on the skin, and the procedure was repeated for another four to five times. Treatments were done thrice at monthly intervals, and patients were followed up for another 3 months. Outcome measures included the mMASI score, physician and patient global assessments, and clinical photography. Both methods of delivering TA into the skin showed significant decreases in the mean mMASI scores from baseline to the end of the follow-up period. The arm treated with microneedling had more improvement but the difference between the two groups was not statistically significant. The authors attributed this finding to the ability of the microneedling device in achieving deeper and more even delivery of the medication [16].

17.4 Conclusion

These aforementioned studies show that vitamin C iontophoresis is safe and effective for the short- and long-term treatment of melasma. Though different forms of vitamin C were used, all yielded positive outcomes. Glutathione iontophoresis is also a safe and effective procedure, which can be added to any regimen for melasma. It is simple and takes only a few minutes to perform and is virtually painless without any downtime. Side effects were mild and transient, and the procedure was well tolerated.

Mesotherapy using tranexamic acid also appears to be safe and promising as an adjunctive treatment for melasma. Based on the above studies, intralesional TA is able to produce relatively fast results without significant side effects. Since small amounts of the drug are directly injected into the dermis, there is very little chance of systemic absorption and therefore systemic side effects.

Both procedures are able to facilitate transdermal delivery of molecules that would otherwise be difficult to transport through the skin at optimum concentrations that result in good clinical improvement. The sample sizes of these studies were small, however, and perhaps larger clinical trials maybe done.

References

1. Sarkar R, Chugh S, Garg VK. Newer and upcoming therapies for melasma. Indian J Dermatol Venereol Leprol. 2012;78(4):417–28.
2. Khan A, Yasir M, Asif M, Chauhan I, Singh A, Sharma R, et al. Iontophoretic drug delivery: history and applications. J App Pharm Sci. 2011;1(3):11–24.
3. Rawat S, Vengurlekar S, Rakesh B, Jain S, Srikarti G. Transdermal delivery by iontophoresis. Indian J Pharm Sci. 2008;70(1):5–10.
4. Rukari TG, Alhat BR. Iontophoresis: an electrically assisted drug delivery system. J Adv Drug Deliv. 2014;1(1):58–70.
5. Taylor MB, Yanaki JS, Draper DO, Shurtz JC, Coglianese M. Successful short-term and long-term treatment of melasma and postinflammatory hyperpigmentation using vitamin C with a full-face iontophoresis mask and a mandelic/malic acid skin care regimen. J Drugs Dermatol. 2013;12(1):45–50.

6. Huh CH, Seo KI, Park JY, Lim JG, Eun HC, Parl KC. A randomized, double-blind, placebo-controlled trial of vitamin C iontophoresis in melasma. Dermatol. 2003;206(4):316–20.
7. Choi YK, Rho YK, Yoo KH, Lim YY, Li K, Kim BJ, et al. Effects of vitamin C vs. multivitamin on melanogenesis: comparative study in vitro and in vivo. Int J Dermatol. 2010;49(2): 218–26.
8. Yoo JM, Park HJ, Choi SW, Kim HO. Vitamin C – iontophoresis in melasma. Korean J Dermatol. 2001;39(3):285–91.
9. Kim S, Oh SY, Lee SH. Comparative study of glycolic acid peeling vs. Vitamin C-iontophoresis in melasma. Korean J Dermatol. 2001;39(12):1356–63.
10. Sobhi RM, Sobhi AM. A single-blinded comparative study between the use of glycolic acid 70% peel and the use of topical nanosome vitamin C iontophoresis in the treatment of melasma. J Cosmet Dermatol. 2012;11(1):65–71.
11. Handog EB, Datuin MS, Singzon IA. An open-label, single-arm trial of the safety and efficacy of a novel preparation of glutathione as a skin-lightening agent in Filipino women. Int J Dermatol. 2016;55(2):153–7.
12. Lee JH, Park JG, Lim SH, Kim JY, Ahn KY, Kim MY, et al. Localized intradermal microinjection of tranexamic acid for treatment of melasma in Asian patients: a preliminary clinical trial. Derm Surg. 2006;32:626–31.
13. Tse TW, Hui E. Tranexamic acid: an important adjuvant in the treatment of melasma. J Cosmet Dermatol. 2013;12(1):57–66.
14. Cho HH, Choi M, Cho S, Lee JH. Role of oral tranexamic acid in melasma patients treated with IPL and low fluence QS Nd:YAG laser. J Dermatolog Treat. 2013;24(4):292–6.
15. Malathi M, Thappa DM. Systemic skin whitening/lightening agents: what is the evidence? Indian J Dermatol Venereol Leprol. 2013;79(6):842–6.
16. Budamakuntla L, Loganathan E, Suresh DH, Shanmugam S, Suryanarayan S, Dongare A, et al. A randomised, open-label, comparative study of tranexamic acid microinjections and tranexamic acid with microneedling in patients with melasma. J Cutan Aesthet Surg. 2013;6(3):139–43.

Chapter 18
Quality of Life in Melasma

Andreas Katsambas and Efthymia Soura

18.1 Introduction

Melasma, being more common on the face (Fig. 18.1a), may also be infrequently seen on the neck and the forearms. Both sexes are affected, but the male population (Fig. 18.1b) may represent up to only 10% of cases [1]. This hyperpigmentation disorder is of varying severity and tends to exhibit seasonal changes. As is the case with most dermatological conditions that involve the face, melasma may be a cause of distress for many patients. Daily life can be influenced through alteration of self-perception, loss of confidence, and worsening of mood that may finally lead to decreased interaction with others and lowering of overall quality of life. In addition, melasma is a condition that requires constant treatment, which may be time consuming and expensive, with frequently moderate results and a high recurrence rate [2]. This may be a source of further aggravation for many patients.

The quality of life measures used for the evaluation of melasma impact on everyday life are summarized. In addition, the way that melasma may influence everyday life is also addressed.

18.2 Melasma and Quality of Life Measures

Quality of life (QoL) is considered to be a broad concept that encompasses subjective evaluations of both positive and negative aspects of life and conveys an overall sense of well-being. Health-related quality of life (HRQoL) is a more specific

A. Katsambas, MD (✉) • E. Soura
1st University Clinic of Dermatology and Venereology, Andreas Sygros Hospital, University of Athens, Athens, Greece
e-mail: katsabas1@ath.forthnet.gr

E.B. Handog, M.J. Enriquez-Macarayo (eds.), *Melasma and Vitiligo in Brown Skin*,
DOI 10.1007/978-81-322-3664-1_18

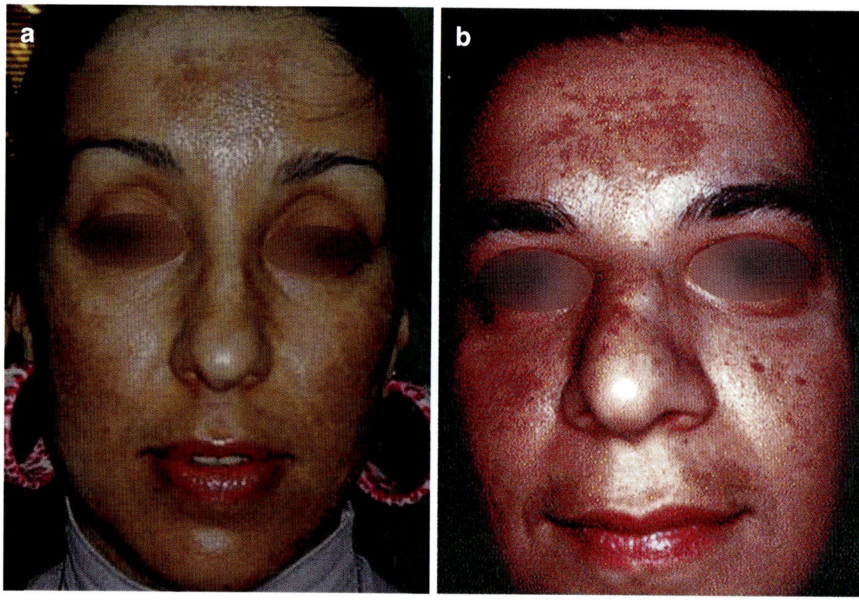

Fig. 18.1 Facial melasma in an adult (**a**) female patient (**b**) male patient

determinant of QoL, which includes those aspects of overall quality of life that can be clearly shown to affect health (physical or mental) [3].

Overall, the instruments used for determining QoL in melasma patients can be divided into two main categories: those that are non-disease-specific and those that are disease-specific.

18.2.1 Non-disease-specific QoL instruments

A number of QoL measures have been used in order to determine the impact of skin disease in patients. These include the Dermatology Life Quality Index (DLQI), the Dermatology Quality of Life Scales (DQoLS), the Family Dermatology Life Quality Index (FDLQI), and the Skindex-29, Skindex-17, and Skindex-16, among others [4]. Out of these, the two most commonly used instruments are the DLQI and the Skindex-16 questionnaires.

The DLQI questionnaire was developed by Finlay and Khan and is comprised of ten items that explore various aspects of an individual's everyday life. These include disease-associated restriction of daily activity, personal feelings, interpersonal relationships, leisure, and treatment efficacy evaluations [5].

The Skindex questionnaire was developed by Chren et al. and was initially comprised of 61 items that explored both the physical and psychosocial impact of dermatological conditions. The design of this instrument focused mainly on assessing the disability caused by the disease rather than the emotional well-being of the patients. In recent years, the Skindex instrument was condensed to a 30-item (Skindex-29) version and later to a 16-item (Skindex-16) version [6]. The newer versions explore many aspects more relevant to the dermatological disease (such as feelings of irritation, stinging, and itching) as well as feelings of embarrassment, frustration, and difficulty in socializing with others. In this way, disease symptoms and emotional and functional well-being can be assessed [7, 8].

18.2.2 Disease-Specific QoL instruments

The main disadvantage of DLQI and Skindex-16 in evaluating QoL in melasma is that these instruments give equal attention to the assessment of physical and psychosocial distress. Melasma, on the other hand, is a disorder that impacts the psychosocial well-being of patients far more than their physical well-being since it is asymptomatic. This diagnostic void is filled by the disease-specific QoL measure, Melasma Quality of Life (MELASQoL) scale.

The MELASQoL measure was initially introduced by Balkrishnan et al. and is comprised of ten items [9]. MELASQoL focuses mainly on questions relevant to melasma HRQoL and uses a combination of items from the Skindex-16 (seven items) and the skin discoloration questionnaire (three items). Each item is rated on a 7-point Likert scale with possible answers ranging from "not bothered at all" (score = 1) to "bothered all the time" (score = 7). Scores are summed up to produce a total score of 7–70, with higher scores corresponding to a lower quality of life. MELASQoL centers mainly on the evaluation of the patient's feelings on skin appearance, emotions of frustration or embarrassment, and the burden of melasma in interpersonal relationships [10]. MELASQoL is the most popular instrument used in the evaluation of QoL in melasma patients, as it has shown high discriminatory power, validity, and internal consistency and has been translated in a number of languages [9].

18.2.3 Overview of Disease Severity Instruments

An interesting characteristic of dermatological QoL measures is that they are highly subjective, and the results obtained depend heavily on the patient's perception of themselves. That said, QoL in dermatologic patients may not be directly correlated with the actual severity of their dermatological condition. For this reason, various instruments that can assess disease severity may be used concomitantly with QoL instruments. These measures are also rather subjective, as the assessment is performed by a dermatologist and not an "objective" instrument, such as a DermaSpectrometer [10]. Nevertheless, they are most commonly used in clinical practice and include the melasma severity scale, the Munsell color chart for melasma, the physician's global assessment, the patient's global assessment scales [11], and the Melasma Area and Severity Index (MASI) score, among others. The MASI score is the most popular disease severity assessment instrument for melasma. Developed by Kimbrough-Green et al., it was based on the Psoriasis Area and Severity Index calculation concept [12]. However, the complex relationship between patient psychological well-being and disease severity is further highlighted by the inability of MASI to capture the considerable emotional and psychological effects of melasma on patients. This is another reason why both types of instruments should be used in order to achieve a more complete approach to patients.

18.3 Melasma and Impact in Quality of Life

A number of studies have been performed in order to assess the impact of melasma in everyday life. In the study by Balkrishnan et al., 102 women were evaluated with the use of MASI, DLQI, Skindex-16, skin discoloration questionnaire, and MELASQoL instruments. It was shown that patients felt that their social life, recreation / leisure, and emotional well-being were severely affected by the condition (mean reported MELASQoL score: 36). Overall, there was a moderate correlation of MASI scores with the MELASQoL scores and a high correlation of MELASQoL scores with the DLQI, the Skindex-16, and the skin discoloration questionnaires [9]. Similar results were reported by Dominguez et al. in a study that included 99 women of Hispanic origin, recruited from an outpatient clinic in Texas. Social life, physical health, and emotional well-being were reported to be influenced by the presence of melasma. In addition, the financial cost of treating the disorder was also reported as a major concern (mean reported MELASQoL score: 42) [13].

In another study by Dogramaci et al., 114 Turkish women were evaluated with the use of MASI and MELASQoL instruments. It was reported that melasma was considered an important source of frustration, decreased patient freedom, and feeling of unattractiveness (mean reported MELASQoL score: 29.9) [14]. Similar results were reported in a recent study by Ikino et al. that included 51 patients from Brazil. The vast majority of patients (94.11 %) felt bothered about their skin appearance, while most expressed feelings of depression, frustration, and embarrassment. In addition, 78.43 % felt unattractive due to the presence of melasma. Interestingly, patients did not feel that melasma had a severe impact on their freedom, social life, or interaction with others (mean reported total MELASQoL score: 34.40) [15]. Almost identical results were reported by other studies that included Brazilian women [16–18]. Overall, young age, mild psychiatric disorders (i.e., anxiety) and lower educational levels of patients were associated with higher MELASQoL scores [19].

MELASQoL has also been used in the evaluation of melasma treatment efficacy. In a study by Cestari et al. that included 300 patients from Brazil, feelings of unattractiveness (43 %), frustration (55 %), embarrassment (57 %), and an influence of the disease on interpersonal relationships (42 %) were reported. However, after treatment with a triple combination cream (hydroquinone, fluocinolone acetonide, and tretinoin) for 8 weeks, the MELASQoL scores of the patients on the treatment arm had improved significantly. More specifically, 12.2 % of patients continued to experience frustration, 9.3 % continued to experience embarrassment, and 5.8 % reported an impact on interpersonal relationships, compared to 59.7 %, 56 %, and 35.3 % of the no treatment arm patients, respectively [20].

Similar results were reported by other studies were QoL instruments other than MELASQoL were used. For instance, in a study from Pakistan where DLQI scores were obtained from 100 patients, it was reported that the presence of melasma was associated with strong feelings of embarrassment and self-consciousness. However, this study differed from other studies in the fact that patients also reported a strong impact of melasma on social interactions with close friends, relatives, or partners and even in the choice of clothing [21].

Melasma-associated embarrassment was also reported as the main complaint in another study from Thailand. However, DLQI scores from patients with melasma were compared to those of patients suffering from other dermatoses, and it was found that melasma patients exhibited lower DLQI scores than psoriasis, acne, and vitiligo patients but higher than patients with viral warts, seborrheic keratosis, moles, and benign skin tumors.

Another aspect of melasma that was investigated was the "willingness to pay" intent. Interestingly, it was reported that patients were willing to spend more on melasma treatments than on clothes and footwear (7.2 % of their total monthly income). These results showcase the grave impact of melasma on QoL [22].

Overall, melasma is considered rare among males. As a result of this, only few males have been involved in studies assessing QoL. In a study by Pichardo et al., it was reported that DLQI scores were higher in a subset of the investigated patients. In general, male patients seem to be less concerned than female patients regarding the presence of melasma [23]. Regardless, inquiry on the impact of melasma on everyday life among male patients must be considered, especially since camouflage make-up is not a practical option for them.

18.4 Conclusion

Melasma is a condition with a noticeable impact on patient everyday life. Most studies have reported similar results with some minor variations. These variations reflect mainly the cultural and economic differences between countries. For instance, social expectations, average wedding age, educational level, and income can differ widely from country to country. However, all studies agree in that melasma influences emotional well-being greatly and that it is associated with feelings of embarrassment, frustration, and unattractiveness. This also shows the similarities between various cultures and further highlights the importance of taking the time to discuss with patients. Assessing the impact of melasma in QoL could lead to achieving better patient compliance, by assisting constructive communication between patients and physicians and by choosing appropriate treatments based on realistic expectations on efficacy and on willingness of patients to conform. In addition, QoL instruments can be used as tools for assessing and comparing treatment efficacies as well as monitoring patients after treatment completion.

References

1. Nicolaidou E, Katsambas AD. Pigmentation disorders: hyperpigmentation and hypopigmentation. Clin Dermatol. 2014;32(1):66–72.
2. Stratigos AJ, Katsambas AD. Optimal management of recalcitrant disorders of hyperpigmentation in dark-skinned patients. Am J Clin Dermatol. 2004;5(3):161–8.
3. McHorney CA. Health status assessment methods for adults: past accomplishments and future challenges. Annu Rev Public Health. 1999;20:309–35.
4. Augustin M, Langenbruch AK, Gutknecht M, Radtke MA, Blome C. Quality of life measures for dermatology: definition, evaluation, and interpretation. Curr Derm Rep. 2012;1(3): 148–59.
5. Finlay AY, Khan GK. Dermatology Life Quality Index (DLQI)—a simple practical measure for routine clinical use. Clin Exp Dermatol. 1994;19(3):210–6.
6. Chren MM, Lasek RJ, Quinn LM, Mostow EN, Zyzanski SJ. Skindex, a quality-of-life measure for patients with skin disease: reliability, validity, and responsiveness. J Invest Dermatol. 1996;107(5):707–13.
7. Chren MM, Lasek RJ, Flocke SA, Zyzanski SJ. Improved discriminative and evaluative capability of a refined version of Skindex, a quality-of-life instrument for patients with skin diseases. Arch Dermatol. 1997;133(11):1433–40.
8. Chren MM, Lasek RJ, Sahay AP, Sands LP. Measurement properties of Skindex-16: a brief quality-of-life measure for patients with skin diseases. J Cutan Med Surg. 2001;5(2): 105–10.
9. Balkrishnan R, McMichael AJ, Camacho FT, Saltzberg F, Housman TS, Grummer S, et al. Development and validation of a health-related quality of life instrument for women with melasma. Br J Dermatol. 2003;149(3):572–7.
10. Pandya A, Berneburg M, Ortonne JP, Picardo M. Guidelines for clinical trials in melasma. Pigmentation Disorders Academy. Br J Dermatol. 2006;156 Suppl 1:21–8.
11. Taylor SC, Torok H, Jones T, Lowe N, Rich P, Tschen E, et al. Efficacy and safety of a new triple-combination agent for the treatment of facial melasma. Cutis. 2003;72(1):67–72.
12. Kimbrough-Green CK, Griffiths CE, Finkel LJ, Hamilton TA, Bulengo-Ransby SM, Ellis CN, Voorhees JJ. Topical retinoic acid (tretinoin) for melasma in black patients. A vehicle-controlled clinical trial. Arch Dermatol. 1994;130(6):727–33.
13. Dominguez AR, Balkrishnan R, Ellzey AR, Pandya AG. Melasma in Latina patients: cross-cultural adaptation and validation of a quality-of-life questionnaire in Spanish language. J Am Acad Dermatol. 2006;55(1):59–66.
14. Dogramaci AC, Havlucu DY, Inandi T, Balkrishnan R. Validation of a melasma quality of life questionnaire for the Turkish language: the MelasQoL-TR study. J Dermatol Treat. 2009;20(2):95–9.
15. Ikino JK, Nunes DH, da Silva VPM, Frode TS, Sens MM. Melasma and assessment of the quality of life in Brazilian women. An Bras Dermatol. 2015;90(2):196–200.
16. Freitag FM, Cestari TF, Leopoldo LR, Paludo P, Boza JC. Effect of melasma on quality of life in a sample of women living in southern Brazil. J Eur Acad Dermatol Venereol. 2008; 22(6):655–62.
17. Tamega AA, Miot LDB, Bonfietti C, Gige TC, Marques MEA, Miot HA. Clinical patterns and epidemiological characteristics of facial melasma in Brazilian women. J Eur Acad Dermatol Venereol. 2013;27(2):151–6.

18. Purim KS, Avelar MF. [Photoprotection, melasma and quality of life in pregnant women]. Rev Bras Ginecol Obstet: Revista da Federacao Brasileira das Sociedades de Ginecologia e Obstetricia. 2012;34(5):228–34.
19. Handel AC, Miot LDB, Miot HA. Melasma: a clinical and epidemiological review. An Bras Dermatol. 2014;89(5):771–82.
20. Cestari TF, Hexsel D, Viegas ML, Azulay L, Hassun K, Almeida ART, et al. Validation of a melasma quality of life questionnaire for Brazilian Portuguese language: the MelasQoL-BP study and improvement of QoL of melasma patients after triple combination therapy. Br J Dermatol. 2006;156(S1):13–20.
21. Ali R, Aman S, Nadeem M. Quality of life in patients of melasma. J Pak Assoc Dermatol. 2013;23(2):143–8.
22. Leeyaphan C, Wanitphakdeedecha R, Manuskiatti W, Kulthanan K. Measuring melasma patients' quality of life using willingness to pay and time trade-off methods in Thai population. BMC Dermatol. 2011;11:16.
23. Pichardo R, Vallejos Q, Feldman SR, Schulz MR, Verma A, Quandt SA, Arcury TA. The prevalence of melasma and its association with quality of life in adult male Latino migrant workers. Int J Dermatol. 2009;48(1):22–6.

Part III
Vitiligo in Brown Skin

Chapter 19
Vitiligo: Definition, Incidence, Etiology

Vinod Kumar Sharma, Neetu Bhari, and Manoj Kumar Tembhre

19.1 Introduction

Depigmentation of the skin occurring without any preceding inflammation characterizes vitiligo. Affecting approximately only 1 % of the total population, the associated stigma and severe psychosocial distress have been noted in patients suffering from this pigmentary condition. Causation may still be unknown but an underlying autoimmune disorder is highly considered. Though, vitiligo is commonly referred to as leukoderma, injury or inflammation precedes the latter. This chapter discusses the definition, incidence, and current understanding of the etiology of vitiligo.

19.2 Definition

Vitiligo is an acquired disease of pigmentation, and a selective and often continuous loss of epidermal melanocytes characterizes vitiligo; mostly affecting the skin, there is occasional involvement of the mucosa and hairs. As early as 1700–1100 BC, cases of vitiligo have already been recorded. It was known in the Indian subcontinent then as "switra," from the Sanskrit word "sveta," which means "white patch." Switra has been mentioned in the ancient classical texts of Ayurveda and in the Persian history, where it was known in the 2200 BC [1].

V.K. Sharma (✉) • N. Bhari
Department of Dermatology and Venereology, All India Institute of Medical Sciences, New Delhi, India
e-mail: aiimsvks@yahoo.com; drntbhari@gmail.com

M.K. Tembhre
Feinstein Institute of Medical Research, NSLIJ, Manhasset, NY, USA
e-mail: manoj_kt143@yahoo.com

E.B. Handog, M.J. Enriquez-Macarayo (eds.), *Melasma and Vitiligo in Brown Skin*,
DOI 10.1007/978-81-322-3664-1_19

The lack of an international consensus regarding the definition and classification of vitiligo hampers international level research and communication. The Vitiligo European Task Force (VETF) has proposed consensus definitions for the disease, but a need for broader international consensus was felt [2]. Recently, the Vitiligo Global Issues Consensus Conference (VGICC) classification was proposed, including the work of seven regional working groups: North and South Africa, North and South/Central America, Europe, Middle East, Continental Asia/Singapore, Japan/Taiwan, and the Pacific [3] (discussed in the Chap. 21).

19.3 Incidence

Vitiligo is known to affect around 0.1–2 % of the population worldwide; in India, its prevalence is about 0.5–2.5 % (range: 0.46–8.8 %) [4–15]. The population frequency of vitiligo in Caucasians has been estimated as 0.38 % [3], and in the United States, the incidence was estimated at 1 % [5, 6]. The annual prevalence of vitiligo determined in Korea was 0.12–0.13 % over a 3-year period of a study by Lee et al. [7].

Usually, both sexes have shown equal predilection, but in some studies done in India and Korea, female preponderance has been reported [6, 7]. This may be because of the higher cosmetic and social concerns in female patients.

Onset of vitiligo occurs in childhood or young adulthood with a peak age at 10–30 years. Around 50 % of cases were reported to appear before 20 years of age and nearly 70–80 % before 30 years [8, 9]. In a study of 692 vitiligo patients from China, the mean age of onset was 23.69 ± 13.83 years [10]. Its onset is rare in old age or infancy. However, late-onset vitiligo was reported from Chandigarh, India, with a mean age of onset of 55 ± 2.3 years [11]. Similarly, childhood vitiligo (age < 12 years) constituted 23.4 % of vitiligo patients in another Indian study [12].

Regarding the type of vitiligo, generalized vitiligo was the most common pattern noted in studies from India and China, followed by focal and segmental patterns [10–12]. In contrast, acrofacial vitiligo was the most common pattern (44.5 %) in another study of 762 cases, highlighting lack of consensus in the classification of the disease [13].

19.4 Etiology

Vitiligo presents as a complex phenomenon that involves a play of multiple factors, many of which are not clearly delineated. In the past decades, extensive research has been devoted to vitiligo, and multiple hypotheses have been postulated to explain its occurrence [14]. Though the framework for vitiligo pathogenesis is available, further research is still essential to elucidate its exact mechanism.

19.4.1 Genetic

Over the past years, considerable development has been made to understand the role of genetics in vitiligo, with several susceptibility genes being identified (Table 19.1). Vitiligo seen in the families of patients is an indication that genetic factors play an important role in the occurrence of the disease. In this genetic hypothesis, vitiligo inheritance is considered as polygenic and multifactorial. Among multi-generation families, inheritance can occur in an autosomal dominant pattern with incomplete penetrance [15]. The relative risk of vitiligo for first-degree relatives has been shown to be increased by seven- to tenfold [16, 17]. Though, the likelihood of vitiligo in monozygotic twins was reported at 23 %, vitiligo concordance among them is unclear, indicating a potential influence of nongenetic environmental factors (e.g., epigenetics).

To understand the role of genetics in the pathogenesis of vitiligo, various scientific approaches are in use, such as (a) genetic linkage, (b) candidate gene association studies, (c) genome-wide association studies (GWAS), (d) DNA sequencing studies, and (e) gene expression studies.

19.4.1.1 Genetic Linkage Studies

The first vitiligo genetic linkage study performed on the major histocompatibility complex (MHC) reported the linkage of various genetic markers located on human leukocyte antigen (HLA) gene locus [18–20]. However, the linkage analysis in families with vitiligo-related systemic lupus erythematosus identified SLEV1 locus [21] and subsequently reported NLRP1 [22] located on chromosome 17, as one of the novel vitiligo susceptibility loci. The genome-wide linkage studies also revealed the various other susceptibility loci in different ethnic populations, e.g., chromosome 1, 7, 8, 9, 11, 13, 19, and 21 (Caucasians) [23, 24] and chromosome 4, 6, and 22 (Chinese) [20, 23–25]; some of these loci are also confirmed by GWAS.

19.4.1.2 Candidate Gene Association Studies

This approach has been first successfully used to identify the single nucleotide polymorphism (SNP) for CTLA-4 gene locus [26] in vitiligo; however, CTLA-4 locus has been associated with various other autoimmune diseases [27]. Recently, Birlea et al. [28] reported a comprehensive list of 33 vitiligo candidate genes (Table 19.1), but only three genes (TSLP, XBP1, FOXP3) were supported by GWAS studies [29].

19.4.1.3 Genome-Wide Association Studies (GWAS)

The first vitiligo GWAS was carried out in a specific population of Northwestern Romania with a high prevalence of vitiligo and other autoimmune diseases, and it found an association of vitiligo with SMOC2 gene located at distal chromosome

Table 19.1 List of genes and their loci associated with vitiligo susceptibility

Chromosome	Gene	Protein	Function	Casual variant	Other autoimmune disease associations
1p36.23	*REREa*	Atrophin-like protein 1	Regulates apoptosis		
1p13.2	*PTPN22*[a]	Lymphoid-specific protein tyrosine phosphatase nonreceptor type 22	Regulates T-cell receptor signaling	R620W	Type 1 diabetes, SLE, Graves' disease, rheumatoid arthritis, Addison's disease, psoriasis, inflammatory bowel disease
2q33.2	*CTLA4*[a]	Cytotoxic T-lymphocyte antigen 4	Inhibits T cells		Type 1 diabetes, Graves' disease, Hashimoto's thyroiditis, inflammatory bowel disease, SLE
3p13	*FOXP1*[a]	Forkhead box P1	Regulates lymphoid cell development		
3q28	*LPP*[a]	LIM domain-containing preferred translocation partner in lipoma	Unknown		Celiac disease, rheumatoid arthritis
5q22.1	*TSLP*[a]	Thymic stromal lymphopoietin	Regulates T-cell and dendritic cell maturation		
6q21.3	MHC[a] class I (*HLA-A*) MHC class IIb MHC class III	Human leukocyte antigen α chain Unknown Unknown	Presents peptide antigens	02:01[a]	Many Many Many
6q27	*CCR6*[a]	C-C chemokine receptor type 6	Regulates B-cell differentiation, function of dendritic and Th17 cells		Inflammatory bowel disease, rheumatoid arthritis, Graves' disease

10p15.1	*IL2RA*[a]	Interleukin-2 receptor α chain	Regulates lymphocyte response to bacteria via IL2		Type 1 diabetes, Graves' disease, multiple sclerosis, rheumatoid arthritis, SLE
11q14.3	*TYR*[a]	Tyrosinase	Key enzyme of melanin biosynthesis	R402Q	
14q12	*GZMB*[a]	Granzyme B	Mediates target cell apoptosis by cytotoxic T cells and natural killer cells, activation-induced cell death of effector Th2 cells		
17p13.2	*NLRP1*[a]	NACHT, LRR, and PYD domains-containing protein 1			Type 1 diabetes, Addison's disease, celiac disease, systemic sclerosis
21q22.3	*UBASH3A*[a]	Ubiquitin-associated and SH3 domain-containing A	Regulates T-cell receptor signaling		Type 1 diabetes
22q12.1	*XBP1*[a]	X-box binding protein 1	Regulates expression of MHC class II genes, IL6, B-cell and plasma cell differentiation		Crohn's disease
22q13.1	*C1QTNF6*[a]	C1q and tumor necrosis factor-related protein 6	Unknown		Type 1 diabetes, rheumatoid arthritis
Xp11.23	*FOXP3*[a]	Forkhead box P3	Regulates regulatory T cells	Casual variant	Defective gene in immunodysregulation polyendocrinopathy enteropathy X-linked (IPEX) syndrome

(continued)

Table 19.1 (continued)

Chromosome	Gene	Protein	Function	Casual variant	Other autoimmune disease associations
12q13.2	IKZF4	Ikaros zinc finger protein	T-cell transcriptional regulator subfamily		
6q15	BACH2	BTB and CNC homology 1	B-cell transcriptional repressor, basic leucine zipper	R620W	
10q25.3	CASP7	Caspase 7	Apoptotic executioner protein		
11p13	CD44	CD44 antigen	T-cell regulator		
11q14.3	TYR	Tyrosinase	Melanin biosynthetic enzyme		
11q21	Gene	None	TYR regulation		

Adapted and modified from Spritz et al. [37]

Numerous studies have indicated that *CTLA4* is only associated with vitiligo in patients who also have other autoimmune diseases, suggesting that apparent association of *CLTA4* with vitiligo is secondary to epidemiological association with these other diseases

[a]Genes with confirmed involvement in generalized vitiligo susceptibility on the basis of GWAS

[b]The MHC class II region is associated with both vitiligo susceptibility and age of onset

6q27 (in the vicinity of IDDM8, a linkage and association signal for type I diabetes mellitus and rheumatoid arthritis). Among the Caucasian and Chinese populations with vitiligo, this gene was also detected in the GWAS done [29–32]. To date, these particular populations carry three large GWAS of vitiligo, while a small gene-centric GWAS of vitiligo was reported in Indian–Pakistani patients [32–36]. These studies collectively identified 30 vitiligo susceptibility loci in Caucasians (Table 19.1). The subsequent parallel studies in the Chinese population have detected nine vitiligo susceptibility loci, suggesting some common susceptibility genes (LPP, the HLA class I gene region, CCR6, IL2RA, IKZF4, and C1QTNF6) between Caucasian and Chinese [37]. There is no major GWAS study performed in the Indian population, which is required for understanding the genetic aspect of vitiligo in this population.

19.4.1.4 DNA Sequencing Studies

The first sequencing study was performed for GTP-cyclohydrolase I gene (GCH1) that reported the association of vitiligo with GCH1 mutations. However, the findings were proven false much later [38, 39]. Over the years, DNA sequencing was performed for many candidate genes (ASIP, MC1R, MYG1/c12orf10, and POMC), but none showed significant differences [40–43].

Recently, the more robust next-generation DNA re-sequencing is being used to identify sequence variation. Sequencing of both HLA-A and TYR in Caucasian vitiligo patients had shown that the predominant HLA-A vitiligo-associated susceptibility allele is HLA-A*02:01:01:01, and the two common non-synonymous substitutions of TYR, S192Y and R402Q, exert both individual and synergistic protective effects [44].

19.4.1.5 Gene Expression Studies

The first gene expression study identified a gene VIT1 (FBXO11), which was down-regulated in vitiligo melanocytes, but its role in vitiligo development remains uncertain [45]. In the recent years, many genome-wide expression studies have been performed reporting many differentially expressed genes in vitiligo patients, but none can be proven to be the causal factor of vitiligo.

To date, there are approximately 36 (confirmed and suggestive) susceptibility loci identified for generalized vitiligo among various ethnic populations. Immunoregulatory proteins are approximately encoded by 90 %, while the 10 % encode melanocyte proteins, suggesting the major involvement of immune parameters and hence strengthening the autoimmune theory of pathogenesis.

19.4.2 Autoimmune Hypothesis

The autoimmune hypothesis is the most popular theory for the non-segmental and generalized type of vitiligo. Stronger evidence for this theory comes from the higher frequency of concomitant autoimmune diseases in vitiligo patients and response of vitiligo to treatment with immunosuppressives [46, 47].

Inflammatory cell infiltrates were noticed at the margin of vitiligo macules [48]. The epidermis-infiltrating T cells revealed an amplification of the CD8/CD4 ratio and IL-2 receptor expression suggesting that melanocyte obliteration could be cytotoxic CD8+ T cell mediated [49].

Many studies have shown the potential role of cytokines in the causation of vitiligo. Vitiligo skin showed significantly increased expression of IL-10, interferon-γ (IFN-γ), and tumor necrosis factor α (TNF-α) when compared to control skin. Levels of Th2 cytokine IL-10 were also found to be increased in lesional skin [50]. This explains the mechanism of action of tacrolimus in vitiligo, which potentially suppresses the Th1 response via the Th2 cytokine IL-10 suppression. Recently, elevated IL-17 levels have been found in both the lesional skin and sera of the vitiligo patients compared to controls, and it showed a positive correlation with the disease duration [51].

Humoral immunity has also been proposed to contribute to the autoimmune hypothesis of vitiligo pathogenesis. In a study by Kemp et al., 23 % of the non-segmental vitiligo patients were positive for tyrosine hydroxylase antibodies, an enzyme essential for melanogenesis pathway [52]. Harning et al., on measuring the levels of antibodies against pigment surface antigens, have shown that IgG- and IgM-based pigment cell antibodies were present in 80 % of active vitiligo patients. No IgG was seen among stable patients and controls, but 21 % of inactive vitiligo patients and 16 % of controls had notable levels of IgM [53]. In later studies, antibodies to MCHRl (melanin-concentrating hormone receptor 1) were found in 16.4 % of vitiligo patients, whereas no reactivity was exhibited in the control sera [54].

Regarding the association of other autoimmune diseases, Ingordo et al. found that 42.5 % of the vitiligo patients had circulating antibodies (antithyroglobulin antibodies in 27.5 %, anti-thyroperoxidase in 22.5 %, and anti-smooth muscle antibody in 17.3 %). However, an overt thyroid disease was seen in only 5 % of the cases [55].

In the recent years, regulatory T (Tregs) cells have gained much attention for their role in vitiligo occurrence. These cells are chief immunoregulatory T cells that maintain the immune system homeostasis by suppression of the proliferation of autoreactive T cells and thereby maintain the immune tolerance to self-antigens. The defect in Treg frequency, function, and homing has been reported, indicating the role of autoimmunity due to the breakdown of body's tolerance mechanism in vitiligo [56].

Thus far, the autoimmune hypothesis is one of the strongest and most attractive hypotheses in the genesis of vitiligo.

19.5 Conclusion

Vitiligo, an acquired depigmentary skin condition with accompanying severe psychosocial distress, affects the adult population with a reported preponderance among females of brown skin. Though, further research is still needed to point its exact mechanism, several hypotheses in the recent years have led to a better understanding in the development of this disorder. At present, genetics and the autoimmune hypotheses are well supported by several well-founded studies.

References

1. Barman S. Switra and its treatment in Veda. Anc Sci Life. 1995;15:71–4.
2. Taïeb A, Picardo M, Members VETF. The definition and assessment of vitiligo: a consensus report of the Vitiligo European Task Force. Pigment Cell Res. 2007;20:27–35.
3. Ezzedine K, Lim HW, Suzuki T, Katayama I, Hamzavi I, Lan CC, et al. Revised classification/nomenclature of vitiligo and related issues: the Vitiligo Global Issues Consensus Conference. Pigment Cell Melanoma Res. 2012;25:E1–13.
4. Howitz J, Brodthagen H, Schwartz M, Thomsen K. Prevalence of vitiligo. Epidemiological survey on the Isle of Bornholm, Denmark. Arch Dermatol. 1977;113:47–52.
5. Halder R, Taliaferro S. Vitiligo. In: Wolff K, Goldsmith L, Katz S, Gilchrest B, Paller A, Lefell D, editors. Fitzpatrick's dermatology in general medicine. 7th ed. New York: McGraw-Hill; 2008. p. 72.
6. Shah H, Mehta A, Astik B. Clinical and sociodemographic study of vitiligo. Indian J Dermatol Venereol Leprol. 2008;74:701.
7. Lee H, Lee MH, Lee DY, Kang HY, Kim KH, Choi GS, et al. Prevalence of vitiligo and associated comorbidities in Korea. Yonsei Med J. 2015;56:719–25.
8. Yaghoobi R, Omidian M, Bagherani N. Vitiligo: a review of the published work. J Dermatol. 2011;38:419–31.
9. Sehgal VN, Srivastava G. Vitiligo: compendium of clinico-epidemiological features. Indian J Dermatol Venereol Leprol. 2007;73:149–56.
10. Mchepange UO, Gao XH, Liu YY, Liu YB, Ma L, Zhang L, et al. Vitiligo in North-Eastern China: an association between mucosal and acrofacial lesions. Acta Dermatol Venereol. 2010;90:136–40.
11. Dogra S, Parsad D, Handa S, Kanwar AJ. Late onset vitiligo: a study of 182 patients. Int J Dermatol. 2005;44:193–6.
12. Handa S, Dogra S. Epidemiology of childhood vitiligo: a study of 625 patients from North India. Pediatr Dermatol. 2003;20:207–10.
13. Agarwal S, Ojha A, Gupta S. Profile of vitiligo in Kumaun region of Uttarakhand India. Indian J Dermatol. 2014;59:209.
14. Njoo MD, Westerhof W. Vitiligo. Pathogenesis and treatment. Am J Clin Dermatol. 2001;2:167–81.
15. Alkhateeb A, Stetler GL, Old W, Talbert J, Uhlhorn C, Taylor M, et al. Mapping of an autoimmunity susceptibility locus (AIS1) to chromosome 1p31.3-p32.2. Hum Mol Gen. 2002;11:661–7.
16. Bhatia PS, Mohan L, Pandey ON, Singh KK, Arora SK, Mukhija RD. Genetic nature of vitiligo. J Dermatol Sci. 1992;4:180–4.
17. Nath SK, Majumder PP, Nordlund JJ. Genetic epidemiology of vitiligo: multilocus recessivity cross – validated. Am J Hum Genet. 1994;55:981–90.

18. Arcos-Burgos M, Parodi E, Salgar M, Bedoya E, Builes J, Jaramillo D, et al. Vitiligo: complex segregation and linkage disequilibrium analyses with respect to microsatellite loci spanning the HLA. Hum Genet. 2002;110:334–42.
19. Zamani M, Spaepen M, Sghar SS, Huang C, Westerhof W, Nieuweboer-Krobotova L, et al. Linkage and association of HLA class II genes with vitiligo in a Dutch population. Br J Dermatol. 2001;145:90–4.
20. Liang Y, Yang S, Zhou Y, Gui J, Ren Y, Chen J, et al. Evidence for two susceptibility loci on chromosomes 22q12 and 6p22 in Chinese generalized vitiligo families. J Invest Dermatol. 2007;127:2552–7.
21. Nath SK, Kelly JA, Namjou B, Lam T, Bruner GR, Scofield RH, et al. Evidence for a susceptibility gene, SLEV1, on chromosome 17p13 in families with vitiligo-related systemic lupus erythematosus. Am J Hum Genet. 2001;69:1401–6.
22. Jin Y, Mailloux CM, Gowan K, Riccardi SL, LaBerge G, Bennett DC, et al. NALP1 in vitiligo-associated multiple autoimmune disease. New Engl J Med. 2007;356:1216–25.
23. Spritz RA, Gowan K, Bennett DC, Fain PR. Novel vitiligo susceptibility loci on chromosomes 7 (AIS2) and 8 (AIS3), confirmation of SLEV1 on chromosome 17, and their roles in an autoimmune diathesis. Am J Hum Genet. 2004;74:188–91.
24. Fain PR, Gowan K, LaBerge GS, Fain PR. A genomewide screen for generalized vitiligo: confirmation of AIS1 on chromosome 1p31 and evidence for additional susceptibility loci. Am J Hum Genet. 2003;72:1560–4.
25. Chen JJ, Huang W, Gui JP, Yang S, Zhou FS, Xiong QG, et al. A novel linkage to generalized vitiligo on 4q13-q21 identified in a genomewide linkage analysis of Chinese families. Am J Hum Genet. 2005;76:1057–65.
26. Kemp EH, Ajjan RA, Waterman EA, Gawkrodger DJ, Cork MJ, Watson PF, et al. Analysis of a microsatellite polymorphism of the cytotoxic T-lymphocyte antigen-4 gene in patients with vitiligo. Br J Dermatol. 1999;140:73–8.
27. Gough SCL, Walker LSK, Sansom DM. CTLA4 gene polymorphism and autoimmunity. Immunol Rev. 2005;204:102–15.
28. Birlea SA, Jin Y, Bennett DC, Herbstman DM, Wallace MR, McCormack WT, et al. Comprehensive association analysis of candidate genes for generalized vitiligo supports XBP1, FOXP3, and TSLP. J Invest Dermatol. 2011;131:371–81.
29. Jin Y, Birlea SA, Fain PR, Gowan K, Riccardi SL, Holland PJ, et al. Variant of TYR and autoimmunity susceptibility loci in generalized vitiligo. New Engl J Med. 2010;362:1686–97.
30. Birlea SA, Fain PR, Spritz RA. A Romanian population isolate with high frequency of vitiligo and associated autoimmune diseases. Arch Dermatol. 2008;144:310–6.
31. Birlea SA, Gowan K, Fain PR, Spritz RA. Genome-wide association study of generalized vitiligo in an isolated European founder population identifies SMOC2, in close proximity to IDDM8. J Invest Dermatol. 2010;130:798–803.
32. Quan C, Ren YQ, Xiang LH, Sun LD, Xu AE, Gao XH, et al. Genome-wide association study for vitiligo identifies susceptibility loci at 6q27 and the MHC. Nat Genet. 2010;42:614–8.
33. Jin Y, Birlea SA, Fain PR, Mailloux CM, Riccardi SL, Gowan K, et al. Common variants in FOXP1 are associated with generalized vitiligo. Nat Genet. 2010;42:576–8.
34. Jin Y, Birlea SA, Fain PR, Ferrara TM, Ben S, Riccardi SL, et al. Genome-wide association analyses identify 13 new susceptibility loci for generalized vitiligo. Nat Genet. 2012;44:676–80.
35. Tang XF, Zhang Z, Hu DY, Xu AE, Zhou HS, Sun LD, et al. Association analyses identify three susceptibility Loci for vitiligo in the Chinese Han population. J Invest Dermatol. 2013;133:403–10.
36. Birlea SA, Ahmad FJ, Uddin RM, Ahmad S, Pal SS, Begum R, et al. Association of generalized vitiligo with MHC class II loci in patients from the Indian subcontinent. J Invest Dermatol. 2013;133:1369–72.
37. Spritz RA. Six decades of vitiligo genetics: genome-wide studies provide insights into autoimmune pathogenesis. J Invest Dermatol. 2012;132:268–73.

38. De la Fuente-Fernandez R. Mutations in GTP-cyclohydrolase I gene and vitiligo. Lancet. 1997;350:640.
39. Bandyopadhyay D, Lawrence E, Majumder PP, Ferrell RE. Vitiligo is not caused by mutations in GTP-cyclohydrolase I gene. Exp Dermatol. 2000;25:152–3.
40. Na GY, Lee KH, Kim MK, Lee SJ, Kim DW, Kim JC. Polymorphisms in the melanocortin-1 receptor (MC1R) and agouti signaling protein (ASIP) genes in Korean vitiligo patients. Pigment Cell Res. 2003;16:383–7.
41. Széll M, Baltás E, Bodai L, Bata-Csörgo Z, Nagy N, Dallos A, et al. The Arg160Trp allele of melanocortin-1 receptor gene might protect against vitiligo. Photochem Photobiol. 2008;84: 565–71.
42. Eskandani M, Hasannia S, Golchai J. Assessment of MC1R and α-MSH genes sequences in Iranian vitiligo patients. Indian J Dermatol. 2010;55:325–8.
43. Philips MA, Kingo K, Karelson M, Rätsep R, Aunin E, Reimann E, et al. Promoter polymorphism – 119C/G in MYG1 (C12orf10) gene is related to vitiligo susceptibility and Arg4Gln affects mitochondrial entrance of Myg1. BMC Med Genet. 2010;11:56.
44. Jin Y, Ferrara T, Gowan K, Holcomb C, Rastrou M, Erlich HA, et al. Next-generation DNA re-sequencing identifies common variants of TYR and HLA-A that modulate the risk of generalized vitiligo via antigen presentation. J Invest Dermatol. 2012;132:1730–3.
45. Le Poole IC, Sarangarajan R, Zhao Y, Stennett LS, Brown TL, Sheth P, et al. 'VIT1', a novel gene associated with vitiligo. Pigment Cell Res. 2001;14:475–84.
46. Amerio P, Tracanna M, De Remigis P, Betterle C, Vianale L, Marra ME, et al. Vitiligo associated with other autoimmune diseases: polyglandular autoimmune syndrome types 3B + C and 4. Clin Exp Dermatol. 2006;31:746–9.
47. Mahmoud BH, Hexsel CL, Hamzavi IH. An update on new and emerging options for the treatment of vitiligo. Skin Therapy Lett. 2008;13:1–6.
48. Le Poole IC, van den Wijngaard RM, Westerhof W, Das PK. Presence of T cells and macrophages in inflammatory vitiligo skin parallels melanocyte disappearance. Am J Pathol. 1996;148:1219–28.
49. Lili Y, Yi W, Ji Y, Yue S, Weimin S, Ming L. Global activation of CD8+ cytotoxic T lymphocytes correlates with an impairment in regulatory T cells in patients with generalized vitiligo. PLoS One. 2012;7, e37513.
50. Taher ZA, Lauzon G, Maguiness S, Dytoc MT. Analysis of interleukin- 10 levels in lesions of vitiligo following treatment with topical tacrolimus. Br J Dermatol. 2009;161:654–9.
51. Bassiouny DA, Shaker O. Role of interleukin-17 in the pathogenesis of vitiligo. Clin Exp Dermatol. 2011;36:292–7.
52. Kemp HE, Emhemad S, Akhtar S, Watson PF, Gawkrodger DJ, Weetman AP. Autoantibodies against tyrosine hydroxylase in patients with non-segmental (generalised) vitiligo. Exp Dermatol. 2010;20:35–40.
53. Harning R, Gui J, Bystryn JG. Relation between the incidence and level of pigment cell antibodies and disease activity in vitiligo. Soc Invest Dermatol. 1991;97:1078–80.
54. Kemp HE, Waterman EA, Häwes BE, O'Neill K, Gottumukkala RV, Gawkrodger DJ, et al. The melanin- concentrating hormone receptor 1, a novel target of autoantibody responses in vitiligo. J Clin Invest. 2002;109:923–30.
55. Ingordo V, Gentile G, Iannazzone SS, Cusano F, Naldi L. Vitiligo and autoimmunity: an epidemiological study in a representative sample of young Italian males. J Eur Acad Dermatol Venereol. 2010;25:105–9.
56. Tembhre MK, Parihar AS, Sharma VK, Sharma A, Chattopadhyay P, Gupta S. Alteration in regulatory T cells and programmed cell death 1-expressing regulatory T cells in active generalized vitiligo and their clinical correlation. Br J Dermatol. 2015;172:940–50.

Chapter 20
Pathogenesis of Vitiligo

Rashmi Sarkar, Sumit Sethi, and Anjali Madan

20.1 Introduction

Vitiligo is a pigmentary disorder where functioning melanocytes undergo selective destruction that leads to the depigmentation of the skin, hair, and mucosal surfaces. It is a complex disease involving the interplay of multiple factors as genetic predisposition and environmental factors. In almost 50% of the patients, vitiligo starts before the age of 20 years, affecting both sexes with equal frequency [1]. The VGICC [2] classifies vitiligo into three types: segmental vitiligo (SV), non-segmental vitiligo (NSV), and unclassifiable vitiligo (UnV).

The pathogenesis of vitiligo has been expounded by several theories over the years. Neural theory was first propagated in the 1950s which were followed by thoughts and theories like neurogenic, genetic, the autoimmune hypothesis, autocytotoxic, microenvironmental, viral, apoptotic, reactive oxygen species (ROS), cell adhesion disorders, multivariate theories, and melanocytorrhagy hypothesis [3].

Most of the earlier hypotheses were one-dimensional and did not have complete basis to explain the pathophysiology of vitiligo. They failed to explain the fundamental basis and were not evidence based, paving the need for contemporary theories that could better explain the disease in toto. Universally agreed upon principles are an absence of functional melanocytes in vitiliginous skin and a loss and destruction of histochemically recognized melanocytes.

R. Sarkar (✉) • A. Madan
Department of Dermatology and Venereology, Maulana Azad Medical College and Associated Hospitals, New Delhi 110 002, India
e-mail: rashmisarkar@gmail.com; anjalimadan85@gmail.com

S. Sethi, MBBS, MD, DNB
Genesis Centre of Dermatology, Janakpuri, New Delhi 110 002, India
e-mail: sethi1587@gmail.com

E.B. Handog, M.J. Enriquez-Macarayo (eds.), *Melasma and Vitiligo in Brown Skin*,
DOI 10.1007/978-81-322-3664-1_20

Various perceptions of the components applicable to the pathophysiology of vitiligo are detailed in this chapter.

20.2 Neural Hypothesis

The neural theory hypothesizes the secretion of a certain neurochemical mediator from nearby nerve endings that is cytotoxic to pigment cells. The following clinical observations support the theory:

1. The presence of a segmental form of vitiligo confined to one section of the body
2. Severe emotional stress precipitating the onset of vitiligo
3. Increased incidence of vitiligo in patients with neurological disorders

The neural theory, proposed in 1959, built around the finding that segmental vitiligo occurs along the nerve dermatomes in the body exhibiting symptoms such as hyperhidrosis and emotional disorders. It was proposed that nervous system dysregulation is seen at local and/or systemic levels, damaging the melanocytes and affecting melanin production, as seen in the vitiligo tissues. Abnormalities of the autonomic nerve system may also exist in vitiligo lesions, that is, decreased parasympathetic tone and an increased adrenergic tone. High levels of neurotransmitters may directly lead to cell cytotoxicity. Indirectly, through local vasoconstriction, cellular hypoxia ensues followed by stress-generated hydrogen peroxide production [4, 5].

20.3 Genetic Hypothesis

Most of the cases of vitiligo are sporadic, but familial clustering has been seen, and according to several studies, 6.25–38 % of patients have a positive family history for vitiligo [5]. Various epidemiologic studies have indicated that vitiligo is polygenic and multifactorial, inherited in a non-Mendelian pattern with incomplete penetrance. Genomically identical monozygotic twins have shown 23 % concordance in developing vitiligo, suggesting a significant nongenetic environmental component. Different phenotypes of vitiligo are linked with specific genetic susceptibility genes and environmental exposures [6].

20.4 The Autoimmune Hypothesis

The autoimmune theory is more commonly associated with generalized vitiligo and focal non-dermatomal vitiligo. Various autoimmune disorders and organ-specific antibodies have been associated with vitiligo. Indirectly, the fact that different topical therapies that work in vitiligo have immune-modulating effects, sustains the notion of an autoimmune pathogenesis of the disease.

20.4.1 *Humoral Immunity*

Antibodies to intracellular pigment cell antigens, nonpigment cell antigens (common tissue antigens), and cell surface pigment cell antigens are the different categories of antibodies in the sera of vitiligo patients. The presence of different antibodies and the nonspecificity for melanocytes suggest that their formation may be a secondary phenomenon, following disruption of the melanocyte/keratinocyte unit and destruction of melanocytes. Nonetheless, melanocytes are known to be more sensitive than fibroblasts or keratinocytes to immune- or toxin-mediated injury, so even these nonspecific antibodies may lethally damage the melanocytes, sparing the surrounding cells [7].

20.4.2 *Cellular Immunity*

Primary or secondary to damage of melanocytes by specific cytotoxic T-cell immune reaction may play a role in their destruction. An increased CD8/CD4 ratio has been observed in the epidermotropic T cells of perilesional skin. These T cells frequently juxtapose the remaining melanocytes and express the skin-homing cutaneous lymphocyte antigen [7, 8].

20.5 Viral Theory

The possible involvement of viruses [i.e., hepatitis C virus (HCV), hepatitis B virus (HBV), Epstein-Barr virus, *Cytomegalovirus* (CMV), and HIV] in the etiopathogenesis or deterioration of vitiligo has been suggested by some authors. Active immune surveillance may result in melanocyte destruction, either by killing cells hosting infectious agents or attacking cells portraying similar antigens (antigen mimicry) [9, 10].

20.6 Melanocytorrhagy Theory

This theory attempts to explain the Koebner phenomenon in vitiligo by proposing a role of weak basal attachments of melanocytes. A minor friction or trauma and/or other stressors (i.e., catecholamines, reactive oxygen species (ROS), or autoimmune elements) can prompt the transepidermal migration and loss of melanocytes. The concept of "melanocytorrhagy" or chronic melanocytes' detachment together with other theories has been used to explain a single integrated hypothesis of vitiligo pathogenesis [11].

20.7 Oxidative Stress Hypothesis

Oxidative stress hypothesis suggests that a lack of balance in the redox (reduction-oxidation) state of the vitiligo affected skin leads to a considerable production of reactive oxygen species, as H_2O_2. Abnormally low level of catalase has been detected in vitiliginous skin, which correlates with high H_2O_2 levels in the epidermis. ROS, through oxidative processes, can damage biological processes coupled with excessive H_2O_2, thus initiating melanocytic failure and apoptosis. Langerhans cells can activate and trigger melanocytes reactive immune response, leading to eradication of skin melanocytes, resulting in depigmentation [12].

20.8 Double Strike Hypothesis

In 2010, Michelsen presented the double strike hypothesis that explains the pathophysiological mechanisms of vitiligo and hypopigmentation associated with melanoma. It states that two different major pathophysiological mechanisms are involved in vitiligo causality: a humoral antibody-based mechanism and a cellular T-cell-based mechanism. In diffuse vitiligo, the antibody-based mechanism dominates, while the cellular mechanism dominates in localized vitiligo [13].

20.9 Intrinsic Theory

It is postulated that an intrinsic defect leads to melanocyte apoptosis in vitiligo. Abnormalities include: (1) circular rough endoplasmic reticulum (RER) profiles, (2) dilated RER, and/or (3) membrane bound-compartments of melanosomes [14].

20.10 Integrated Theory (Convergence Theory)

Patients present in a variety of clinical types and state different histories of onset of disease, which makes it appealing to believe that the etiology of vitiligo varies among individual patients. A "convergence theory" suggests that stress, genetic factors, mutations, infection, accumulation of toxic compounds, altered cellular environment, autoimmunity, and impaired melanocyte migration and/or proliferation can all play a role in pathogenesis of vitiligo. Vitiligo seems like a syndromic entity with a multicausal etiology rather than a single disease [5, 10] (Fig. 20.1).

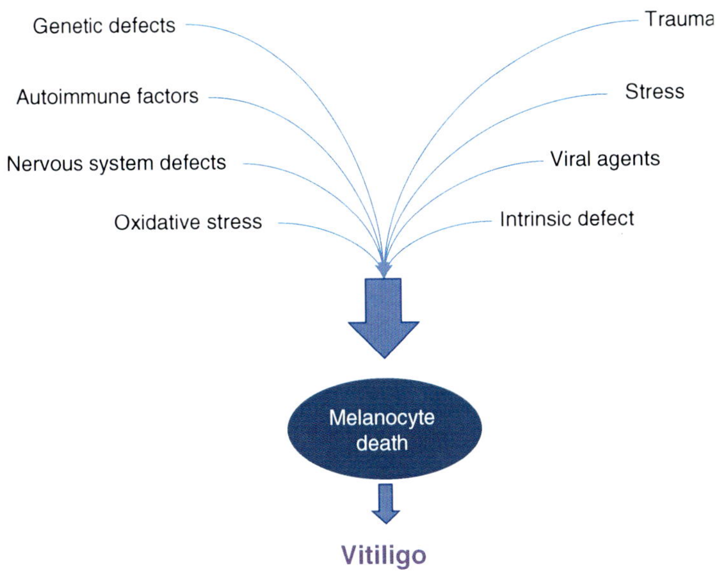

Fig. 20.1 Factors leading to melanocyte death

20.11 Conclusion

Though the exact causation of vitiligo still eludes us, it is safe to assume that several different pathophysiologic mechanisms may be involved. Best supported is the autoimmune hypothesis because of the numerous genetic associations and linkage studies, in combination with abnormal cellular and humoral immunity. However, the exact contribution of the aberrant immune responses in vitiligo pathogenesis has not yet been permanently established. The neural, humoral, cytotoxic, and oxidative stress hypotheses have modest evidence. The concept of melanocytorrhagy and decreased melanocyte survival still has to be convincingly demonstrated. Because all these ideas show promise, it seems probable that vitiligo, in reality, may be a final end result of a variety of anomalies that exhibit a common phenotype. The triggers underlying vitiligo pathogenesis may vary depending on the type and distribution of vitiligo patches. Further research works are necessary to clarify the interaction of all the abovementioned mechanisms and factors for a better comprehension of the pathophysiology of vitiligo and subsequent successful management.

References

1. Taïeb A, Picardo M. Clinical practice. Vitiligo. N Engl J Med. 2009;360:160–9.
2. Ezzedine K, Lim HW, Suzuki T, Katayama I, Hamzavi I, Lan CC, et al. Revised classification/nomenclature of vitiligo and related issues: the Vitiligo Global Issues Consensus Conference. Pigment Cell Melanoma Res. 2012;25(3):E1–13.

3. Picardo M, Taieb A. Pathophysiology overview. In: Picardo M, Taieb A, editors. Vitiligo. Berlin/Heidelberg: Springer; 2010. p. 149–54.
4. Lerner AB. Vitiligo. J Invest Dermatol. 1959;32(2, Part 2):285–310.
5. Njoo MD, Westerhof W. Vitiligo. Pathogenesis and treatment. Am J Clin Dermatol. 2001; 2(3):167–81.
6. Alikhan A, Felsten LM, Daly M, Petronic-Rosic V. Vitiligo: a comprehensive overview part I. Introduction, epidemiology, quality of life, diagnosis, differential diagnosis, associations, histopathology, etiology, and work-up. J Am Acad Dermatol. 2011;65(3):473–91.
7. Ongenae K, Van Geel N, Naeyaert JM. Evidence for an autoimmune pathogenesis of vitiligo. Pigment Cell Res. 2003;16(2):90–100.
8. Kemp EH, Waterman EA, Weetman AP. Autoimmune aspects of vitiligo. Autoimmunity. 2001;34(1):65–77.
9. Halder RM, Chappell JL. Vitiligo update. Semin Cutan Med Surg. 2009;28(2):86–92.
10. Le Poole IC, Das PK, van den Wijngaard RM, Bos JD, Westerhof W. Review of the etiopathomechanism of vitiligo: a convergence theory. Exp Dermatol. 1993;2(4):145–53.
11. Gauthier Y, Cario Andre M, Taieb A. A critical appraisal of vitiligo etiologic theories. Is melanocyte loss a melanocytorrhagy? Pigment Cell Res. 2003;16:322–32.
12. Glassman SJ. Vitiligo, reactive oxygen species and T-cells. Clin Sci. 2011;120:99–120.
13. Michelsen D. The double strike hypothesis of the vitiligo pathomechanism: new approaches to vitiligo and melanoma. Med Hypotheses. 2010;74:67–70.
14. Boissy RE, Liu YY, Medrano EE, Nordlund JJ. Structural aberration of the rough endoplasmic reticulum and melanosome compartmentalization in long-term cultures of melanocytes from vitiligo patients. J Invest Dermatol. 1991;97:395–404.

Chapter 21
Vitiligo Classification and Clinical Presentations

Andreas D. Katsambas and Electra Nicolaidou

21.1 Introduction

Progressive loss of functional melanocytes characterizes vitiligo, presenting as well-circumscribed white macules and patches on the skin. Affecting 0.1–2 % of the general population worldwide, highest prevalence of 8.8 % was noted in Gujarat, India [1].

Vitiligo can be a psychologically devastating disease, especially for patients with darker skin phototypes, such as those with brown or black skin [2]. This chapter will focus on the most recent classification of the various forms of the disease, with emphasis on vitiligo presentation among patients with brown skin.

21.2 Classification

There is a need for a classification system that can both guide prognosis and lead to a more homogenous reporting in vitiligo research. With this goal in mind, the Vitiligo Global Issues Consensus Conference (VGICC), held in 2011 in Bordeaux,

A.D. Katsambas, MD (✉)
1st Department of Dermatology and Venereology, National and Kapodestrian University of Athens, School of Medicine, Andreas Sygros Hospital Hospital for Skin and Venereal Diseases, Athens, Greece

1st University Clinic of Dermatology and Venereology, Andreas Sygros Hospital, University of Athens, Athens, Greece
e-mail: katsabas1@ath.forthnet.gr

E. Nicolaidou
1st Department of Dermatology and Venereology, National and Kapodestrian University of Athens, School of Medicine, Andreas Sygros Hospital Hospital for Skin and Venereal Diseases, Athens, Greece

E.B. Handog, M.J. Enriquez-Macarayo (eds.), *Melasma and Vitiligo in Brown Skin*, DOI 10.1007/978-81-322-3664-1_21

resulted in a consensus on vitiligo classification and nomenclature [3]. The two main categories are shown in Table 21.1, as non-segmental vitiligo (NSV) and segmental vitiligo (SV).

21.2.1 Vitiligo/NSV

The term *vitiligo* includes different usually multifocal clinical subtypes that are all clearly distinct from *SV*. The depigmented macules and patches vary in size from a few to several centimeters in diameter and involve both sides of the body with a tendency toward symmetrical distribution. *Vitiligo/NSV* can be *generalized*, *acrofacial*, *universal*, *mucosal*, and *mixed* (associated with SV). Rare types of *vitiligo/NSV* include *vitiligo punctata* and *hypochromic vitiligo/vitiligo minor*.

21.2.1.1 Generalized Vitiligo

This is the most common form of the disease. It is characterized by lesions involving the face, trunk, and extremities, usually in a symmetrical pattern (Fig. 21.1).

Table 21.1 Main types of vitiligo, according to VGICC classification [3]

1. Vitiligo/non-segmental vitiligo (NSV)
1.1 Generalized
1.2 Acrofacial
1.3 Universal
1.4 Mucosal
1.5 Mixed
2. Segmental vitiligo (SV)

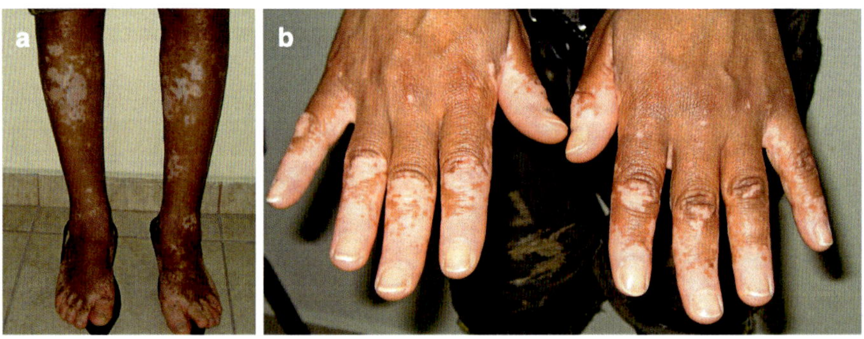

Fig. 21.1 Generalized vitiligo: symmetrical lesions on the shins and feet (**a**) and hands (**b**)

21.2.1.2 Acrofacial Vitiligo

Acrofacial vitiligo is limited to the face, head, hands, and feet (Fig. 21.2). Depigmentation of the distal fingers and facial orifices is usually present. Acrofacial vitiligo may evolve into typical generalized vitiligo.

21.2.1.3 Universal Vitiligo (Vitiligo Universalis)

In *universal vitiligo*, more than 80 % of the body surface area is depigmented (Fig. 21.3). It is the most extensive form of the disease, and hair involvement is also common. Some pigmentation may be still present, especially in sun-exposed areas. *Universal vitiligo* can be the end point of a progressive *generalized vitiligo* that has evolved to nearly complete depigmentation of the skin and hair.

21.2.1.4 Mucosal Vitiligo

Mucosal vitiligo is characterized by involvement of the oral and/or genital mucosae (Fig. 21.4). It is included in *vitiligo/NSV* when it is associated with skin involvement. If the skin lesions are not present, *mucosal vitiligo* is classified as *undetermined/unclassified* vitiligo.

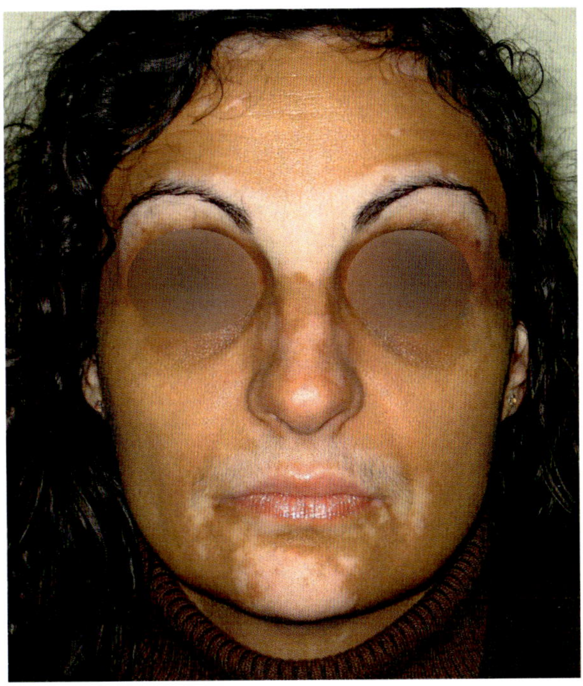

Fig. 21.2 Acrofacial vitiligo: lesions on the face (lesions on the hands were also present)

21.2.1.5 Mixed Vitiligo

Mixed vitiligo refers to *segmental vitiligo* which has been followed by *vitiligo/NSV* with a delay of at least 6 months [4]. In patients with *mixed vitiligo*, the "segmental" part of the disease is usually more resistant to treatment. Risk factors for the progression of *segmental* to *mixed vitiligo* include the presence of halo nevi and leukotrichia [5].

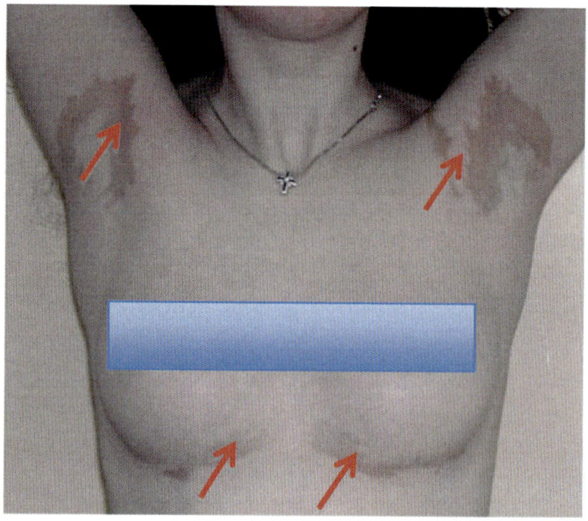

Fig. 21.3 Universal vitiligo: note the few remaining islands with normal pigmentation (*arrows*)

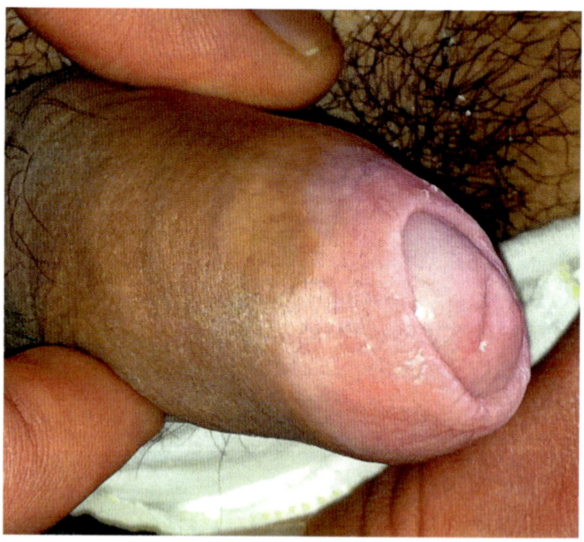

Fig. 21.4 Mucosal vitiligo: lesions on the prepuce and glans penis

21.2.1.6 Rare Types

Vitiligo punctata refers to multiple, small (confetti-like), sharply demarcated depigmented macules (Fig. 21.5).

Hypochromic vitiligo/vitiligo minor is characterized by the presence of hypopigmented lesions alone or in association with completely depigmented lesions [6]. This type of *vitiligo/NSV* has been very sparsely reported, and it seems to be limited to dark-skinned individuals. Histological examination should be performed to rule out hypopigmented mycosis fungoides (Fig. 21.6).

21.2.2 Segmental Vitiligo

In *segmental vitiligo*, one or more vitiligo lesions are distributed on a unilateral segment of the body. The lesions usually (but not always) respect the midline (Fig. 21.7).

Mono-segmental vitiligo is the most common form of SV. Rarely, multiple segmental lesions are noted either unilaterally or bilaterally. The onset of these multiple lesions can be simultaneous or not.

Segmental vitiligo may progress to *mixed vitiligo*, if lesions that correspond to *vitiligo/NSV* appear in a patient with segmental disease.

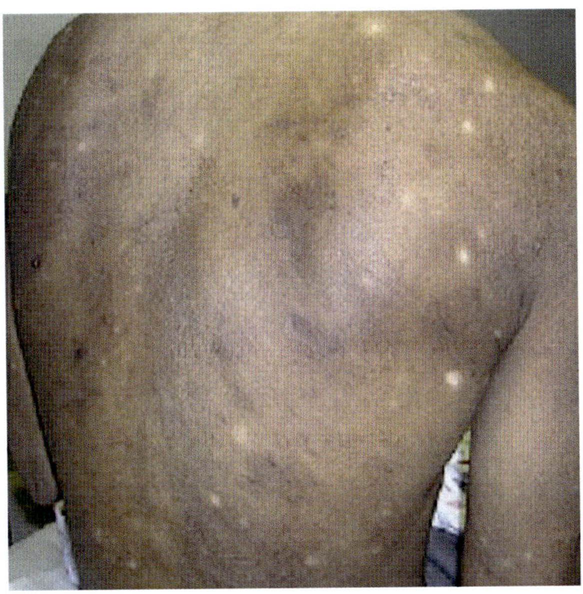

Fig. 21.5 Vitiligo punctate: confetti-like lesions

21.2.3 Undetermined/Unclassified Vitiligo

Focal vitiligo refers to one or more acquired lesions that do not fit a segmental distribution. This form may evolve into either *SV* or *vitiligo/NSV*.

Mucosal vitiligo is classified as *undetermined/unclassified vitiligo* when oral and/or genital mucosal lesions occur without skin involvement. If skin involvement exists, *mucosal vitiligo* is included in *vitiligo/NSV*.

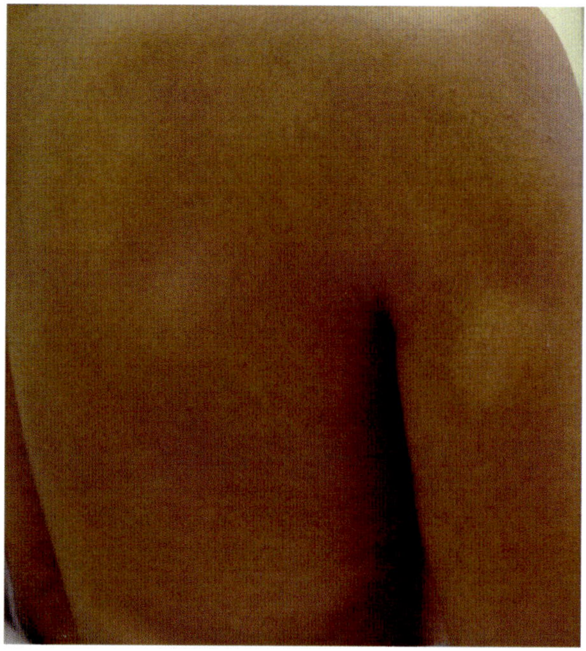

Fig. 21.6 Mycosis fungoides lesions resembling hypochromic vitiligo

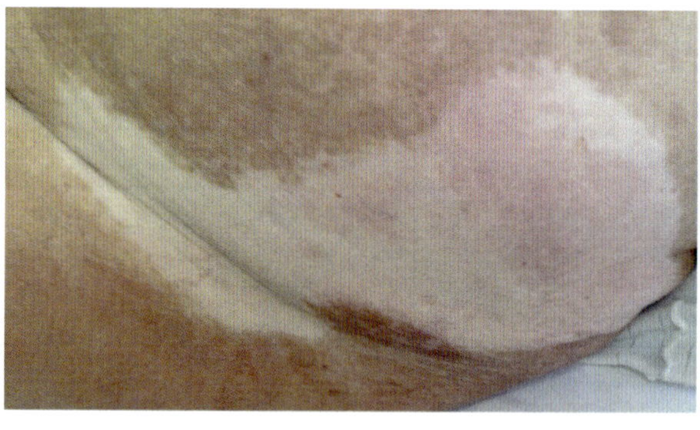

Fig. 21.7 Segmental vitiligo (erythema inside the vitiligo lesion is caused by atopic dermatitis)

21.3 Clinical Presentations

Vitiligo usually presents with sharply demarcated, totally amelanotic (milk-white) macules and patches surrounded by normal skin. Lesions can be round, oval, or completely irregular in shape, and they range from millimeters to several centimeters in diameter. In patients with brown or black skin, the contrast between the lesional and normal skin is striking. The lesions are usually asymptomatic. Pruritus has been reported in rare cases.

Lesions can appear anywhere on the body, and they are usually symmetric. Typical sites include the face, nipples, axillae, dorsal surface of the hands, anogenital region, elbows, knees, shins, and dorsal surface of feet [7]. The disease seems to favor sites that are subjected to repeated trauma, friction, or pressure.

Leukotrichia may be associated with vitiligo lesions. On the scalp, vitiligo often presents as localized patches of white hair (poliosis) (Fig. 21.8). Scattered white hairs or even total depigmentation of all scalp hair can also occur.

The onset of the disease is usually insidious. Most patients become aware of the lesions during the spring or summer, when the contrast between the normal and lesional skin is greater due to the tan produced by sun exposure. In a recent clinical study that included more than 1,000 patients from Gujarat, India, the lower limb was the most common site of initial disease presentation (41.5 % of patients), followed

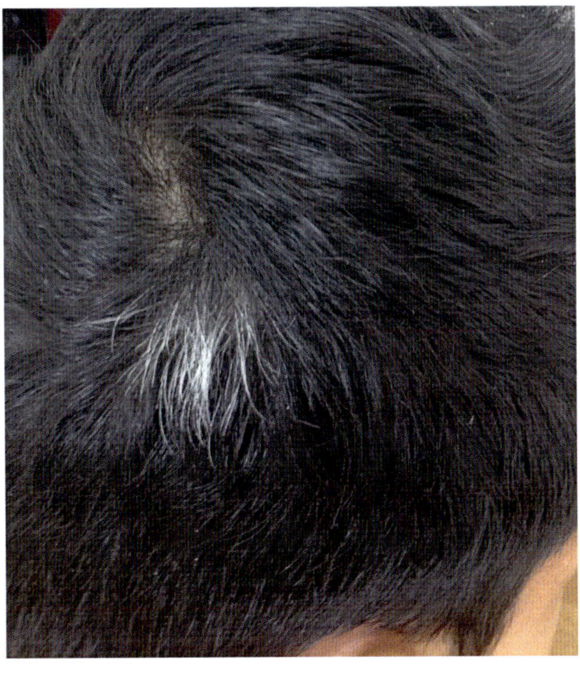

Fig. 21.8 Leukotrichia in vitiligo patient

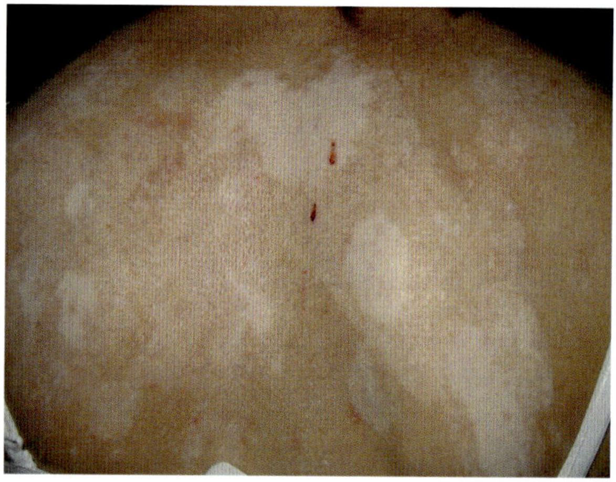

Fig. 21.9 Trichrome vitiligo: is a zone between the normal and lesional skin with an intermediate degree of pigmentation

by the scalp, face, upper limb, and trunk [1]. In another study from India that included 625 children with vitiligo, the most common site of onset was the head and neck, followed by the lower limbs, trunk, upper limbs, and mucosa [8]. The head and neck was the most common site of initial disease presentation in another study from India that included 182 patients with disease onset after 50 years of age [9].

The most common form of vitiligo is the *generalized* form of *vitiligo/NSV*. In the study from Gujarat, India, generalized vitiligo was present in 58 % of patients, followed by acrofacial (28 %), segmental (7 %), universal (7 %), and mucosal form [1]. Generalized vitiligo was also the most prevalent form in the study that included pediatric population with 78 % of patients, followed by focal (14.4 %), segmental (4.6 %), and acrofacial form (1.6 %) [8], as well as in the study that included patients with disease onset after 50 years of age with 84 % of patients, followed by focal (5.5 %), segmental (4.4 %), and acrofacial (3.8 %) [9]. The course of *vitiligo/NSV* is unpredictable. It may regress spontaneously, stabilize for a long period of time, show a slow progression, or exacerbate acutely. When the disease is progressive, new lesions may appear or/and the old ones may enlarge centrifugally.

Vitiligo lesions are often described as *active* or *stable*. A *stable* lesion is one that has not changed in the past 12 months [3]. A variant of *active* disease is *trichrome* vitiligo, in which there is a zone of varying width between the normal and lesional skin with a uniform intermediate degree of pigmentation, which gives the impression of "three color" (Fig. 21.9). The number of melanocytes has also been found to be intermediate in this zone [10].

Segmental vitiligo is characterized by a different clinical presentation and different prognosis, compared to *vitiligo/NSV*. Clinically, in *segmental vitiligo*, one or more lesions are distributed on a unilateral segment of the body. SV spreads within the segment over a period of 1–2 years and then the disease is usually stabilized. It is more common in patients with disease onset in childhood, compared to patients with disease onset during adolescence or adulthood [11]. The reported rate (4.6 %) of segmental vitiligo among children with brown skin [8] is lower, compared to children from other ethnic groups [11].

Halo nevus, an acquired melanocytic nevus surrounded by a halo of depigmentation, may also be present in vitiligo patients. It may be solitary or multiple and can occur alone or in combination with vitiligo. The exact relation between halo nevi and vitiligo remains to be elucidated [12, 13]. Halo nevi were present in 4.4 % of children [8] and 3.8 % of adult patients [12] with vitiligo from India. Higher rates, up to 31 %, have been reported in white patients [12].

21.4 Conclusion

The new VGICC classification system attempts to meet the need for a classification system that can both guide prognosis and lead to a more homogenous reporting in vitiligo research.

In vitiligo patients with brown skin, the striking difference between the lesional and healthy skin can impose a huge burden, as far as quality of life is concerned. The most common type of vitiligo in patients with brown skin is the generalized form. Rates of segmental vitiligo seem lower in patients with brown skin, compared to patients from other ethnic groups

References

1. Vora RV, Patel BB, Chaudhary AH, Mehta MJ, Pilani AP. A clinical study of vitiligo in a rural set up of Gujarat. Indian J Community Med. 2014;39:143–6.
2. Sangma LN, Nath J, Bhagabati D. Quality of life and psychological morbidity in vitiligo patients: a study in a teaching hospital from North-East India. Indian J Dermatol. 2015;60:142–6.
3. Ezzedine K, Lim HW, Suzuki T, Katayama I, Hamzavi I, Lan CCE. Revised classification/nomenclature of vitiligo and related issues: The Vitiligo Global Issues Consensus Conference. Pigment Cell Melanoma Res. 2012;25:E1–13.
4. Ezzedine K, Gauthier Y, Leaute-Labreze C, Marquez S, Bouchtnei S, Jouary T, et al. Segmental vitiligo associated with generalized vitiligo (mixed vitiligo): a retrospective case series of 19 patients. J Am Acad Dermatol. 2011;65:965–71.
5. Ezzedine K, Diallo A, Leaute-Labreze C, Seneschal J, Prey S, Ballanger F, et al. Halo naevi and leukotrichia are strong predictors of the passage to mixed vitiligo in a subgroup of segmental vitiligo. Br J Dermatol. 2012;166:539–44.
6. Ezzedine K, Mahe A, van Geel N, Cardot-Leccia N, Gauthier Y, Descamps V, et al. Hypochromic vitiligo: delineation of a new entity. Br J Dermatol. 2015;172:716–21.
7. Alikham A, Felsten LM, Daly M, Petronic-Rosic V. Vitiligo: a comprehensive overview. J Am Acad Dermatol. 2011;65:473–91.
8. Handa S, Dogra S. Epidemiology of childhood vitiligo: a study of 625 patients from North India. Pediatr Dermatol. 2003;20:207–10.
9. Dogra S, Parsad D, Handa S, Kanwar AJ. Late onset vitiligo: a study of 182 patients. Int J Dermatol. 2005;44:193–6.
10. Hann SK, Kim YS, Yoo JH, Chun YS. Clinical and histopathologic characteristics of trichrome vitiligo. J Am Acad Dermatol. 2000;42:589–96.
11. Nicolaidou E, Antoniou C, Miniati A, Lagogianni E, Matekovits A, Stratigos A, et al. Childhood- and later-onset vitiligo have diverse epidemiologic and clinical characteristics. J Am Acad Dermatol. 2012;66:954–8.

12. Van Geel N, Vandenhaute S, Speeckaert R, Brochez L, Mollet I, De Cooman L, Lambert J. Prognostic value and clinical significance of halo naevi regarding vitiligo. Br J Dermatol. 2011;164:743–9.
13. Patrizi A, Bentivogli M, Raone B, Dondi A, Tabanelli M, Neri I. Association of halo nevus/I and vitiligo in childhood: a retrospective observational study. J Eur Acad Dermatol Venereol. 2013;27:e148–52.

Chapter 22
Dermoscopy in Vitiligo

Devinder Mohan Thappa, Laxmisha Chandrashekar, and Munisamy Malathi

22.1 Introduction

Vitiligo, an acquired, idiopathic disorder characterized by circumscribed depigmented macules with convex borders, is primarily a clinical diagnosis without the need for diagnostic tools. The presence of clinically evident leukotrichia further enhances diagnostic accuracy and also signifies poorer prognosis especially in segmental vitiligo. However, diagnostic difficulties arise occasionally when focal vitiligo needs to be differentiated from chemically induced leukoderma, tinea versicolor, pityriasis alba, halo nevus, depigmented nevus, and postinflammatory hypopigmentation (PIH). Moreover, in many circumstances a diagnosis of early localized vitiligo cannot be definitely made, based on clinical examination alone. Since vitiligo is associated with significant emotional disturbances, a reliable early diagnosis is essential to initiate appropriate counseling and early treatment. In such conditions, dermoscopy, the dermatologist's stethoscope, might play a role in obviating the need for a skin biopsy for histopathological confirmation, especially in children.

D.M. Thappa (✉) • L. Chandrashekar • M. Malathi
Dermatology and Sexually Transmitted Diseases Department,
Jawaharlal Institute of Postgraduate Medical Education and Research (JIPMER),
Puducherry 605006, India
e-mail: dmthappa@gmail.com; laxmishac@gmail.com; mmalthi.dr@live.com

E.B. Handog, M.J. Enriquez-Macarayo (eds.), *Melasma and Vitiligo in Brown Skin*,
DOI 10.1007/978-81-322-3664-1_22

22.2 Role of Dermoscopy in Vitiligo

Dermoscopy (digital epiluminescence microscopy or "dermatoscopy"), by magnifying the clinical image manifold, allows for the appreciation of subtle features invisible to the naked eye. To date, dermoscopy has been reported to be beneficial in certain circumstances in vitiligo:

- Diagnosis of early vitiligo [1]
- Assessment of the stage of the disease (evolution, stability, or repigmentation) [2, 3]
- Assessment of treatment response by detecting clinically inapparent leukotrichia especially in the segmental variant [4]
- Diagnosis of blue vitiligo [5] and nail trichrome vitiligo [6]
- Differentiation of guttate vitiligo from idiopathic guttate hypomelanosis [7]

22.3 Dermoscopic Patterns Described in Vitiligo

Dermoscopy facilitates the recognition of vitiligo, by revealing characteristic depigmentation patterns. A pattern of hypopigmentation with residual perifollicular pigmentation (Fig. 22.1) has been described as a specific pattern in vitiligo by Chuh and Zawar [1]. The residual perifollicular pigmentation is a well-described phenomenon in vitiligo seen in active lesions, as well as lesions in spontaneous remission or after treatment. This is because, in the early phase of the disease, the melanocytes in

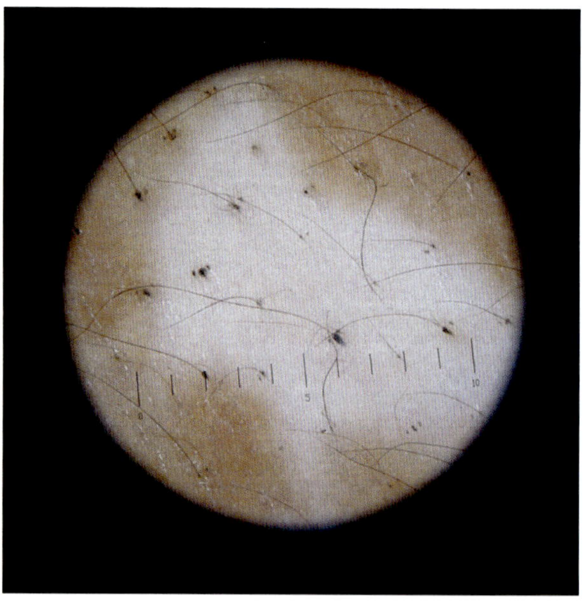

Fig. 22.1 Retention of perifollicular pigmentation in early lesion of vitiligo

the interfollicular compartment are lost, followed by loss of melanocytes in the perifollicular compartment. However, this specific sign seen in vitiligo has also been reported in idiopathic guttate hypomelanosis [7].

22.4 Dermoscopic Findings in the Diagnosis of Early Vitiligo

Thatte and Khopkar [3] in their recent study have reported the following dermoscopic findings in evolving vitiligo: reduced/absent (Fig. 22.2), reversed pigmentary network (Fig. 22.3), perifollicular and perilesional hyperpigmentation (Fig. 22.4), and a diffuse white glow under UV light. The predominant findings noted were reduced (40 %), absent (30 %), and reversed pigmentary network (20 %).

Reversed pigmentary network, a well-described finding in the dermoscopy of melanoma and melanocytic nevus, refers to a white or depigmented net-like pattern with pigmentation. It is similar to the salt and pepper pattern reported by Chandrashekar [2]. In vitiligo, there is a gradual loss of melanocytes and melanin which allows the light to directly pass into the dermis without being reflected by the melanocytes and melanin. This leads to a window through which light passes into the dermis and is reflected by dermal collagen.

In the initial stages of evolving vitiligo, this leads to an area of relative hyperpigmentation produced by the pale area corresponding to the papillary dermis in the normal reticulate pattern of pigmentation. The appearance of "reversed pigmentary network pattern" in evolving vitiligo is thus seen.

Identification of leukotrichia in nonlesional skin on dermoscopy may also be considered as an earlier dermoscopic marker of impending vitiligo. In a recent

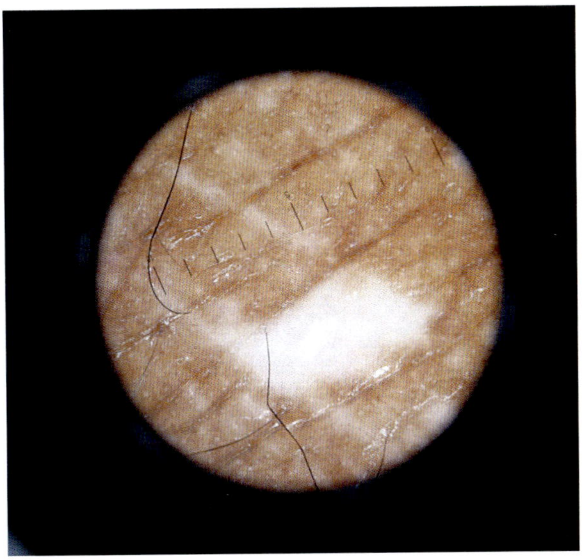

Fig. 22.2 Absence of pigment network with Koebner phenomenon in an early lesion of vitiligo

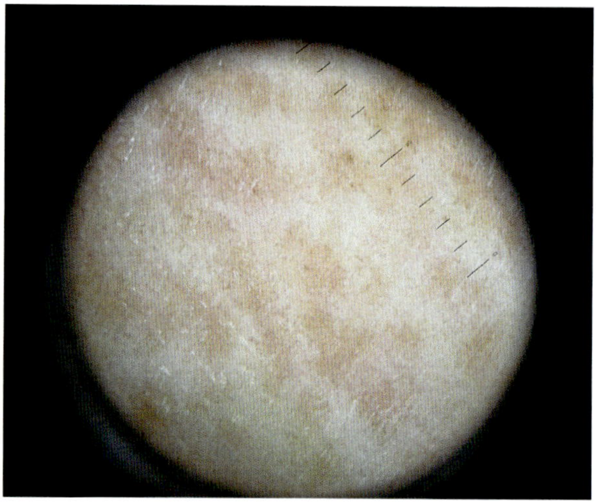

Fig. 22.3 Reversed pigmentary network in an early lesion of vitiligo

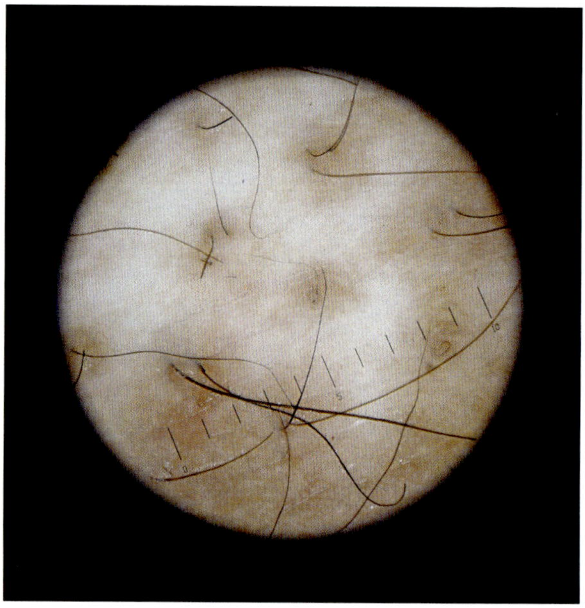

Fig. 22.4 Perifollicular pigmentation with reduced pigment network in an early lesion of vitiligo

report by Sonthalia et al. [8], perifollicular depigmentation and evolving leukotrichia in areas of clinically unaltered pigmentation has been suggested as an early predictive sign of impending vitiligo.

22.5 Dermoscopic Features to Assess the Stage of Vitiligo

Assessing the stability of vitiligo when considering vitiligo surgery is another area where the dermoscope comes as a handy tool. There are various well-described clinical signs of progressive activity like confetti macules, koebnerization, onset of new

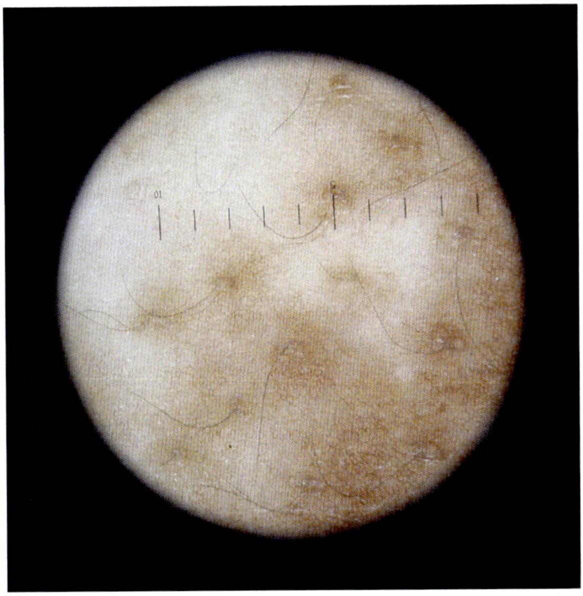

Fig. 22.5 Perifollicular hyperpigmentation in a case of stable repigmenting vitiligo

macules, and trichrome. In a Chinese study [9], it was reported that residual perifollicular pigmentation was observed in 91.94 % of patients with progressive vitiligo when compared to 62.86 % of those with stable vitiligo. There was no residual perifollicular pigmentation observed in nonvitiligo depigmented lesions. The presence of telangiectasia, early reservoirs of pigmentation, and perilesional hyperpigmentation was reported to be related to the stage of vitiligo and treatment history of patients.

Chandrashekar [2] has reported various signs associated with stable and progressive vitiligo. The various dermoscopic findings associated with stability and repigmentation of vitiligo are marginal and perifollicular hyperpigmentation (Fig. 22.5), reticular pigmentation (well-defined pigment network within the depigmented macule), and marginal reticular pigmentation (well-defined pigment network at the margins of the macule) (Fig. 22.6). The various dermoscopic findings associated with progressive vitiligo include polka dot or confetti-like (depigmented dots distributed in a polka dot pattern) (Fig. 22.7), comet tail (micro-Koebner phenomenon) (Fig. 22.8), starburst or nebulous (Fig. 22.9), trichrome vitiligo (three zones, brown, tan, and white) (Fig. 22.10), and salt and pepper pattern.

22.6 Dermoscopic Features to Assess Treatment Response by Detecting Clinically Inapparent Leukotrichia

Prominent rarefaction and pigment reduction in terminal hair shafts might suggest impending leukotrichia [8]. In segmental vitiligo, detection of leukotrichia (Fig. 22.11) with the help of dermoscopy might be a useful predictor of treatment

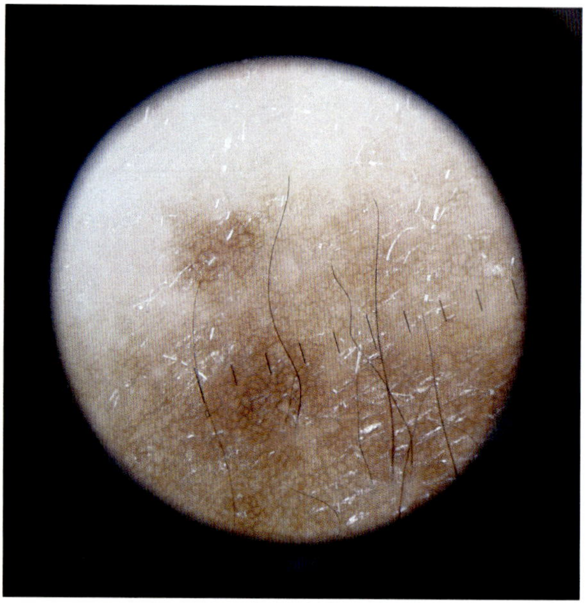

Fig. 22.6 Marginal reticular hyperpigmentation in a stable vitiligo

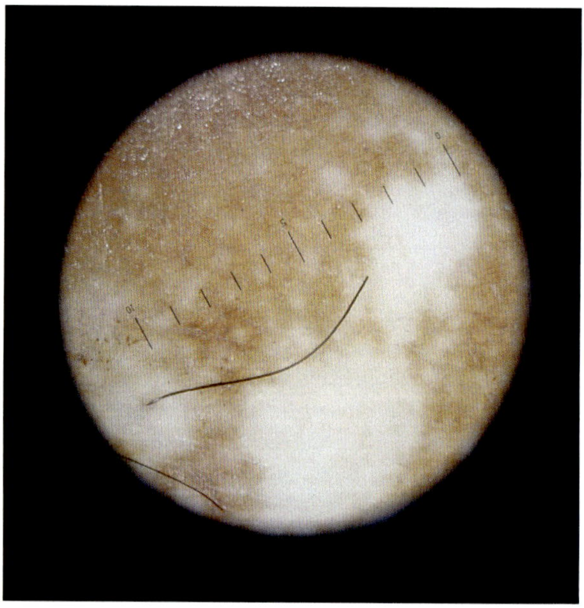

Fig. 22.7 Polka dots (confetti macules) in active lesions of vitiligo

response and decision on treatment modalities, as the presence of leukotrichia suggests poor response to treatment [4]. Repigmentation of vitiligo macules associated with leukotrichia may be minimal or absent because the loss of hair melanocytes is usually permanent, and repigmentation may not be possible with medical therapy.

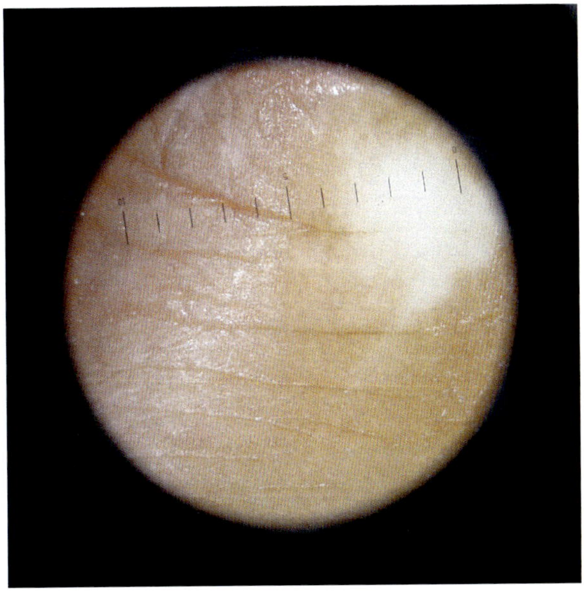

Fig. 22.8 Absent pigmentary network with comet tail-like projection (micro-Koebner phenomenon)

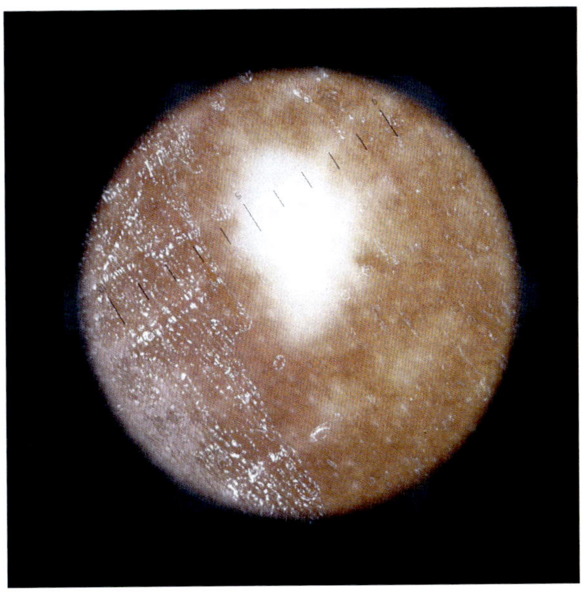

Fig. 22.9 Starburst appearance with absent pigmentary network in progressive vitiligo

22.7 Dermoscopic Features in the Diagnosis of Blue Vitiligo

Blue vitiligo is a distinct rare variant of vitiligo. It is characterized by a blue-gray appearance corresponding histologically with the absence of epidermal melanocytes and presence of numerous dermal melanophages. This occurs due to PIH following

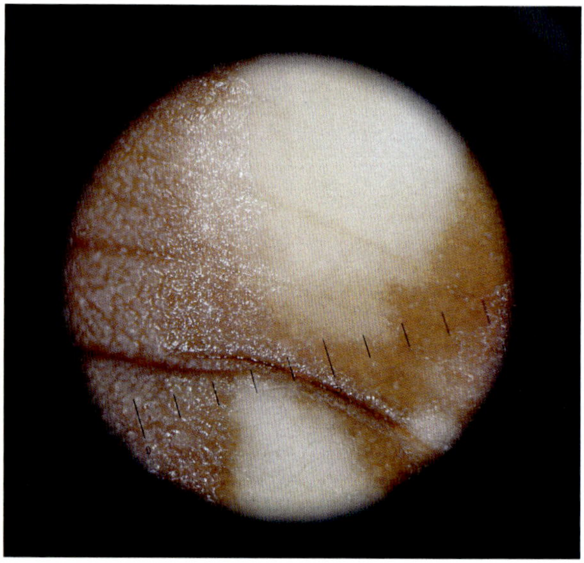

Fig. 22.10 Trichrome sign with three shades seen in a case of progressive vitiligo

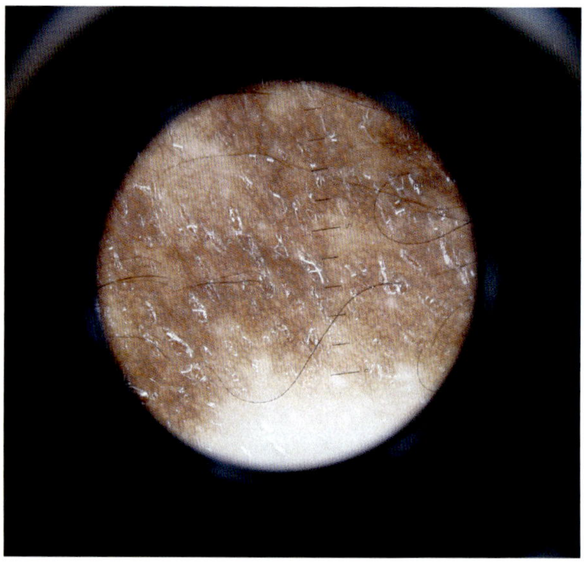

Fig. 22.11 Leukotrichia with marginal reticular hyperpigmentation in a case of stable vitiligo

psoralen chemotherapy. The blue color could be due to enhanced absorption and scattering of visual light by deep dermal melanin. The dermoscopic findings that aid in the diagnosis of this rare condition include a linear depigmented macule in the center with multiple blue dots (representing the dermal melanin) (Fig. 22.12) at the interface between the blue macule and hypopigmented macule, absence of epidermal melanin on the side of the blue macule, and reticular pigmentation with a few depigmented macules and scattered blue dots over the side of the hypopigmented macule [5].

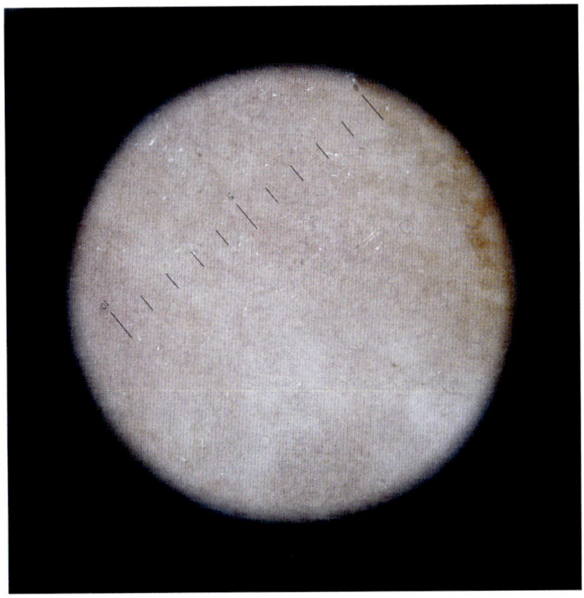

Fig. 22.12 Absent pigmentary network with multiple blue dots in a case of blue vitiligo

22.8 Dermoscopic Features in the Diagnosis of Nail Trichrome Vitiligo

Trichrome vitiligo, a marker of disease activity, is characterized by macules with an intermediate zone of hypochromia located between the achromic center and the peripheral unaffected skin. Though clinically evident, it is better appreciated with a dermoscope. Trichrome vitiligo of the nail unit presenting with brown, light brown, and achromic areas has been reported to be better identified with a dermoscope, indicating disease progression [6].

22.9 Dermoscopic Features Differentiating Guttate Vitiligo from Idiopathic Guttate Hypomelanosis

Sometimes, it might be difficult to differentiate a guttate vitiligo from idiopathic guttate hypomelanosis by clinical examination, especially in darker races. But differentiating the two conditions is of prognostic and therapeutic significance. Errichetti and Stinco reported the detection of cloudy or cloudy sky-like pattern in idiopathic guttate hypomelanosis. Guttate vitiligo shows a dense/glowing white shade and possible follicular hyperpigmentation but typically lacks a hyperpigmented patchy network [10].

22.10 Conclusion

Noninvasive investigations like dermoscopy have a role in vitiligo when the diagnosis is uncertain, as in the early disease, and for objective evaluation of treatment response. However, dermoscopy in vitiligo is in its infancy with only few published case reports and series, thus warranting the need for standardization of nomenclature for uniform reporting and validation of findings.

References

1. Chuh AA, Zawar V. Demonstration of residual perifollicular pigmentation in localized vitiligo—a reverse and novel application of digital epiluminescence dermoscopy. Comput Med Imaging Graph. 2004;28:213–7.
2. Chandrashekhar L. Dermoscopy: a tool to assess stability in vitiligo. In: Khopkar U, editor. Dermoscopy and trichoscopy in diseases of the brown skin: Atlas and Short Text. New Delhi: Jaypee Brothers Medical Publishers; 2012. p. 112–3.
3. Thatte SS, Khopkar US. The utility of dermoscopy in the diagnosis of evolving lesions of vitiligo. Indian J Dermatol Venereol Leprol. 2014;80:505–8.
4. Lee DY, Kim CR, Park JH, Lee JH. The incidence of leukotrichia in segmental vitiligo: implication of poor response to medical treatment. Int J Dermatol. 2011;50:925–7.
5. Chandrashekar L. Dermatoscopy of blue vitiligo. Clin Exp Dermatol. 2009;34:e125–6.
6. Di Chiacchio NG, Ferreira FR, de Alvarenga ML, Baran R. Nail trichrome vitiligo: case report and literature review. Br J Dermatol. 2013;168:668–9.
7. Bambroo M, Pande S, Khopkar US. Dermoscopy in the differentiation of idiopathic guttate hypomelanosis (IGH). In: Khopkar U, editor. Dermoscopy and trichoscopy in diseases of the brown skin: Atlas and Short Text. New Delhi: Jaypee Brothers Medical Publishers; 2012. p. 97–103.
8. Sonthalia S, Sarkar R, Arora R. Novel dermoscopic findings of perifollicular depigmentation and evolving leukotrichia in areas of clinically unaltered pigmentation: an early predictive sign of impending vitiligo. Pigment Int. 2014;1:28–30.
9. Meng RuSong M, Guang Z, RuiKang C, Xiao M, ZhiGuo J. Application of polarized light dermoscopy in the early diagnosis of vitiligo and its differential diagnosis from other depigmented diseases. Chin J Dermatol. 2009;42:810–3.
10. Errichetti E, Stinco G. Dermoscopy of idiopathic guttate hypomelanosis. J Dermatol. 2015;42:1118–9.

Chapter 23
The Histopathology of Vitiligo in Brown Skin

Johannes F. Dayrit

23.1 Importance of Histopathology in Vitiligo

The diagnosis of vitiligo based on clinical grounds is often straightforward when presentation is classical. However, when the presentation is atypical, cases should be referred for expert assessment by a dermatologist [1]. More commonly observed differential diagnoses of vitiligo in brown skin include chemical leukoderma, idiopathic guttate hypomelanosis, pityriasis alba, hypopigmented mycosis fungoides, and tuberculoid leprosy. Histopathology can confirm the diagnosis of vitiligo and can assist to differentiate it from other disorders in ambiguous cases [2].

In the assessment of histopathological findings of vitiligo in pigmented skin, it is important to remember that there is no variation in melanocyte concentration and density among races [3]. Melanosomes in pigmented skin, however, are noted to be distributed throughout the entire epidermis, with dense clusters in the basal layer and heavy pigmentation in the stratum corneum. In fair white skin, only few melanosomes are observed in the basal layer and the stratum malphigi [4–6].

The exact reason of melanocyte loss in vitiligo remains unclear and debatable, but more recent observations have implicated the role of cellular immunity in the pathogenesis [7].

J.F. Dayrit
Department of Dermatology, Research Institute for Tropical Medicine, Metro Manila, Philippines

Department of Internal Medicine, De La Salle University Medical Center, Cavite, Philippines
e-mail: yohannmdderm@gmail.com

E.B. Handog, M.J. Enriquez-Macarayo (eds.), *Melasma and Vitiligo in Brown Skin*,
DOI 10.1007/978-81-322-3664-1_23

23.2 Epidermis

A biopsy of vitiliginous skin (Fig. 23.1a) shows thinning of the epidermis in 53 % of cases [8], absence of melanocytes in the basal cell layer, and complete loss of melanin pigments (Fig. 23.1b). The advancing edge of the lesion may show larger melanocytes, often vacuolated with giant melanosomes and increased number of dendrites. Occasionally, a lymphocyte is present next to a melanocyte showing early apoptosis [9, 10] (Fig. 23.2a, b). Effacement of the dermoepidermal junction is present in 39 % of cases [8].

In a recent study done by Wang et al. [11] in 20 patients diagnosed with non-segmental vitiligo, the immunohistochemical marker Melan-A was used to quantify melanocytes in normal-appearing lesional skin, depigmented lesional skin, and the leading edge skin from vitiligo lesions. Abundant expression of Melan-A was observed in pigmented lesional skin, highlighting melanized keratinocytes and melanocytes found at the dermoepidermal junction (DEJ). By comparison,

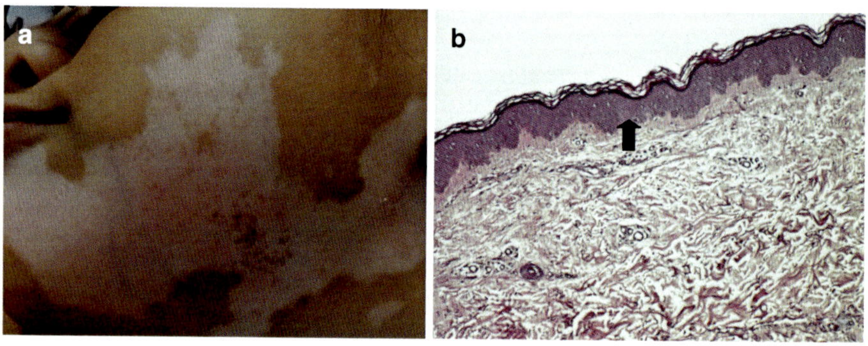

Fig. 23.1 Clinical picture of vitiligo in a Filipino (**a**) and histopathology (**b**) showing absence of melanocytes and melanin in the basal cell layer (*arrow*) (H & E, × 40)

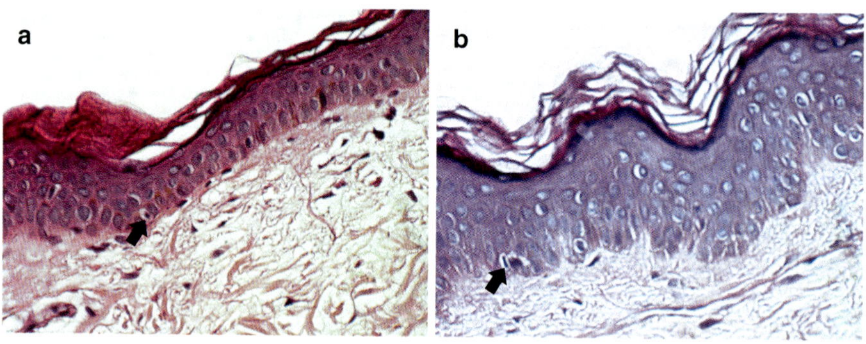

Fig. 23.2 (**a**) Melanocytes showing apoptosis (*arrow*) may be seen in some biopsies with either follicular repigmentation or at the edge of the lesion; (**b**) A lymphocyte (*arrow*) is present next to an apoptotic melanocyte (H & E, ×400)

melanocytes were absent, and no positivity was observed in depigmented lesional skin samples. However, staining of the leading edge of depigmented vitiligo skin showed fewer Melan-A-positive cells (Fig. 23.3a), which are apoptotic and show distorted cellular morphology (Fig. 23.3b, c).

The number of epidermal Langerhans cells is greater in the leading edge and lesional skin as compared to non-lesional skin, shown through the use of immunohistochemical markers CD207/Langerin and CD11c. The Langerhans cells reside in the lower half of the epidermis in contrast to non-lesional pigmented skin where they are uniformly distributed in the stratum malphigi. More mature and activated Langerhans cells are found in the leading edge vitiligo skin compared to non-lesional and depigmented lesional skin as demonstrated by the markers HLA-DR+ and DC-LAMP+ [11].

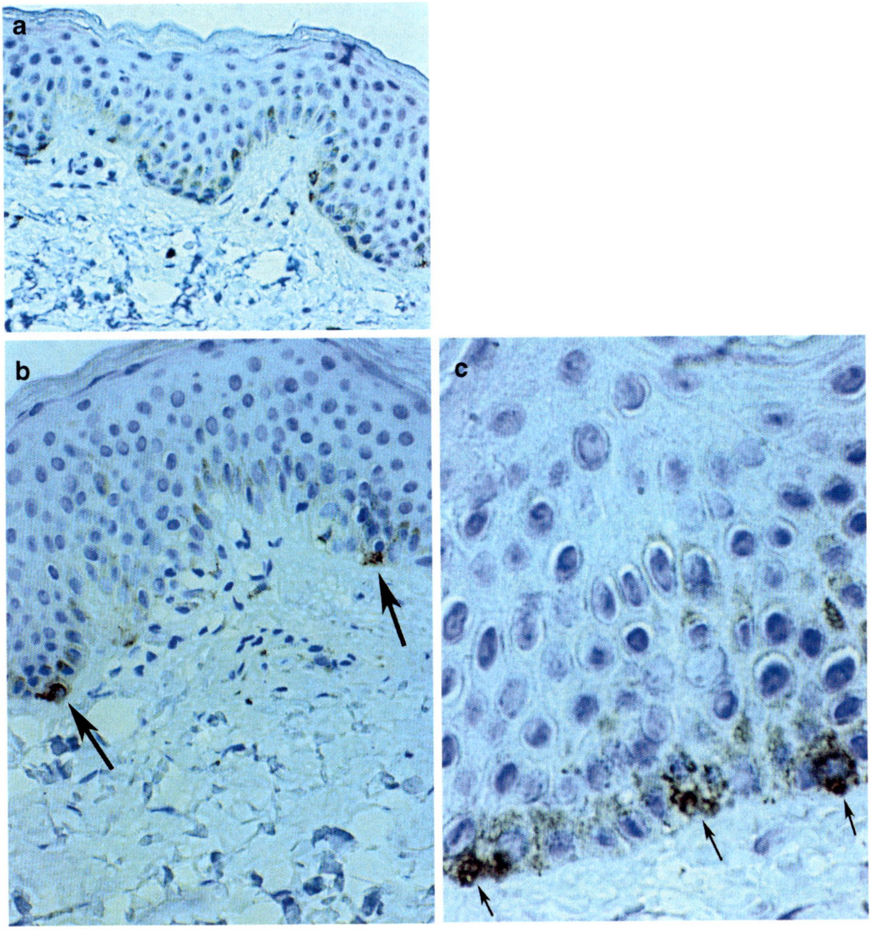

Fig. 23.3 Immunohistochemistry of the leading edge of depigmented vitiligo skin shows markedly decreased number of Melan-A-positive melanocytes in the basal cell layer (**a**) and highlights apoptotic melanocytes showing distorted morphology (*arrows*, **b**, **c**) (Melan-A stain ×400)

23.3 Dermis

A review of 74 vitiligo specimens revealed (1) perivascular mononuclear inflammatory cell infiltrates in 30 %, (2) sweat gland degeneration in 72 %, (3) sebaceous gland/hair follicle degeneration in 38 %, and (4) nerve degeneration in 78 % [8] (Fig. 23.4a). A mild lymphocytic infiltrate in the upper dermis is a common finding [12] (Fig. 23.4b).

By immunohistochemistry, the pan T-cell marker CD3+ and the cytotoxic CD8+ cells are observed in depigmented lesional skin, further suggesting T-cell-mediated cytotoxicity as one of the mechanisms for melanocyte killing. Also, majority of T cells are found to be both CD3+ and CD4 + (>60 %) [11]. At the leading edge skin of vitiligo lesions, the CD3+ cells are located in the papillary and upper reticular dermis where they form aggregates and are frequently observed to be hugging the basal cell layer or directly infiltrating the epidermis [11]. These cells correspond to the perivascular and focally lichenoid infiltrate of lymphocytes located close to the epidermis (Fig. 23.5a, b).

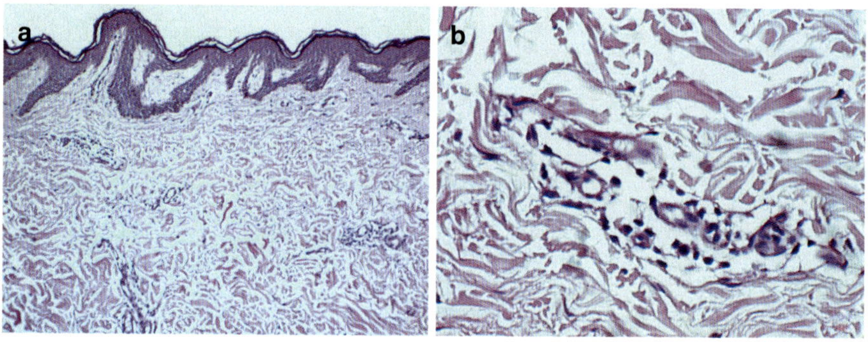

Fig. 23.4 (**a**) The dermis reveals decreased number of adnexal structures (H & E ×40) and (**b**) a mild predominantly lymphocytic inflammatory infiltrate (H & E ×400)

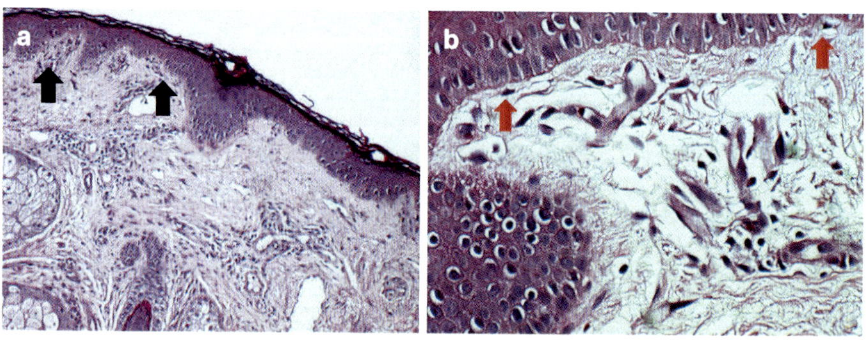

Fig. 23.5 (**a**) A biopsy on the advancing edge of the lesion shows mononuclear cells in the papillary dermis, either in clumps (*black arrows*, H & E ×40) or as single cells moving toward the epidermis (*red arrows*, H & E ×400)

23.4 Special Stains Used in Vitiligo

Useful special stains which can detect both active and dormant melanocytes include HMB45, Mel-5, and NKI/beteb. DOPA detects active melanocytes, and a pan-melanoma cocktail HMB45 + tyrosinase + MART-1 (Melan-A) can maximize yield [13–15].

For research purposes, T-cell CD markers CD3 and CD8 are used to highlight and quantify infiltrating and dermal lymphocytes. CD 207/Langerin, integrin CD11c, HLA-DR, DC-LAMP, and CD83 are additional immunohistochemical stains used to quantify and detect the activity of Langerhans and dermal dendritic cells.

23.5 Differential Diagnosis

23.5.1 Idiopathic Guttate Hypomelanosis (IGH)

IGH is characterized by 2–5 mm hypopigmented or porcelain-white macules usually seen on sun-exposed extremities of the elderly (Fig. 23.6a). Histopathologically, IGH is characterized by hyperkeratosis of the stratum corneum, atrophic epidermis with flattened rete ridges, decreased melanin content, and reduced melanocytes in the basal layer (Fig. 23.6b). In a study by Kim et al. [16] comparing lesional and normal skin, hyperkeratosis was a common feature in patients with IGH, but atrophic epidermis and flattened rete ridges were not. There was also a significantly decreased amount of melanin pigment and detectable melanocytes in the epidermal layers of IGH skin compared to normal skin. The decrease in pigmentation in IGH therefore could be due to decreased number and dysfunction of degenerative melanocytes in addition to a decreased number of melanosomes in some melanocytes.

IGH is thus characterized histopathologically by hyperkeratosis, decreased melanin, and melanocytes, in contrast to vitiligo where a complete loss of melanin pigment and absence of melanocytes are seen [9].

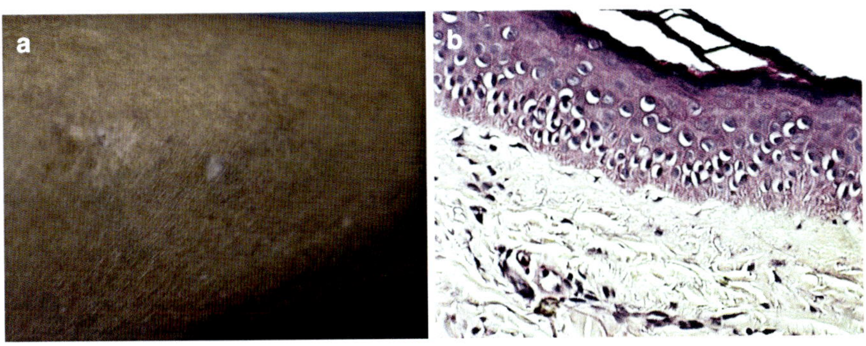

Fig. 23.6 (**a**) Clinical picture of idiopathic guttate hypomelanosis in brown skin and (**b**) histopathological findings of flattened rete ridges and markedly decreased number of melanocytes and melanin in the basal cell layer (H & E ×100)

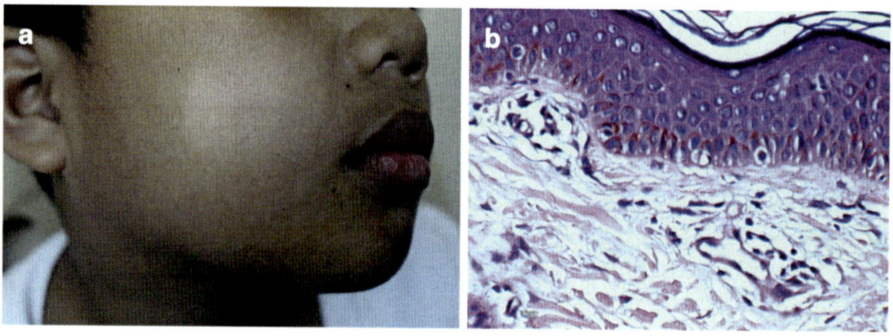

Fig. 23.7 (**a**) Pityriasis alba in a Filipino boy presenting as a hypopigmented patch on the cheeks and (**b**) histopathological findings of spongiosis and normal number of melanocytes in the basal cell layer (H & E ×400)

23.5.2 Pityriasis Alba (PA)

Pityriasis alba (PA) is characterized by variably hypopigmented slightly scaling patches seen on the face, neck, and shoulders of patients with or without atopic dermatitis (Fig. 23.7a). According to In et al. [17], biopsy specimens of patients assessed with PA revealed spongiosis with exocytosis, hyperkeratosis, and acanthosis in the epidermis; dermal perivascular lymphocytic infiltrates were seen, but not common. The main findings of PA are in the pilar apparatus and include follicular plugging, follicular spongiosis, and atrophic sebaceous glands. There were no significant differences in the number of melanocytes between lesional and normal skin, which both show a normal number of melanocytes in the basal cell layer (Fig. 23.7b). Electron microscopy also revealed degenerative changes in some melanocytes and a reduced number of melanosomes in the keratinocytes from lesional skin.

PA therefore is characterized histopathologically by follicular plugging, follicular spongiosis, atrophic sebaceous glands, degenerative changes in melanocytes, and reduced number of melanosomes, in contrast to vitiligo where a complete loss of melanin pigment and absence of melanocytes are seen [9].

23.5.3 Hypopigmented Mycosis Fungoides

Hypopigmented mycosis fungoides is a rare variant of MF commonly presenting in young and adolescent patients with darker skin types [18] (Fig. 23.8a). Clinically, lesions may mimic vitiligo, atopic dermatitis, postinflammatory hypopigmentation, leprosy, tinea versicolor, or pityriasis alba [19]. A high level of clinical suspicion is needed to make a diagnosis of this condition. Histologically, lesions present with epidermotropism of solitary or clusters of lymphocytes (Pautrier microabscesses) (Fig. 23.8b, c) which is predominantly CD4+ or in some cases CD8+ [20]. Other key diagnostic features include hydropic degeneration of basal cells, partial loss of

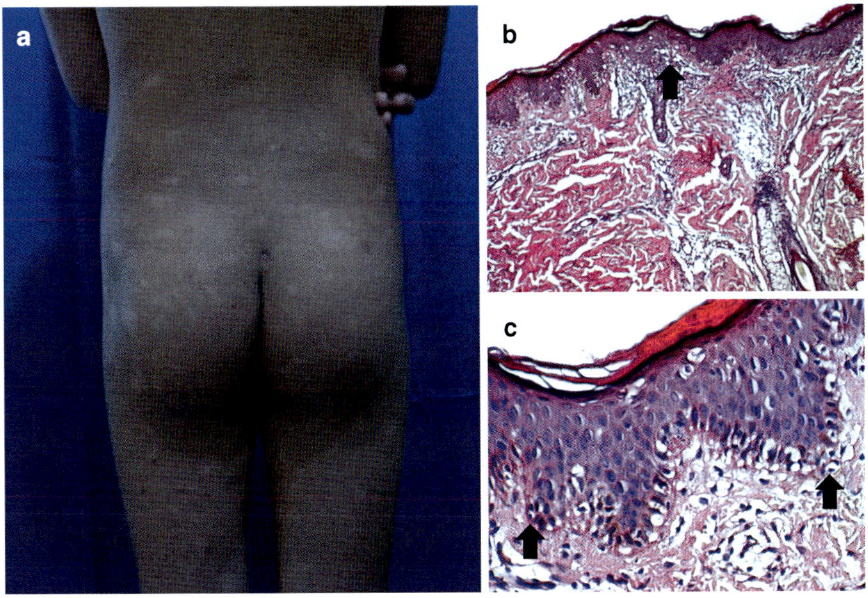

Fig. 23.8 (**a**) Hypopigmented mycosis fungoides in an 8-year-old Filipino girl with (**b**) epidermotropism of medium-sized, haloed lymphocytes in the lower part of the epidermis (H & E ×40). (**c**) The lymphocytes present as either clumps or "string of pearls" (*arrows*) and the underlying collagen appears wiry (H & E ×400)

pigment with preservation of melanocyte, and presence of lymphocytes within the papillary dermis [21]. Though the pathogenesis of this type of MF is not fully elucidated, the hypopigmentation may be attributed to the cytotoxic effect of the T-suppressor lymphocytes on melanocytes [19]. Patients have shown good response with topical mechlorethamine, PUVA, and UVB [18].

23.5.4 Indeterminate and Tuberculoid Leprosy

Hansen disease is a chronic infection caused by *Mycobacterium leprae* affecting mainly the skin and peripheral nerves. The disease is highly infective but with low virulence and a long incubation period [22]. The indeterminate type is the earliest form and most often overlooked clinically. Lesions present as single or multiple hypopigmented or faintly erythematous macules usually on the extremities with normal or impaired sensation [23]. Lesions of tuberculoid leprosy may be hypopigmented and resemble clinically indeterminate lesions (Fig. 23.9a). The presence of palpable induration, patches of erythema, and more prominent anesthesia, anhidrosis, and nerve enlargement distinguishes indeterminate lesions from tuberculoid lesions clinically. The characteristic histopathological findings include a superficial and deep dermal infiltrate around blood vessels, dermal appendages, and nerves

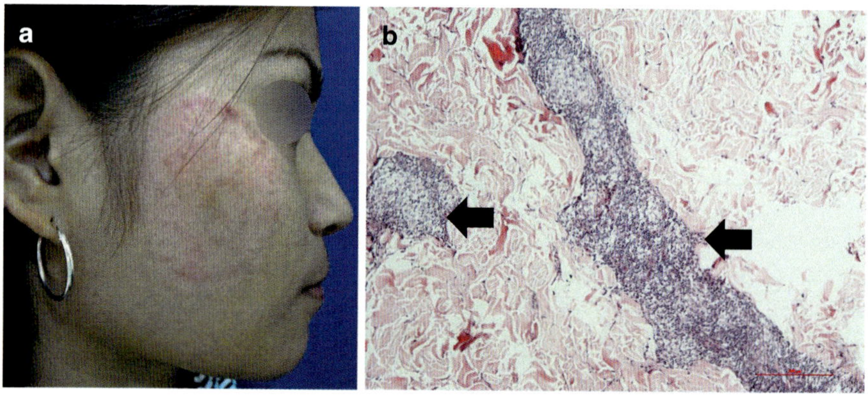

Fig. 23.9 (**a**) Clinical picture of tuberculoid leprosy presenting as a single, hypopigmented, and hypoesthetic patch on the cheek; (**b**) histopathology shows nodular and elongated epithelioid granulomas (*arrows*) surrounding adnexal structures and nerves (H & E ×100)

(Fig. 23.9b), composed predominantly of lymphocytes with few macrophages. Less than 5 % of the dermis is involved by the infiltrate. Scanty acid-fast bacilli may be seen in the perineural infiltrate, arrectores pilorum muscles, and the dermal nerves [24]. There is a decreased pigment in the basal cell layer and in some cases reduction in melanocytes was also reported. The pathogenesis of the hypopigmentation is still unknown [23].

23.6 Conclusion

Limited research and publications have been done on the histopathology of vitiligo in brown skin. A nonspecific diagnosis of postinflammatory pigmentary alteration (PIPA) is often issued in reports, which does not exactly validate the clinical impression of the dermatologist and may even be a source of controversy in some cases. Immunohistochemical studies should likewise be conducted to highlight the cellular immune elements which potentially drive the unique inflammatory responses, which eventually lead to apoptosis and loss of melanocytes.

References

1. Gawkordger DJ, Ormerod AD, Shaw L, Mauri-Sole I, Whitoon ME, Watts MJ, et al. Guideline for the diagnosis and management of vitiligo. Br J Dermatol. 2008;159:1051–76.
2. Montes LF, Abulafia J, Wilborn WH, Hyde BM, Montes CM. Value of histopathology in vitiligo. Int J Dermatol. 2003;42:57–61.
3. Szabo G. The number of melanocytes in human epidermis. Br Med J. 1954;1(4869):1004–2. 1016–17.

4. Kotrajaras R, Kligman AM. The effect of topical tretinoin on photodamaged facial skin: the Thai experience. Br J Dermatol. 1993;129:30.
5. Montagna W, Carlisle K. The architecture of black and white facial skin. J Am Acad Dermatol. 1991;24:929–37.
6. Herzberg AJ, Dinehart SM. Chronologic aging in black skin. Am J Dermatopathol. 1989;11:319–28.
7. Van den Boorn JG, Konijnenberg D, Dellemijn TA, van der Veen JP, Bos JD, et al. Autoimmune destruction of skin melanocytes by perilesional T cells from vitiligo patients. J Invest Dermatol. 2009;129(9):2220–32.
8. Gokhale BB, Mehta LN. Histopathology of vitiliginous skin. Int J Dermatol. 1983;22:477–80.
9. Weedon D. Disorders of pigmentation. In: Weedon D, editor. Skin pathology. 2nd ed. London: Churchill Livingstone; 2002. p. 323–4.
10. Kim YC, Kim YJ, Kang HY, Sohn S, Lee ES. Histopathologic features in vitiligo. Am J Dermatopathol. 2008;30:112–6.
11. Wang CQF, Cruz-Inigo AE, Fuentes-Duculan J, Moussai D, Gulati N, Sullivan-Whalen M, et al. TH17 cells and activated dendritic cells are increased in vitiligo lesions. PLoS One. 2011;6(4), e18907.
12. Horn TD, Abanmi A. Analysis of the lymphocytic infiltrate in a case of vitiligo. Am J Dermatopathol. 1997;19:400–2.
13. Alikhan A, Felsten LM, Daly M, Petronic-Rosic V. Vitiligo: a comprehensive overview. J Am Acad Dermatol. 2011;65:473–91.
14. Ortonne JP. Vitiligo and other disorders of hypopigmentation. In: Bolognia J, Jorizzo J, Rapini R, editors. Dermatology. Philadelphia: Mosby Elsevier; 2008. p. 178–9.
15. Bhawan J. Mel-5: a novel antibody for differential diagnosis of epidermal pigmented lesions of the skin in paraffin-embedded sections. Melanoma Res. 1997;7:43–8.
16. Kim SK, Kim EH, Kang HY, Lee ES, Sohn S, Kim YC. Comprehensive understanding of idiopathic guttate hypomelanosis: clinical and histopathological correlation. Int J Dermatol. 2010;49:162–6.
17. In SI, Yi SW, Kang HY, Lee ES, Sohn S, Kim YC. Clinical and histopathological characteristics of Pityriasis alba. British Association of Dermatologists. Clin Exp Dermatol. 2008;34: 591–7.
18. Akaraphanth R, Douglass MC, Lim HW. Hypopigmented mycosis fungoides: treatment and a 61/2-year follow up of 9 patients. J Am Acad Dermatol. 2000;42:33–9.
19. Ardigo M, Borroni G, Muscardin L, Kerl H, Cerroni L. Hypopigmented mycosis fungoides in Caucasian patients: a clinicopathologic study of 7 cases. J Am Acad Dermatol. 2003;49: 264–70.
20. Shabrawi-Caelen L, Cerroni L, Medeiros LJ, McCalmont TH. Hypopigmented mycosis fungoides: frequent expression of a CD8+ T-cell phenotype. Am J Surg Pathol. 2002;26:450–7.
21. El-Darouti MA, Marzouk SA, Azzam O, Fawzi MM, Abdel-Halim MR, Zayed AA, et al. Vitiligo vs. hypopigmented mycosis fungoides (histopathological and immunohistochemical study, univariate analysis). Eur J Dermatol. 2006;16(1):17–22.
22. Moschella SL. An update on the diagnosis and treatment of leprosy. J Am Acad Dermatol. 2004;51(3):417–26.
23. Weedon D, et al. Bacterial and rickettsial infection. In: Weedon D, editor. Skin pathology. London: Churchill Livingstone; 2002. p. 630–1.
24. Takahashi MD, Andrade HF, Wakamatsu A, Siqueira S, De Brito T. Indeterminate leprosy: histopathologic and histochemical predictive parameters involved in its possible change to paucibacillary or multibacillary leprosy. Int J Lepr Other Mycobact Dis. 1991;59:12–9.

Chapter 24
Differential Diagnosis of Vitiligo in Brown Skin

Ma. Teresita G. Gabriel, Gracia B. Teodosio, and Nani Kumala Dewi Tasmin

24.1 Introduction

Various conditions have similar clinical presentation with vitiligo. Alikhan et al. classified the different differential diagnosis of vitiligo into occupational iatrogenic chemical leukoderma, genetic syndromes, malformations, idiopathic, infections, neoplastic, and postinflammatory hypopigmentation [1]. Listed in Table 24.1 are the mimickers of vitiligo, as we see it among people with brown skin. Good history taking, a thorough physical examination, and the judicious use of histopathology generally yield a straightforward diagnosis.

24.2 Genetic Syndromes

24.2.1 Piebaldism

Piebaldism is an autosomal dominant disorder in tyrosine kinase transmembrane receptor of the melanocyte. This congenital condition is characterized by an extensive, symmetrically distributed depigmented areas. It has been reported in all races with equal sex distribution [2]. Midfrontal poliosis (Fig. 24.1) is seen in 80–90 % of cases. Depigmentation, however, may cover minimal to extensive areas of the entire body. Histopathology reveals a decreased number or total absence of melanocytes and melanin.

M.T.G. Gabriel, MD (✉) • G.B. Teodosio • N.K.D. Tasmin
Department of Dermatology, Research Institute of Tropical Medicine,
Alabang, Muntinlupa City, Philippines
e-mail: dermatologyritm@gmail.com; nkdewi.md@gmail.com

E.B. Handog, M.J. Enriquez-Macarayo (eds.), *Melasma and Vitiligo in Brown Skin*,
DOI 10.1007/978-81-322-3664-1_24

Camouflage or surgical grafting may be helpful and autologous noncultured epidermal cell transplantation has been reported with good result [2, 3].

Table 24.1 Mimickers of vitiligo among people with brown skin

Classification	Disease
Occupational leukoderma	Phenols and other derivatives
Genetic syndromes	Piebaldism
	Tuberous sclerosis
	Hypomelanosis of Ito
Malformations	Nevus anemicus
	Nevus depigmentosus
Idiopathic	Idiopathic guttate hypomelanosis
	Lichen sclerosus et atrophicus
Infections	Tinea versicolor
	Leprosy
	Syphilis
Neoplastic	Mycosis fungoides
	Halo nevus
Postinflammatory hypopigmentation	Pityriasis alba
	Atopic dermatitis/allergic contact dermatitis
	Phototherapy-induced hypopigmentation
	Hypopigmented scar
	Psoriasis
	Discoid lupus erythematosus
	Scleroderma
	Topical drug-induced depigmentation

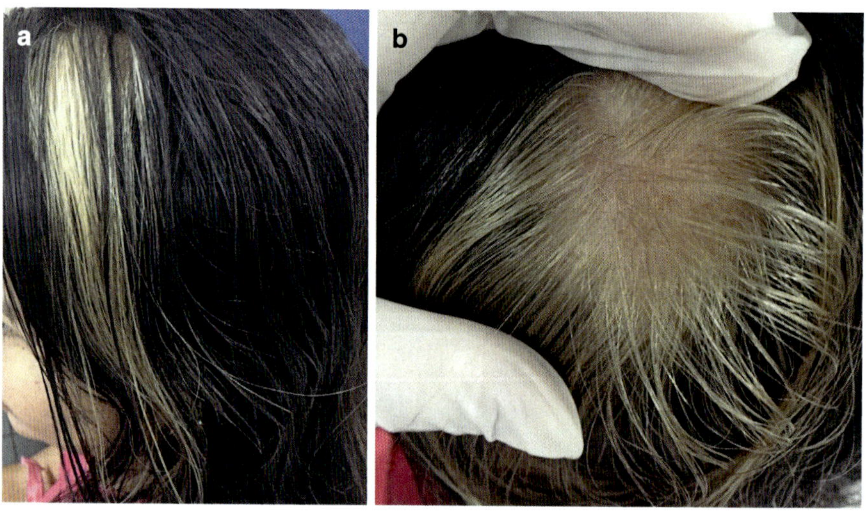

Fig. 24.1 Midfrontal poliosis in a Filipina with piebaldism

24.2.2 Tuberous Sclerosis

Tuberous sclerosis complex (TSC) is an autosomal dominant multisystem neurocutaneous syndrome with characteristic features of multiple hamartomas distributed throughout the skin, central nervous system (CNS), eye, heart, kidney, liver, and lungs. Two-thirds of cases are sporadic. The true incidence of this condition is unknown but reports were between 1 in 5,800 and 1 in 10,000 [4].

There are two different types of hypopigmented macules in TSC: medium- to large-sized hypopigmented macules and tiny confetti-like macules. The ash-leaf macule/spot, which can be mistaken for a vitiligo lesion, is the most characteristic type of hypopigmented lesion in TSC. It is lance-ovate shaped, often linear, usually 1.0–12 cm in diameter, with one end rounded and the other sharp tipped (Fig. 24.2). This typical lesion predilects the trunk and buttocks.

The confetti-like lesions (Fig. 24.2, *arrows*) are characterized by tiny 1–3 mm white spots, symmetrically distributed, typically over the extremities. The hypopigmentation is enhanced by Wood's lamp examination. Histopathology reveals reduction in the number of melanocytes and a decrease in melanosome size and epidermal melanin.

There are notable cutaneous findings in TSC, not evident in vitiligo. Facial angiofibromas are benign hamartomas pathognomonic of TSC, which appear as multiple smooth, firm, pink, 1–5-mm papules over the nasolabial folds, cheeks, and chin (Fig. 24.3a). Shagreen patch is a connective tissue nevus appearing as skin-colored to yellow plaques with irregular pebbled surface and is typically located over the back and buttocks (Fig. 24.3b). Periungual fibromas or angiofibromas are seen as conical, pink, firm projections from the proximal nail folds of fingers and toes which usually arise during puberty.

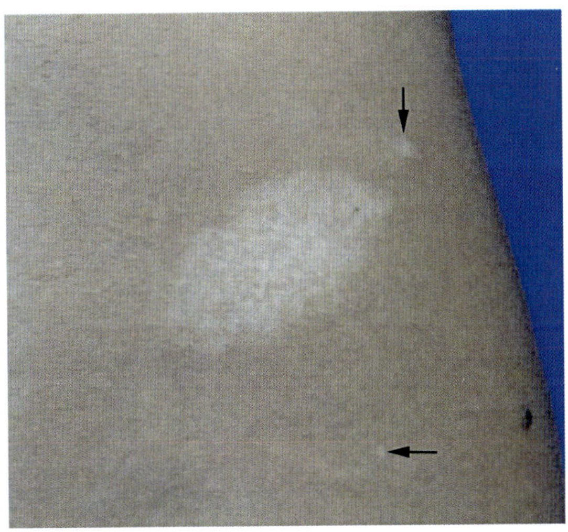

Fig. 24.2 Hypomelanotic patch in TSC: notice the large ash-leaf spot and small confetti-like lesions (*arrows*) on the left thigh of a Filipino patient

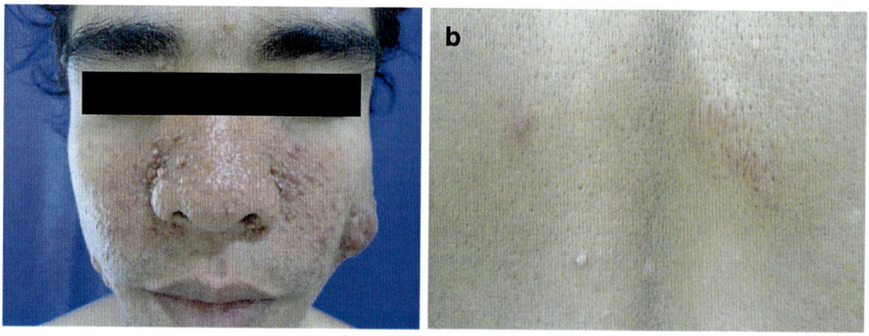

Fig. 24.3 Filipino male with facial angiofibromas on the nasolabial folds (**a**) and shagreen patches on the back (**b**)

Extracutaneous manifestations, if present in TSC, differentiate it further from vitiligo:

- CNS: Tumors producing seizures such as cortical tubers, periventricular calcification, subependymal hamartomas, astrocytomas, infantile spasms, and mental retardation.
- Eye: Retinal hamartomas (phakomas) are seen in 50 % of patients with tuberous sclerosis which appear as gray to yellow plaques on the retina.
- Heart: Cardiac rhabdomyoma.
- Kidney, liver, thyroid, testes, and GIT: Hamartomas of mixed cell type.
- Others: Angiomyolipoma, multiple renal cysts, enamel pits, gingival fibromas, phalangeal cysts, periosteal thickening, and pulmonary cysts.

The management of TSC is presently symptomatic. However, some recent therapeutic trials of mammalian target of rapamycin (mTOR) pathway antagonists such as rapamycin (sirolimus) showed potential therapeutic options for TSC patients [4].

24.3 Malformations

24.3.1 Nevus Anemicus

Nevus anemicus (Fig. 24.4) usually presents at birth with an irregularly shaped hypochromic patch, varying from one to several centimeters in size. The contrast with the surrounding non-lesional skin disappears upon application of pressure [5]. Highly sensitive α-adrenergic receptors of endothelial cells in the affected areas lead to vasoconstriction of small vessels; E-selectin expression is reported to be decreased [6]. Emotional stress and physical activities are shown to be trigger factors. The lesion is usually found on the trunk but the face and extremities may be affected. No abnormal findings are noted on histopathologic evaluation, differentiating it from vitiligo. No treatment is needed for this condition.

Fig. 24.4 Nevus anemicus on the back of a 25-year-old Filipino male. Histopathology showed normal skin findings

Fig. 24.5 Nevus depigmentosus, isolated variant, present at birth in a Filipino patient

24.3.2 Nevus Depigmentosus

Nevus depigmentosus presents as a well-circumscribed irregularly bordered hypopigmented macule or patch that becomes visible from birth or during the first year of life. It presents as hypopigmentation rather than depigmentation, in contrast to vitiligo. It remains stable in its relative size and distribution throughout life. A defect in the transfer of melanosomes from melanocytes to keratinocytes has been reported [7]. There are three clinical variants: isolated (solitary and well-defined lesion) (Fig. 24.5), segmental (unilateral, band-shaped, Blaschkoid distribution lesions), and systematized form (extensive, whorls, and streaks of hypopigmentation following the lines of Blaschko). Nevus depigmentosus is usually not associated with any systemic manifestations. However, the variants manifesting with the Blaschkoid pattern have been associated with developmental disorder and epilepsy. Histopathology reveals marked reduction of melanin with variable melanocyte count (normal to decreased).

Camouflage may be required. Surgical grafting has been reported with poor to good repigmentation; recurrence was noted during follow-up [3].

24.4 Idiopathic

24.4.1 Idiopathic Guttate Hypomelanosis

Idiopathic guttate hypomelanosis (IGH) is a common, benign, idiopathic leukodermic dermatosis, which manifests as asymptomatic, small, 0.2–1.6 cm, achromic, or hypopigmented macules on the sun-exposed areas of the upper and lower extremities (Fig. 24.6). Patients usually have associated signs of photoaging, including atrophy, lentigines, and xerosis. This condition is commonly seen among the elderly, over the age of 50, with female predisposition [8].

The pathogenesis of IGH is not completely understood, but a multifactorial etiology is more likely to be involved, such as senile degeneration, sunlight exposure, and trauma. On histopathology, slight basket-weave hyperkeratosis with epidermal atrophy and flattening of the rete ridges is seen. There is a decrease in melanocytes and epidermal melanin with irregular distribution of pigment granules.

Vitiligo differs from IGH in terms of both age of onset and the size and distribution of lesions. Together with sun protection, reassurance is required in most

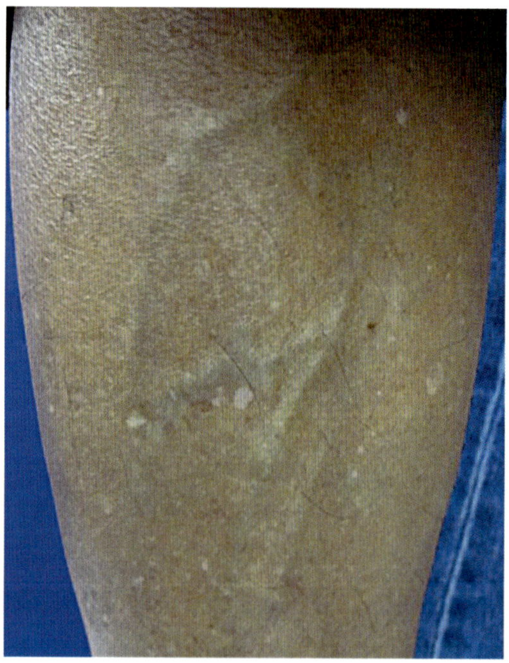

Fig. 24.6 Idiopathic guttate hypomelanosis on the right forearm of a 65-year-old male gardener

patients with IGH. Topical tretinoin, steroids, and calcineurin inhibitors have been proposed to improve the lesions of IGH. However, careful destruction using trichloroacetic acid, liquid nitrogen, or superficial dermabrasion is the most effective treatment [9, 10]. Some reports also showed promising result with fractional CO_2 laser [11].

24.5 Infections

24.5.1 Leprosy (Hansen's Disease)

Leprosy is a chronic mycobacterial infection of the skin and peripheral nerves that is caused by *Mycobacterium leprae*. According to the World Health Organization (WHO), endemic countries for leprosy are India, Brazil, Indonesia, Nigeria, Ethiopia, Bangladesh, and other countries in Southeast Asia, Africa, and Western Pacific region [12]. The Ridley-Jopling classification divided the disease into tuberculoid (TT), borderline (BT, BB, BL), and lepromatous leprosy (LL). The WHO supports only two spectrums, based on the number of acid-fast bacilli (AFB) found in the tissues: paucibacillary (PB) and multibacillary (MB) leprosy. The lesions of leprosy may manifest as solitary to multiple hypopigmented patches (Fig. 24.7) with hypoesthesia and sometimes accompanied by enlargement of peripheral nerve or palsy. Histopathological examination reveals granulomatous dermal infiltrate of predominant foamy histiocytes in perivascular, periadnexal, and perineural areas with or without grenz zone. A definite diagnosis of leprosy requires demonstration of a consistent peripheral nerve abnormality or AFB in tissues. Slit-skin smear

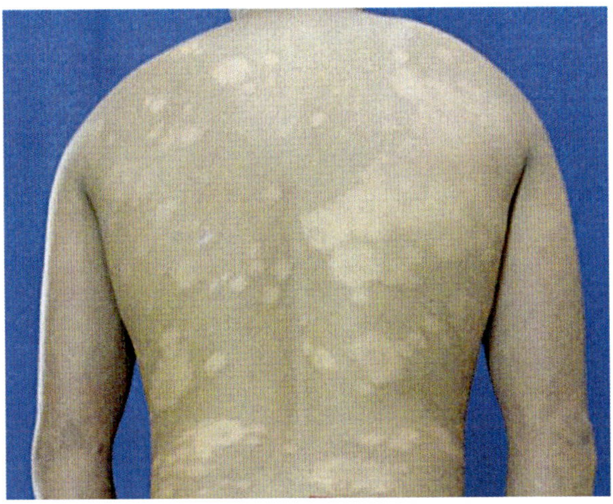

Fig. 24.7 Multiple hypoesthetic hypopigmented patches in a 36-year-old Filipino male with lepromatous leprosy

examination with modified Ziehl-Neelsen stain will help to demonstrate the AFB. Absence of hypoesthesia, nerve abnormalities, and distinct histopathology findings clearly distinguish vitiligo from leprosy.

The WHO recommended the use of multidrug therapy program for treating PB (rifampicin, dapsone) and MB (rifampicin, clofazimine, and dapsone) leprosy with satisfactory results. However, with the emergence of resistant cases, treatment failures have been reported. Options for these cases are the use of other bactericidal agents as clarithromycin, minocycline, and ofloxacin.

24.5.2 Tinea Versicolor

Tinea versicolor is a superficial fungal infection caused by dimorphic, lipophilic organisms in the genus *Malassezia*, formerly known as *Pityrosporum*. This saprophytic yeast, known to be a normal commensal organism of the skin, may be converted to its parasitic form, resulting in the manifestation of the disease. Predisposing factors are genetic predisposition, warm humid environments, immunosuppression, and malnutrition.

Multiple hypopigmented macules or patches with fine dust-like superficial scaling seen in tinea versicolor (Fig. 24.8) differentiate it from vitiligo. The trunk, upper back, abdomen, and proximal extremities are mostly affected. Wood's lamp examination reveals a yellowish fluorescence. Histopathology discloses mild hyperkeratosis and acanthosis of the epidermis with a mild dermal perivascular infiltrate. Periodic acid-Schiff (PAS) stain helps to detect the organism. On potassium hydroxide (KOH) 10 % examination of skin scrapings, the characteristic fungal spores and cigar-butt hyphae appear as "spaghetti and meatballs."

Several topical antifungal agents may prove useful in the management of tinea versicolor: zinc pyrithione, ciclopirox olamine, sodium sulfacetamide, selenium sulfide 2.5 %, ketoconazole 2 %, terbinafine solution 1 %, and sertaconazole [13].

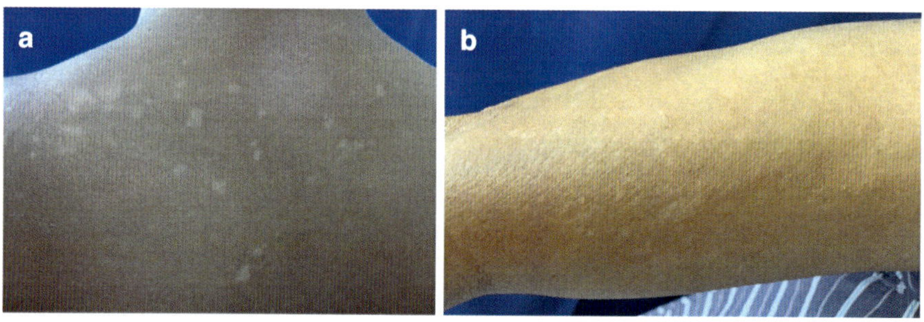

Fig. 24.8 Tinea versicolor on Filipino male patients, presenting as hypopigmented lesions with fine scales on the upper back (**a**) and arm (**b**)

24.6 Neoplastic

24.6.1 Mycosis Fungoides

Mycosis fungoides (MF) is the most common type of cutaneous T-cell lymphoma, usually arising in mid-to-late adulthood. The stages are categorized based on the typical cutaneous manifestations such as patch, plaque, and tumor stages. The early patch stage is more frequently observed among the younger population and darker-skinned individuals. The lesions present as multiple, irregular with indistinct border, hypopigmented macules and patches occasionally associated with pruritus (Fig. 24.9). Distribution of lesions is more common in sun-protected areas [14]. Lymph nodes and visceral organs can be involved in the advanced stage. Characteristic histopathologic findings in MF are atypical lymphocytic cells with cerebriform nuclei, epidermotropism, and Pautrier's abscess. Melanin may be reduced or absent with mild or marked pigmentary incontinence. Inflammatory nonspecific response to cell injury leads to the degeneration of melanocytes and abnormal melanogenesis, leading to the development of hypopigmented MF lesions. At its early stage, the histopathology can be nonspecific and can be similar with other inflammatory disorders. Immunohistochemistry and clonal T-cell receptor arrangement are helpful in establishing the diagnosis.

Patch stage MF is highly responsive to PUVA and narrowband UVB phototherapy, although recurrences were reported after discontinuation of therapy [15].

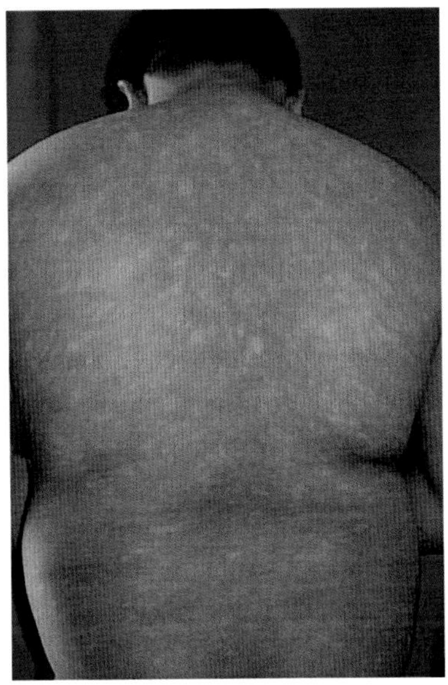

Fig. 24.9 Hypopigmented patches of mycosis fungoides in a 46-year-old Filipino male. Histopathology revealed the presence of Pautrier's microabscesses

24.6.2 Halo Nevus

Halo nevus (HN) is a nevomelanocytic nevus (NMN) encircled by a depigmentation area. It usually appears before adulthood and occurs spontaneously in 1 % of population, without sex and race preponderance [16]. The halo appearance indicates regression of the central nevus, which is produced by an immunologic reaction. It is commonly associated with benign acquired melanocytic nevi, nonmelanocytic tumors, basal cell carcinomas, and even metastatic melanoma [17]. The association of halo nevus with vitiligo remains unclear. However, the incidence of halo nevus in vitiligo is higher than the normal population (3.75 %) [16].

This nevus usually manifests as > 5 mm centrally located brown papular NMN with an oval to round sharply marginated hypomelanosis (Fig. 24.10). Wood's lamp examination usually reveals depigmentation of the halo. Progression of lesion may be divided into three stages: (1) development of a white halo surrounding a preexisting MN, which may be preceded by faint erythema (months); (2) disappearance of the MN (months to years); and (3) repigmentation of the halo area (months to years).

Aouthmany et al. have reported that 51 % of HN remained stable. There was partial nevus regression and persistence of halo in 14.3 %, complete involution of the nevus with persistent halo depigmentation in 4.1 %, some repigmentation of the halo in 8.2 %, and complete repigmentation in 22.4 % of HN cases [16].

Histopathology examination on the halo area shows decrease or total absence of melanin and melanocytes. There is a dense lymphocytic infiltrate within the dermis surrounding surviving nevus cells in nests or singly among the lymphocytes with evidence of cell damage or apoptosis.

Majority of HN lesions are benign. Therefore, reassurance and observation are recommended to avoid discomfort and scarring from surgical intervention [16]. Excision of the nevus is indicated if there are atypical features such as color variegation and irregular borders [18].

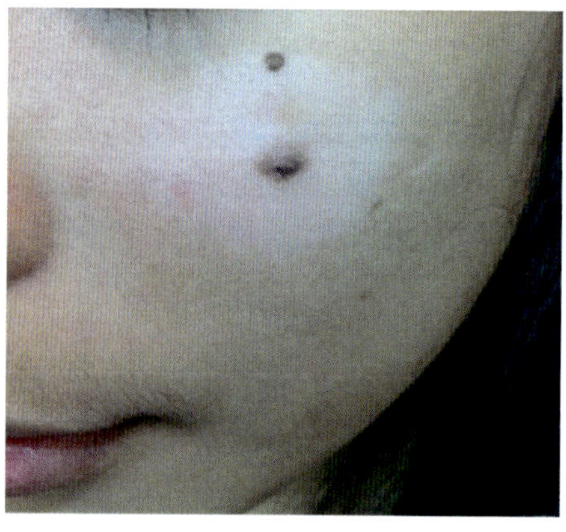

Fig. 24.10 Halo nevus on the left cheek of a 23-year-old Filipino female

24.7 Postinflammatory Hypopigmentation

24.7.1 From Preceding Inflammatory Skin Disorders

Hypopigmentation (Fig. 24.11) may be seen following several inflammatory processes such as psoriasis, atopic and nummular dermatitis, and bacterial and fungal infections. Lesions are seen on the sites of previous inflammation. The borders of the lesions are usually irregular and ill to well defined. Melanocytes are normal in number but melanin production is decreased.

Resultant hypopigmentation is usually reversible. Reassurance, application of emollients, and phototherapy are usually helpful.

24.7.2 Pityriasis Alba

Pityriasis alba (PA) is a common pigmentary disorder that is associated with atopic dermatitis. This condition, mostly observed in children and young adults, affects all skin types but is more prominent in darker-skinned individuals. The hypopigmentation seen is more apparent in summer and fades during winter. The etiology is still poorly understood, but dryness of the skin may have an important role in the development of postinflammatory hypopigmentation in this condition [19]. Sun exposure, frequent bathing, and hot baths are highly associated with the development of pityriasis alba.

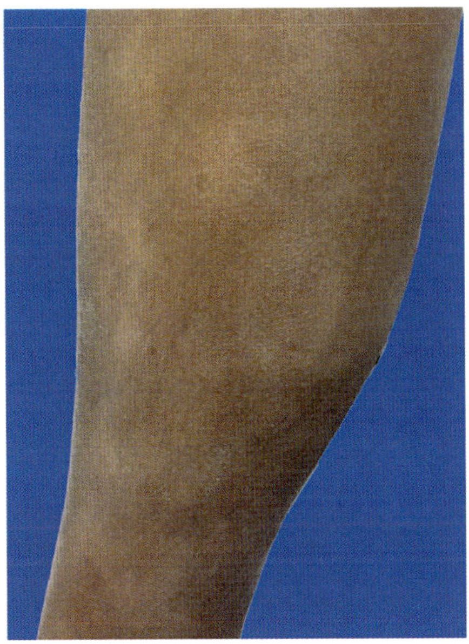

Fig. 24.11 Postinflammatory hypopigmentation on the left leg of a Filipino male patient with atopic dermatitis

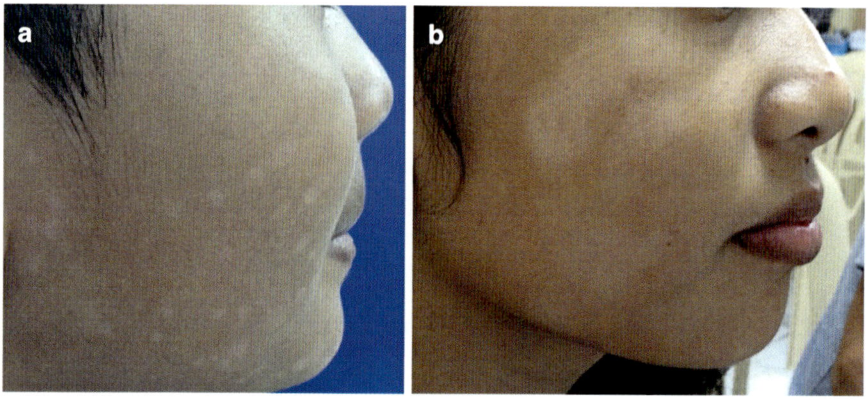

Fig. 24.12 Pityriasis alba clinically seen as multiple macules on the face in a Filipino boy (**a**) and patches in a 20-year-old Filipina (**b**)

PA presents with round, oval to irregular-shaped, ill-defined hypopigmented macules (Fig. 24.12a) and patches (Fig. 24.12b) with slight or no pruritus. Early lesions can be pinkish with elevated borders and progressively become hypopigmented with powdery white scales. Any skin area can be affected, but the face and neck regions are the most frequent sites. Histopathology shows hyperkeratosis, some parakeratosis, and markedly reduced melanin in basal cell layers of the epidermis, with normal melanocyte count. Slight perivascular lymphocytic infiltrate and edema of the upper dermis are usually noted. In Wood's lamp examination, the lesions are not totally amelanotic in contrast to vitiligo.

Pityriasis alba is a self-limited disease, but topical steroids and emollients are helpful in early lesions. Avoiding sun exposure, use of sunscreens, and reducing the frequency and temperature of baths should be recommended [19].

24.7.3 Discoid Lupus Erythematosus

Discoid lupus erythematosus (DLE) is a discoid variant of chronic cutaneous lupus erythematosus (CCLE) with potential scarring and disfigurement. DLE, the most common variant of CCLE, is found in 15–30% of systemic lupus erythematosus (SLE) patients. The age of onset is usually between 20 and 40 years of age with female preponderance. DLE can affect all races but it is more prevalent among people with color [20]. Pathogenesis of DLE is not completely understood, but reports suggested the involvement of factors such as ultraviolet irradiation, autoantibody generation, T cell, dendritic cells, and other immune cell dysfunction.

Clinical presentation of DLE is asymptomatic to painful, erythematous to violaceous, scaly papules and plaques with follicular plugging and can progress to cause disfiguring, scarred, atrophic, and dyspigmented plaques with alopecia. In patients with colored skin, marked hypopigmentation (Fig. 24.13) and hyperpigmentation are usually seen, and the clinical manifestations are more severe. The face (eyebrows, eyelids, nose, and lips), scalp, ears, V-area of the neck, and extensor aspects

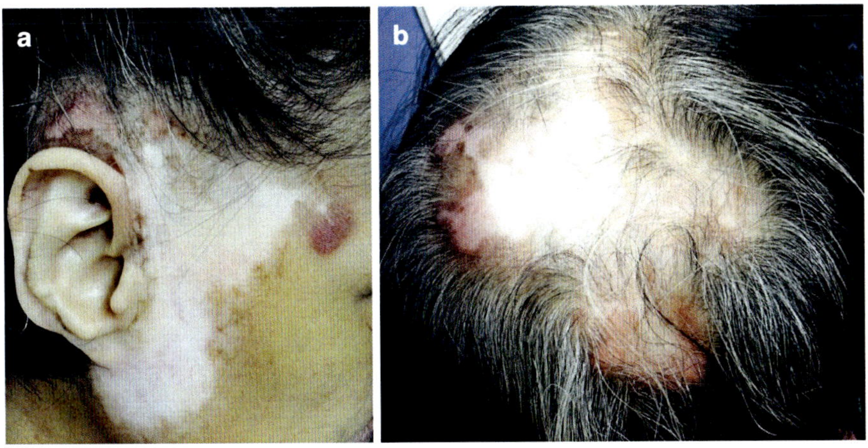

Fig. 24.13 Filipino patients with DLE – hypopigmented lesion on the preauricular area (**a**) and scalp (**b**)

of the arms are usually affected. Histopathology examination reveals hyperkeratosis, follicular plugging, epidermal atrophy, vacuolar degeneration of basal cell layer, apoptotic keratinocytes, and a dense perivascular and periadnexal infiltrate. Thickening of basement membrane, pigment incontinence, and dermal mucin deposition may also be seen.

Triggering factors include oral medications (i.e., procainamide, hydralazine, isoniazid, minocycline, and acebutolol), smoking, and UV exposure. The first-line treatment for DLE lesions is topical and intralesional corticosteroids and hydroxychloroquine. Topical calcineurin inhibitors are also reported to be useful in DLE. In severe and recalcitrant cases, systemic therapies, such as corticosteroids, retinoids, dapsone, methotrexate, cyclosporine, and mycophenolate mofetil, may be required [9].

24.7.4 Scleroderma

Scleroderma is an inflammatory connective tissue disorder characterized by excessive accumulation of collagen in the dermis. It may extend to the subcutaneous tissue and fascia, producing thickening and hardening of the skin. The lesions may be circumscribed, linear, deep, or generalized. The initial erythematous to violaceous indurated plaques with violaceous borders may gradually become ivory in color. Hypopigmentation can develop in chronic sclerosis with perifollicular pigmentary retention (salt-and-pepper appearance) which is highly suggestive of systemic scleroderma and can be the early sign preceding the sclerosis [21, 22]. Sites of predilection for hypopigmented lesions are the anterior chest, legs, forearms, hands (Fig. 24.14), and distal fingers. Contracture, cosmetic, or functional deformity, limb length discrepancy, and associated systemic disease (arthritis, pulmonary hypertension, chronic renal insufficiency) may develop and cause significant morbidity.

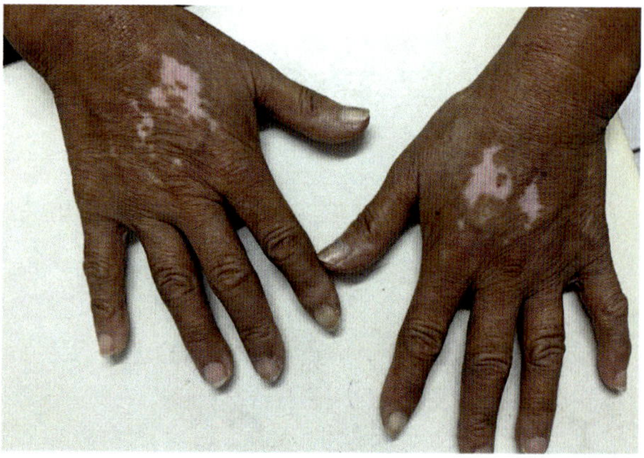

Fig. 24.14 Hypopigmented patches on both dorsal aspects of the hands in a 53-year-old Filipino patient with scleroderma. There is associated induration of the upper extremities. Histopathologic findings were consistent with scleroderma

Histopathology reveals atrophy of epidermis, decreased epidermal melanin, and dermal fibrosis with thickening of collagen bundles sometimes extending to subcutaneous tissue. Sung et al. reported some cases of juvenile localized scleroderma with vitiligo-like hypopigmented lesions. Immunohistochemistry with Melan-A and Fontana-Masson staining revealed a decrease in melanocyte count at the dermoepidermal junction (DEJ). CD3 and CD8 were increased at the DEJ of hypopigmented scleroderma lesion, suggesting this to be the cause of immune-mediated loss of melanocytes in vitiligo. Hypopigmented scleroderma lesion can be distinguished from vitiligo by immunostaining evaluation, showing decrease in CD34 at the fibrotic area and increase in FXIIIA at the papillary and/or reticular dermis.

Treatment of active localized lesions of scleroderma includes high-potent topical steroid or tacrolimus. PUVA, methotrexate, and systemic steroids are reserved for deep, generalized, and systemic scleroderma [23].

24.8 Conclusion

There are various diseases that mimic vitiligo ranging from genetic conditions to malformations, infections, occupational, neoplastic, as well as idiopathic causes and disorders giving rise to postinflammatory hypopigmentation. It is imperative to get a complete history, perform a detailed physical examination to include associated signs and symptoms, and correlate with histopathologic examination to reach an accurate diagnosis. Important ancillary procedures may aid in confirming the diagnosis.

References

1. Alikhan A, Felsten LM, Daly M, Petronic-Rosic V. Vitiligo: a comprehensive overview. J Am Acad Dermatol. 2011;65:473–91.
2. Oiso N, Fukai K, Kawada A, Suzuki T. Piebaldism. J Dermatol. 2013;40:330–5.

3. Van Geel N, Wallaeys E, Goh BK, De Mil M, Lambert J. Long term results of non-cultured epidermal cellular grafting in vitiligo, halo nevi, piebaldism and nevus depigmentosus. Br J Dermatol. 2010;163:1186–93.
4. Schwartz RA, Fernandez G, Kotulska K, Jozwiak S. Tuberous sclerosis complex: advances in diagnosis, genetics, and management. J Am Acad Dermatol. 2007;57:189–202.
5. Marque M, Roubertie A, Jaussent A, Carneiro A, Meunier L, Guillot B, et al. Nevus anemicus in neurofibromatosis type 1: a potential new diagnostic criterion. J Am Acad Dermatol. 2013;69:768–75.
6. Mizutani H, Ohyanagi S, Umeda Y, Shimizu M, Kupper TS. Loss of cutaneous delayed hypersensitivity reactions in nevus anemicus: evidence for close concordance of cutaneous delayed hypersensitivity and endothelial E-selectin expression. Arch Dermatol. 1997;133:617–20.
7. Kim SK, Kang HY, Lee ES, Kim YC. Clinical and histopathologic characteristics of nevus depigmentosus. J Am Acad Dermatol. 2006;55:423–8.
8. Shin MK, Jeong KH, Oh IH, Choe BK, Lee MH. Clinical features of idiopathic guttate hypomelanosis in 646 subjects and association with other aspects of photoaging. Int J Dermatol. 2011;50:798–805.
9. Passeron T, Ortonne JP. Atlas of pigmentary disorder. Switzerland: Springer International Publishing; 2014. p. 175, 153.
10. Rerknimitr P, Disphanurat W, Achariyakul M. Topical tacrolimus significantly promotes repigmentation in idiopathic guttate hypomelanosis: a double-blind, randomized, placebo-controlled study. J Eur Acad Dermatol Venereol. 2013;27:460–4.
11. Shin J, Kim M, Park SH, Oh SH. The effect of fraction carbon dioxide lasers on idiopathic guttate hypomelanosis: a preliminary study. J Eur Acad Dermatol Venereol. 2013;27:e243–6.
12. World Health Organization. Global leprosy: update on the 2012 situation. Wkly Epidemiol Rec. 2013;88:365–79.
13. Kundu RV, Garg A. Yeast infections: Candidiasis, Tinea (Pityriasis) Versicolor, and Malassezia (Pityrosporum) Folliculitis. In: Goldsmith LA, Katz SI, Gilchrest BA, Paller AS, Leffel DJ, Wolff K, editors. Fitzpatrick's dermatology in general medicine. 8th ed. New York: McGraw-Hill Companies, Inc; 2012. p. 2308–10.
14. Akaraphanth R, Douglass MC, Lim HW. Hypopigmented mycosis fungoides: treatment and 61/2 year follow-up of 9 patients. J Am Acad Dermatol. 2000;42:33–9.
15. Kanokrungsee S, Vachiramon V. Hypopigmented mycosis fungoides treated with narrowband UVB: A10-year retrospective study. J Am Acad Dermatol. 2011;64(2 Suppl 1):AB114.
16. Aouthmany M, Weinstein M, Zirwas MJ, Brodell RT. The natural history of halo nevi: a retrospective case series. J Am Acad Dermatol. 2012;67:582–6.
17. James WD, Berger TG, Elston DM. Melanocytic nevi and neoplasms. In: James WD, Berger TG, Elston DM, editors. Andrews' diseases of the skin: clinical dermatology. London: Saunders Elsevier; 2011. p. 680.
18. Wolff K, Johnson RA. Fitzpatrick's color atlas & synopsis of clinical dermatology. 6th ed. New York: McGraw-Hill; 2009. p. 183–4.
19. Lin RL, Janniger CK. Pityriasis alba. Cutis. 2005;76:21–4.
20. Jones TE, Drenkard C, Bao GB, Lim S, Parker S. Incidence of discoid lupus erythematosus without systemic lupus: data from the Georgia lupus registry. J Am Acad Dermatol. 2013;68(4):AB71. p. 5935.
21. Sung JJ, Chen TS, Gilliam AC, McCalmont TH, Gilliam AE. Clinicohistopathological correlations in juvenile localized scleroderma: studies on a subset of children with hypopigmented juvenile localized scleroderma due to loss of epidermal melanocytes. J Am Acad Dermatol. 2011;65:364–73.
22. Rai VM, Balachandran C. Pseudovitiligo in systemic sclerosis. Dermatol Online J. 2005;11:41.
23. Zwischenberger BA, Jacobe HT. A systematic review of morphea treatments and therapeutic algorithm. J Am Acad Dermatol. 2011;65:925–41.

Chapter 25
Comorbidities in Vitiligo

Rahul Mahajan and M. Ramam

25.1 Introduction

Vitiligo occurs due to a complex interaction among genetic, environmental and immunologic factors. This ultimately leads to melanocyte damage resulting in the characteristic depigmented lesions. The prevalence of vitiligo varies from 0.5 to 3 % in different regions of the world [1]. Although the disease is typically asymptomatic and nonfatal, the profound cosmetic disfigurement it produces has a significant negative impact on the patient's quality of life. This often leads to a sense of humiliation and loss of self-esteem. The disease has been classified variably on the basis of age of onset (into early/prepubertal or late/post-pubertal onset) and on the extent of involvement. Half of all patients develop the disease before 20 years of age [2].

Many patients with vitiligo exhibit other dermatologic as well as systemic diseases. However, the association of comorbidities and vitiligo is complex and multifactorial. The linkage is subject to a number of biases and confounding factors such as age of onset, lifestyle factors, impaired health-related quality of life, depression and therapeutic interventions. Table 25.1 enumerates the various diseases commonly associated with vitiligo. Some of these associations can be explained on the basis of shared immunopathogenesis of the two diseases; others are mere co-occurrences as random events. The present chapter focuses on the various disease associations of vitiligo.

R. Mahajan • M. Ramam (✉)
Department of Dermatology and Venereology, All India Institute of Medical Sciences, New Delhi, India
e-mail: drrahulpgi@yahoo.com; mramam@hotmail.com

E.B. Handog, M.J. Enriquez-Macarayo (eds.), *Melasma and Vitiligo in Brown Skin*,
DOI 10.1007/978-81-322-3664-1_25

Table 25.1 Diseases associated with vitiligo

1. Autoimmune disorders	
1.1 Systemic diseases	Hashimoto thyroiditis Myasthenia gravis Graves' disease Sjögren's syndrome Systemic lupus erythematosus (SLE) Inflammatory bowel disease (IBD) Rheumatoid arthritis
1.2 Dermatoses	Alopecia areata
1.3 Autoimmune syndromes	Autoimmune polyendocrinopathy-candidiasis-ectodermal dysplasia (APECED) syndrome Schmidt syndrome Alezzandrini syndrome Vogt-Koyanagi-Harada disease Mitochondrial encephalomyopathy, lactic acidosis and stroke-like episodes (MELAS) syndrome
2. Atopic disorders	Atopic dermatitis Hay fever Asthma
3. Inflammatory dermatoses	Psoriasis
4. Psychiatric disorders	Depression Anxiety Sleep disturbances Alexithymia
5. Malignancy	Melanoma Nonmelanoma skin cancers (NMSC) Mycosis fungoides (MF)
6. Miscellaneous associations	Ocular abnormalities Hearing abnormalities Baboon syndrome *H. pylori* infection Kallin syndrome Nevi such as congenital melanocytic nevus, halo nevi and nevus depigmentosus Striae distensae Leprosy

25.2 Epidemiology

Paediatric-onset vitiligo may be associated with a higher prevalence of allergic diseases and a lower prevalence of thyroid diseases [3]. In adults, Schallreuter et al. found a high prevalence of thyroid diseases and presence of thyroid autoantibodies and a higher prevalence of congenital nevi (6.2 % compared with 2.8 % in a normal healthy population) among 321 individuals with vitiligo [4].

In another large 15-year retrospective population-based study, non-stratified analysis showed a significant association between vitiligo and psoriasis, atopic dermatitis and several autoimmune diseases such as alopecia areata, Hashimoto thyroiditis, myasthenia gravis, Graves' disease, Sjögren's syndrome and systemic lupus erythematosus (SLE) [5]. However, when adjusted for age and gender, increased risks of SLE, Sjögren's syndrome, myasthenia gravis and rheumatoid arthritis were observed only in certain age groups. In a similar study from the United States, 23 % of the vitiligo patients had one of the following autoimmune disorders: thyroid-related diseases (11.7 %), psoriasis (7.6 %), rheumatoid arthritis (2.9 %), alopecia areata (2.4 %), inflammatory bowel disease (IBD) (2.4 %), SLE(2.4 %) and type I diabetes mellitus (0.8 %). In addition, 41 % had elevated antinuclear antibody levels [6].

In a large retrospective study of 1416 vitiligo patients by Kanwar et al. from India, vitiligo was associated with other cutaneous and systemic diseases in 116 (8.2 %) patients [7]. These were classified as autoimmune and non-autoimmune diseases and both these groups were further subdivided into systemic and primary dermatologic diseases. Autoimmune diseases were present in 3.2 % of the patients and included primary dermatologic diseases (0.2 %) and systemic diseases (3 %) like hypothyroidism, hyperthyroidism and diabetes mellitus. Non-autoimmune diseases were present in 5 % of the patient population and included unrelated primary dermatologic diseases (2.6 %) such as melasma, acanthosis nigricans, cutaneous amyloidosis, lichen sclerosus et atrophicus and systemic diseases (2.4 %) like hypertension and polycystic ovary disease. However, they did not find any significant association of vitiligo with any of these disorders.

In another study from South India, Shankar et al. found among vitiligo patients a high incidence of autoantibodies (22.5 %), vitamin B12 deficiency (30 %), hypothyroidism (11.3 %), elevated absolute eosinophil count (16.3 %), hypoacusis (10 %) and retinal changes (8.8 %) [8].

25.3 Vitiligo and Other Autoimmune Disorders

Vitiligo is considered an autoimmune disease due to the presence of autoantibodies against melanocytes in patients' sera [9], the detection of organ-specific antibodies in the patients' sera and frequently in first-degree relatives and the association of the disease with HLA-DR4 and HLA-DR1. There is a production of autoantibodies directed against melanocyte antigens, and their titres may correlate with the activity and extent of the disease [10]. Moreover, altered cellular immunity is present, in addition to and in combination with a humoral response [11]. Equally important is the observation regarding the associations of vitiligo with other autoimmune conditions.

In a study assessing the association between vitiligo and autoimmune diseases in Caucasian probands and their families [12], the frequencies of six autoimmune disorders were significantly elevated in vitiligo probands and their first-degree relatives: vitiligo, autoimmune thyroid disease, pernicious anaemia, Addison's disease, SLE and probably IBD. Such association can best be explained by an overall genetic susceptibility to autoimmunity.

The link of vitiligo with autoimmune thyroid disorders is the best established. They may be present in as many as one-fourth of vitiligo patients with disease onset during childhood [13–15], although the onset of the two diseases may be separated by more than a decade [16]. One study identified thyroid disease in 18.5 % of 15,126 vitiligo patients [17]. Conversely, vitiligo is more common in those with autoimmune thyroid disorders [18].

Patients with non-segmental vitiligo are more likely to have autoimmune disorders than those with segmental vitiligo [19]. In a study from Japan by Tanioka et al., one-fourth of the patients with non-segmental vitiligo had associated comorbidities [20]. Among the associations, autoimmune diseases were the most common in 43 % of patients, with autoimmune thyroid disease noted in 7.4 %. Other autoimmune associations included myasthenia gravis, Sjögren's syndrome and autoimmune nephritis. Another study from Japan found autoimmune diseases in 20.3 % of patients with generalized vitiligo [21]. In a study comparing paediatric-onset and later-onset vitiligo, longer duration of disease and a positive family history of thyroid disease were associated with the presence of thyroid disease only in the childhood-onset group [3].

A higher incidence of thyroid microsomal antibody is found in vitiligo patients and their family members. In a multicentre study from Italy [22], at least one circulating autoantibody was detected in 61 (41.8 %) of 146 subjects. Other autoantibodies observed in this study included anti-thyroperoxidase (25.6 %), anti-thyroglobulin (23.4 %), antinuclear antibodies (16.8 %) and anti-gastric parietal cell antibodies (7.8 %). Another controlled study of 226 vitiligo patients found an increased incidence of antinuclear (12.4 %), antimicrosomal (7.1 %) and anti-smooth muscle antibodies (25.7 %) [23].

Vitiligo may be associated with several autoimmune syndromes. In a small case series assessing the association between vitiligo and multiple autoimmune syndrome, type III multiple autoimmune disease was diagnosed in all the 11 patients observed [24]. Vitiligo and thyroid disorders were noticed in seven and ten patients, respectively. Autoimmune polyendocrinopathy-candidiasis-ectodermal dysplasia (APECED)/autoimmune polyendocrine syndrome type 1 (APS1)/ polyglandular autoimmune syndrome type 1 (PGA1) presents with a combination of Addison's disease, hypoparathyroidism, ectodermal dysplasia and/or chronic mucocutaneous candidiasis. Other manifestations may include alopecia areata, vitiligo, gastrointestinal symptoms, gonadal failure and ocular and dental anomalies [25]. A study of 68 patients with APECED found that 13 had vitiligo [25].

Schmidt syndrome/APS2 is an autosomal dominant disorder with variable expressivity [26]. Like APECED, it presents with polyglandular failure (Addison's disease, hypothyroidism and type I diabetes mellitus) and occasionally vitiligo and/or hypogonadism [27]. Vogt-Koyanagi-Harada disease is a systemic T-cell-mediated disorder characterized by uveitis, aseptic meningitis, dysacusis, alopecia, poliosis, tinnitus and vitiligo (8–100 %) [28–30]. Alezzandrini syndrome presents with unilateral facial vitiligo, poliosis, deafness and tapetoretinal degeneration [31, 32]. Mitochondrial encephalomyopathy, lactic acidosis and stroke-like episodes (MELAS) syndrome is a mitochondrial disorder that presents with central nervous system abnormalities, neurosensory hearing loss, diabetes mellitus and cardiomyopathy. Vitiligo may be seen in 11 % (3/28) of MELAS patients [33].

25.4 Vitiligo and Atopy

Patients with vitiligo, especially those with early-onset disease, have a significantly higher risk for atopic dermatitis. The probable pathophysiologic factors linking these two dermatoses could be common genetic factors, melanocyte destruction due to the inflammation seen in atopic dermatitis or koebnerization due to scratching. Silverberg and Silverberg found a higher prevalence of atopic disorders in patients with vitiligo compared to the general adult population [34]. They suggested that a history of atopic disease may be helpful to predict the progression of vitiligo to widespread disease. Kuriyama et al. conducted a prospective observational study to investigate the leukoderma-related clinical manifestations and bioparameters in atopic dermatitis and found that 8/52 (15.4 %) of patients had leukoderma. There is a female preponderance, a more severe eczema, a lower frequency of allergic rhinitis and a higher frequency of prurigo lesions in patients who have concurrent atopic dermatitis and vitiligo [35].

In a recent systematic review and meta-analysis, 16 studies of vitiligo were included [36]. In the pooled analysis of the studies, patients with vitiligo had significantly higher odds of atopic dermatitis than control patients without these disorders. Subgroup analysis found higher odds of atopic dermatitis in patients with early-onset vitiligo (<12 years) compared to those with late-onset vitiligo (*OR*, 3.54; 95 % *CI*, 2.24–5.63, $p < .001$).

25.5 Vitiligo and Inflammatory Dermatoses

Concurrent occurrence of vitiligo and psoriasis has been frequently noted. Yazdanpanah et al. reported that among the 219 and 154 patients suffering from psoriasis and vitiligo, respectively, 12 patients (0.19 %) had psoriasis and vitiligo simultaneously [37]. The simultaneous occurrence in the psoriasis group was 5.48 % and in the vitiligo group was 7.79 %. Of the 717 vitiligo patients seen at the Mayo Clinic over a 5-year period, 29 (4.04 %) had concurrent psoriasis [38]. Dermoscopic findings include dilated capillaries and red globules of psoriasis against a background of depigmentation, aptly called as "the red in white sea" sign [39].

Arunachalam et al., investigated the implications of disease association between vitiligo and psoriasis [40]. The presence of vitiligo and even mild psoriasis is significantly correlated with a family history of cardiovascular disease. Multivariate analysis demonstrated that inflammation or pruritus in vitiligo macules (*OR* 2.56, $p = 0.047$) and a family history of cardiovascular disease (*OR* 4.07, $p = 0.02$) were the most significant predictors of patients having both psoriasis and vitiligo, while the presence of organ-specific autoantibodies (*OR* 0.24, $p = 0.007$) was significantly associated with patients having only vitiligo.

25.6 Vitiligo and Psychiatric Diseases

Since vitiligo carries a significant social stigma in many parts of the world, it is not surprising that patients with this disease have a higher psychological morbidity. Psychological disturbances are common in patients with vitiligo and were found in 31 % of adult Sudanese patients [41]. These disturbances were mild in 17.2 % and severe in 13.8 %.

Psychological morbidity in vitiligo has frequently been compared with other chronic skin conditions, most notably psoriasis. In a study from India, 30 adult patients with psoriasis and vitiligo were studied [42]. The prevalences of psychiatric morbidity as assessed by the standardized Hindi version of the General Health Questionnaire (GHQ-H) were found to be significantly higher in vitiligo patients (53.3 % versus 16.22 %). The prevalence of depression was also much higher in the vitiligo cohort (23.3 % versus 10 %), while anxiety was observed in 3.3 % in both groups. In another study from India, Mattoo et al. found similar rates of psychiatric morbidity among patients with psoriasis (33.6 %) and vitiligo (24.7 %) [43].

Alexithymia is a personality trait characterized by difficulties in differentiating and describing feelings. Recently, alexithymia has been associated with numerous dermatologic conditions including vitiligo. In a case-control study, Picardi et al. suggested that vulnerability to vitiligo is not increased by stressful events except for unpredictable and uncontrollable aversive events which occurred three times more frequently in cases than controls [44]. Based on the Toronto Alexithymia Scale (TAS-20), and the Multidimensional Scale of Perceived Social Support, alexithymia, insecure attachment and poor social support appear to increase susceptibility to vitiligo, possibly through deficits in emotion regulation or reduced ability to cope effectively with stress.

25.7 Vitiligo and Malignancy

The development of nonmelanoma skin cancer (NMSC) in patients with vitiligo is still debated. Due to the loss of melanocytes and of melanin, it has been postulated that patients with vitiligo have an increased risk of developing melanoma. Evidence supporting the concept that vitiligo has a higher incidence of melanoma and vice versa is limited [45]. In addition, a slightly higher incidence of NMSC has been reported in those with vitiligo [46, 47]. In contrast, the development of vitiligo in patients with metastatic melanoma may be associated with a favourable prognosis [48]. The immunologic mechanisms that lead to melanocyte destruction in vitiligo may also destroy malignant pigment cells.

Several mechanisms have been proposed to explain the negative association between vitiligo and skin cancer. This includes stricter sun protection likely to be undertaken by patients with vitiligo, a protective immunologic response as described above, lack of melanocytes within vitiligo lesions, overexpression of the p53 tumour suppressor gene which may protect against NMSC and overproduction of pro-inflammatory cytokines, such as interleukin-1 and tumour necrosis factor alpha (TNF-α) which stimulate the production of superoxide dismutase and glutathione peroxidase thus reducing the risk of skin cancer [49]. Teulings et al. reported a decreased risk of melanoma and NMSC in patients with vitiligo. They observed that adjusted for confounders, patients with vitiligo had a threefold lower probability of developing melanoma (adjusted *OR* 0.32; 95 % *CI* 0.12–0.88) and NMSC (adjusted *OR* 0.28; 95 % *CI* 0.16–0.50) [50]. In another study, the same authors suggested that although vitiligo occurs only in a low percentage of patients with melanoma treated with immunotherapy, induction of vitiligo lesions suggests a clear survival benefit and is important as an indicator of effective anti-melanoma immunity and improved survival [51].

Less commonly, vitiligo has been associated with cutaneous T-cell lymphoma (CTCL). Herrmann et al. analysed case records of 25 patients with CTCL and concomitant vitiligo [52]. They observed a younger age, stage IIB–IV disease and presence of a CD8+CD4- mycosis fungoides phenotype to be associated with the development of vitiligo. Increased risk of vitiligo was associated with the use of methotrexate and CD4 antibody therapies, which may indirectly indicate advanced disease.

25.8 Miscellaneous

Vitiligo has been associated with ophthalmologic and auditory findings. Up to 20 % of patients with vitiligo have hearing loss which is caused by functional disorders of intermediate cells (melanocytes) of the stria vascularis [53, 54]. Ocular abnormalities may be present in up to 40 % including choroidal anomalies, uveitis [55], iritis [56, 57] and some degree of fundal pigment disturbance [58]. Biswas et al. studied 100 vitiligo patients, of whom 23 % showed hypopigmented spots on the iris, 9 % retinal pigment epithelium hypopigmentation, 5 % uveitis and 11 % with chorioretinal degeneration. The remaining 34 % of patients had no ocular findings [59]. In another study, Baskan et al. studied 45 patients with vitiligo and found nearly 23 % to be having ocular findings that included anterior segment (iris) involvement, ring-like peripapillary atrophy around the optic nerve, atrophy of pigment epithelium, focal hypopigmented spots and diffuse hypopigmentation [60]. The presence of periorbital vitiligo and genital lesions was significantly related to the ocular findings.

In a recent study, vitiligo was associated with *H. pylori* infection [61]. The frequency of *H. pylori* infection was 64.7 % in the patient group and 33.3 % in the control group ($p = 0.012$). Vitiligo has been reported in association with Kallin syndrome, a variant of epidermolysis bullosa simplex (EBS). It has also been reported with baboon syndrome. Association of vitiligo with hypovitaminosis D has been evaluated, and no association was found in a recent study [62]. However, vitamin D deficiency may be seen in young males, male gender with short duration of vitiligo and non-use of phototherapy.

Finally, studies evaluating the association between vitiligo and metabolic syndrome have thrown up conflicting results. While studies by Karadag et al. and Pietrzak et al. have supported such an association, these observations were contradicted by Rodríguez-Martín et al., who found that patients with vitiligo had a better lipid profile, with higher levels of HDL and lower triglyceride, in comparison with the control group [63]. The role of melanocytes in the pathogenesis of metabolic syndrome may be important. As oxidative stress plays a vital role in the pathogenesis of both the metabolic syndrome and the vitiligo, looking for such an association appears interesting.

25.9 Conclusion

In a proportion of patients, vitiligo is more than skin deep and can be associated with other dermatologic and systemic diseases. The association with autoimmune disorders, most notably thyroid disorders, seems to be strong, especially in patients with early-onset non-segmental vitiligo with a family history of autoimmune disease. However, it is not recommended to screen all patients for autoantibodies, as their mere presence does not require intervention. It is best to reserve the tests for those who have clinical signs and symptoms of associated disease. Early-onset non-segmental vitiligo has a strong association with atopic disorders as well. Psychological morbidity should be looked for, as it is both common and amenable to psychosocial interventions that can significantly improve quality of life. Evidence of association with other disorders is less robust. Finally, there is evidence that vitiligo may confer some protection against melanoma and nonmelanoma skin cancers.

References

1. Taieb A, Picardo M. The definition and assessment of vitiligo: a consensus report of the Vitiligo European Task Force. Pigment Cell Res. 2007;20:27–35.
2. Kyriakis KP, Palamaras I, Tsele E, Michailides C, Terzoudi S. Case detection rates of vitiligo by gender and age. Int J Dermatol. 2009;48:328–9.
3. Nicolaidou E, Antoniou C, Miniati A, Lagogianni E, Matekovits A, Stratigos A, et al. Childhood- and later-onset vitiligo have diverse epidemiologic and clinical characteristics. J Am Acad Dermatol. 2012;66:954–8.
4. Schallreuter KU, Lemke R, Brandt O, Schwartz R, Westhofen M, Montz R, et al. Vitiligo and other diseases: coexistence or true association? Hamburg study on 321 patients. Dermatology. 1994;188:269–75.

5. Chen YT, Chen YJ, Hwang CY, Lin MW, Chen TJ, Chen CC, et al. Comorbidity profiles in association with vitiligo: a nationwide population-based study in Taiwan. J Eur Acad Dermatol Venereol. 2015;29:1362–9.
6. Sheth VM, Guo Y, Qureshi AA. Comorbidities associated with vitiligo: a ten-year retrospective study. Dermatol. 2013;227:311–5.
7. Kanwar AJ, Mahajan R, Parsad D. Effect of age at onset on vitiligo. J Cutan Med Surg. 2013;17:253–8.
8. Shankar DSK, Shashikala K, Madala R. Clinical patterns of vitiligo and its associated comorbidities: a prospective controlled cross-sectional study in South India. Indian Dermatol Online J. 2012;3:114–8.
9. Moellman GE, Kross P, Halaban R. On the subject of serum antibodies to melanocytes. J Invest Dermatol. 1985;84:333–4.
10. Baharav E, Merimski O, Shoenfeld Y, Zigelman R, Gilbrud B, Yecheskel G, et al. Tyrosinase as an autoantigen in patients of vitiligo. Clin Exp Immunol. 1996;105:84–8.
11. Ongenae K, Van Geel N, Naeyaert JM. Evidence for an autoimmune pathogenesis of vitiligo. Pigment Cell Res. 2003;16:90–100.
12. Alkhateeb A, Fain PR, Thody A, Bennett DC, Spritz RA. Epidemiology of vitiligo and associated autoimmune diseases in Caucasian probands and their families. Pigment Cell Res. 2003;16:208–14.
13. Pagovich OE, Silverberg JI, Freilich E, Silverberg NB. Thyroid abnormalities in pediatric patients with vitiligo in New York City. Cutis. 2008;81:463–6.
14. Iacovelli P, Sinagra JL, Vidolin AP, Marenda S, Capitanio B, Leone G, et al. Relevance of thyroiditis and of other autoimmune diseases in children with vitiligo. Dermatol. 2005;210:26–30.
15. Kakourou T, Kanaka-Gantenbein C, Papadopoulou A, Kaloumenou E, Chrousos GP. Increased prevalence of chronic autoimmune (Hashimoto's) thyroiditis in children and adolescents with vitiligo. J Am Acad Dermatol. 2005;53:220–3.
16. Dittmar M, Kahaly GJ. Polyglandular autoimmune syndromes: immunogenetics and long-term follow-up. J Clin Endocrinol Metab. 2003;88:2983–92.
17. Frati R, Frati C, Sassano PP, Antonaci A. Vitiligo, autoimmune thyroiditis: a rare thyroid cancer arising with bone metastases on maxillofacial area. J Exp Clin Cancer Res. 1999;18:85–7.
18. Shong YK, Kim JA. Vitiligo in autoimmune thyroid disease. Thyroidol. 1991;3:89–91.
19. Zhang Z, Xu SX, Zhang FY, Yin XY, Yang S, Xiao FL, et al. The analysis of genetics and associated autoimmune diseases in Chinese vitiligo patients. Arch Dermatol Res. 2009;301:167–73.
20. Tanioka M, Yamamoto Y, Katoh M, Takahashi K, Miyachi Y. Vitiligo vulgaris and autoimmune diseases in Japan: a report from vitiligo clinic in Kyoto University Hospital. Dermatoendocrinol. 2009;1:43–5.
21. Narita T, Oiso N, Fukai K, Kabashima K, Kawada A, Suzuki T. Generalized vitiligo and associated autoimmune diseases in Japanese patients and their families. Allergol Int. 2011;60:505–8.
22. Ingordo V, Cazzaniga S, Raone B, Digiuseppe MD, Musumeci ML, Fai D, et al. Circulating autoantibodies and autoimmune comorbidities in vitiligo patients: a multicenter Italian study. Dermatol. 2014;228:240–9.
23. Hann SK, Im S, Kim HI, Kim HS, Lee YJ, Park YK. Increased incidence of antismooth muscle antibody in Korean vitiligo patients. J Dermatol. 1993;20:679–83.
24. Klisnick A, Schmidt J, Dupond JL, Bouchou K, Rousset H, Thieblot P, et al. Vitiligo in multiple autoimmune syndrome: a retrospective study of 11 cases and a review of the literature. Rev Med Interne. 1998;19:348–52.
25. Ahonen P, Myllarniemi S, Sipila I, Perheentupa J. Clinical variation of autoimmune polyendocrinopathy-candidiasis-ectodermal dystrophy (APECED) in a series of 68 patients. N Engl J Med. 1990;322:1829–36.

26. Spritz RA, Gowan K, Bennett DC, Fain PR. Novel vitiligo susceptibility loci on chromosomes 7 (AIS2) and 8 (AIS3), confirmation of SLEV1 on chromosome 17, and their roles in an autoimmune diathesis. Am J Hum Genet. 2004;74:188–91.
27. Butler MG, Hodes ME, Conneally PM, Biegel AA, Wright JC. Linkage analysis in a large kindred with autosomal dominant transmission of polyglandular autoimmune disease type II (Schmidt syndrome). Am J Med Genet. 1984;18:61–5.
28. Tsuruta D, Hamada T, Teramae H, Mito H, Ishii M. Inflammatory vitiligo in Vogt-Koyanagi-Harada disease. J Am Acad Dermatol. 2001;44:129–31.
29. Sukavatcharin S, Tsai JH, Rao NA. Vogt-Koyanagi-Harada disease in Hispanic patients. Int Ophthalmol. 2007;27:143–8.
30. Tesavibul N, Sansanayuth W. Vogt-Koyanagi-Harada disease in Thai patients. J Med Assoc Thai. 2005;88(S9):S26–30.
31. Ortonne JP. Vitiligo and other disorders of hypopigmentation. In: Bolognia J, Jorizzo J, Rapini R, editors. Dermatology. Philadelphia: Mosby Elsevier; 2008. p. 928.
32. Hoffman MD, Dudley C. Suspected Alezzandrini's syndrome in a diabetic patient with unilateral retinal detachment and ipsilateral vitiligo and poliosis. J Am Acad Dermatol. 1992;26:496–7.
33. Karvonen SL, Haapasaari KM, Kallioinen M, Oikarinen A, Hassinen IE, Majamaa K. Increased prevalence of vitiligo, but no evidence of premature ageing, in the skin of patients with bp 3243 mutation in mitochondrial DNA in the mitochondrial encephalomyopathy, lactic acidosis and stroke-like episodes syndrome (MELAS). Br J Dermatol. 1999;140:634–9.
34. Silverberg JI, Silverberg NB. Association between vitiligo and atopic disorders: a pilot study. JAMA Dermatol. 2013;149:963–86.
35. Kuriyama S, Kasuya A, Fujiyama T, Tatsuno K, Sakabe J-I, Yamaguchi H, et al. Leukoderma in patients with atopic dermatitis. J Dermatol. 2015;42:215–8.
36. Mohan GC, Silverberg JI. Association of vitiligo and alopecia areata with atopic dermatitis: a systematic review and meta-analysis. JAMA Dermatol. 2015;151:522–8.
37. Yazdanpanah MJ, Banihashemi M, Pezeshkpoor F, Moradifar M, Feli S, Esmaeili H. Evaluation between association of psoriasis and vitiligo. J Cutan Med Surg. 2015;19:140–3.
38. Powell FC, Dicken CH. Psoriasis and vitiligo. Acta Derm Venereol. 1983;63:246–9.
39. Chandrashekar L. Red in white sea sign. J Eur Acad Dermatol Venereol. 2009;23:368.
40. Arunachalam M, Dragoni F, Colucci R, Berti S, Crocetti E, Galeone M, et al. Non-segmental vitiligo and psoriasis comorbidity – a case–control study in Italian patients. J Eur Acad Dermatol Venereol. 2014;28:433–7.
41. Osman AM, Elkordufani Y, Abdullah MA. The psychological impact of vitiligo in adult Sudanese patients. Afr J Psychiatry (Johannesbg). 2009;12:284–6.
42. Sharma N, Koranne RV, Singh RK. Psychiatric morbidity in psoriasis and vitiligo: a comparative study. J Dermatol. 2001;28:419–23.
43. Mattoo SK, Handa S, Kaur I, Gupta N, Malhotra R. Psychiatric morbidity in vitiligo and psoriasis: a comparative study from India. J Dermatol. 2001;28:424–32.
44. Picardi A, Pasquini P, Cattaruzza MS, Gaetano P, Melchi CF, Baliva G, et al. Stressful life events, social support, attachment security and alexithymia in vitiligo. A case–control study. Psychother Psychosom. 2003;72:150–8.
45. Schallreuter KU, Levenig C, Berger J. Vitiligo and cutaneous melanoma. A case study. Dermatologica. 1991;183:239–45.
46. Hexsel CL, Eide MJ, Johnson CC, Krajenta R, Jacobsen G, Hamzavi I, et al. Incidence of nonmelanoma skin cancer in a cohort of patients with vitiligo. J Am Acad Dermatol. 2009;60:929–33.
47. Seo SL, Kim IH. Squamous cell carcinoma in a patient with generalized vitiligo. J Am Acad Dermatol. 2001;45:S227–9.
48. Bystryn JC, Rigel D, Friedman RJ, Kopf A. Prognostic significance of hypopigmentation in malignant melanoma. Arch Dermatol. 1987;123:1053–5.

49. Hammoud SM, Kruis RW, Sigurdsson V. Prediction of the occurrence of melanoma and non-melanoma skin cancer in patients with vitiligo. Acta Derm Venereol. 2016;96(1):106–7.
50. Teulings HE, Overkamp M, Ceylan E, Nieuweboer-Krobotova L, Bos JD, Nijsten T, et al. Decreased risk of melanoma and nonmelanoma skin cancer in patients with vitiligo: a survey among 1307 patients and their partners. Br J Dermatol. 2013;168(1):162–71.
51. Teulings HE, Limpens J, Jansen SN, Zwinderman AH, Reitsma JB, Spuls PI, et al. Vitiligo-like depigmentation in patients with stage III-IV melanoma receiving immunotherapy and its association with survival: a systematic review and meta-analysis. J Clin Oncol. 2015;33:773–81.
52. Herrmann JL, Syklawer E, Tarrillion M, Duvic M, Hughey LC. Concomitant mycosis fungoides and vitiligo: how mycosis fungoides may contribute to melanocyte destruction. Dermatol. 2015;230:143–9.
53. Hong CK, Lee MH, Jeong KH, Cha CI, Yeo SG. Clinical analysis of hearing levels in vitiligo patients. Eur J Dermatol. 2009;19:50–6.
54. Gopal KV, Rama Rao GR, Kumar YH, Appa Rao MV, Vasudev P. Vitiligo: a part of a systemic autoimmune process. Indian J Dermatol Venereol Leprol. 2007;73:162–5.
55. Flynn GE. Bilateral uveitis, poliosis, and vitiligo; with an hereditary factor. Am J Ophthalmol. 1952;35:568–72.
56. Albert DM, Nordlund JJ, Lerner AB. Ocular abnormalities occurring with vitiligo. Ophthalmol. 1979;86:1145–60.
57. Albert DM, Sober AJ, Fitzpatrick TB. Iritis in patients with cutaneous melanoma and vitiligo. Arch Ophthalmol. 1978;96:2081–4.
58. Cowan Jr CL, Halder RM, Grimes PE, Chakrabarti SG, Kenney Jr JA. Ocular disturbances in vitiligo. J Am Acad Dermatol. 1986;15:17–24.
59. Biswas G, Barbhuiya JN, Biswas MC, Islam MN, Dutta S. Clinical pattern of ocular manifestations in vitiligo. J Indian Med Assoc. 2003;101:478–80.
60. Bulbul Baskan E, Baykara M, Ercan I, Tunali S, Yucel A. Vitiligo and ocular findings: a study on possible associations. J Eur Acad Dermatol Venereol. 2006;20:829–33.
61. Rifaioğlu EN, Aydoğan F, Bülbül Şen B, Şen T, Ekiz Ö. Investigation into the frequency of Helicobacter pylori infection with carbon 14 urea breath test in patients with vitiligo. Turk J Med Sci. 2014;44:1051–4.
62. Khurrum H, AlGhamdi KM. The relationship between the serum level of vitamin D and vitiligo: a controlled study on 300 subjects. J Cutan Med Surg. 2016;20(2):139–45.
63. Pietrzak A, Bartosińska J, Hercogová J, Lotti TM, Chodorowska G. Metabolic syndrome in vitiligo. Dermatol Ther. 2012;25(S1):S41–3.

Chapter 26
Topical Medications in Vitiligo

Koushik Lahiri and Anupam Das

26.1 Introduction

Vitiligo is a fairly common dermatosis resulting into significant deterioration in the quality of life [1]. With recent advances in the field of medical sciences, numerous treatment options have emerged for the management of the distressing condition. The basic objectives are to minimize disease progression, attain repigmentation, and achieve cosmetically pleasing results [1]. It is crucial to understand each and every therapeutic modality with respect to the mechanism of action, indications, and contraindications. In this chapter, the topical medications available to treat vitiligo are discussed (Table 26.1).

26.2 Topical Corticosteroids (TCS)

Topical steroids are the first-line drugs for the management of vitiligo. They are responsible for reduction of macrophages and T lymphocytes in vitiliginous patches [9], they likewise reduce the complement-mediated destruction of melanocytes [10]. In children and adults with limited, extrafacial involvement, once-daily application of potent steroids is advisable for not more than 3 months [11]. The response

K. Lahiri (✉)
WIZDERM and Department of Dermatology, Apollo Gleneagles Hospitals, Greenwood Nook, Coral Isle, 14 RB, 369/2 Purbachal, Kalikapur, E M Bypass, Kolkata 700078, India
e-mail: doctorlahiri@gmail.com

A. Das
Department of Dermatology, KPC Medical College and Hospital, Kolkata, India
e-mail: anupamdasdr@gmail.com

E.B. Handog, M.J. Enriquez-Macarayo (eds.), *Melasma and Vitiligo in Brown Skin*, DOI 10.1007/978-81-322-3664-1_26

Table 26.1 Summary of various topical agents used in the treatment of vitiligo

Drug	Mechanism of action	Level of evidence
Corticosteroids	Modulate the immune response by reducing the macrophages and T cells Reduce autoantibodies Inhibit complement-mediated melanocyte destruction	IA
Calcineurin inhibitors	Reduce the tissue counts of IFN-γ, IL-1, IL-2, IL-3, IL-4, IL-5, GM-CSF, TNF-α Enhance melanocyte and melanoblast proliferation	IA (children) IIA (adults)
Vitamin D3 analogs	Target the local immune response in vitiligo, by acting on specific T-cell activation Inhibit the transition of T cells from early to late G1 phase Inhibit the expression of TNF-α IFN-γ Modulate melanocyte maturation and differentiation Upregulates melanogenesis through pathways activated by vitamin D ligand receptors (endothelin receptor and c-kit) [2]	IIA (monotherapy), IB if combined with topical steroids
Photochemotherapy	Psoralens stimulate melanogenesis; photoconjugation of psoralens in melanocyte DNA leads to mitosis, replication and proliferation of melanocytes, increased number of melanosomes, and subsequent apocopation PUVA stimulates the activity of cAMP; leads to increased synthesis of tyrosine, the precursor of melanin; induces a suppressor T-cell response which releases IL-10 suppressing the autoimmune stimulus responsible for the destruction of melanocytes PUVA induces basic fibroblast growth factor (bFGF) and hepatocyte growth factor, leading to re-growth and migration of follicular melanocytes to stratum basale [3–5]	PUVA: IV Khellin: III
L-Phenylalanine	Stimulates melanogenesis in vitiliginous patches	IIB

(continued)

Table 26.1 (continued)

Drug	Mechanism of action	Level of evidence
Monobenzyl ether of hydroquinone (MBEH)	Reacts with tyrosinase to form a reactive quinone product that binds to cysteine residues in tyrosinase proteins to form hapten-carrier complexes causing destruction of melanocytes Induces lysosomal degradation of melanosomes by autophagy A contact sensitizer inducing a delayed-type hypersensitivity response [6]	IV
Antioxidants	Increase catalase activity leading to a decrease in reactive oxygen species Inhibit ROS-mediated destruction of melanocytes	IB
5-Fluorouracil	Direct stimulation of melanocyte proliferation Inhibits agents or cytotoxic cells which destroy melanocytes Immunomodulator stabilizing the vitiligo disease [7]	IV
Piperine	Stimulates the proliferation of melanocytes [8]	IV
Prostaglandin E2	Increases melanocyte proliferation and density	IB
Capsaicin and curcumin	Inhibit apoptosis of melanocytes Reduce the generation of ROS and lipid peroxidation Improve mitochondrial activity Enhance survival of melanocytes	IB

to this therapy is better in children as compared to adults. Moreover, lesions over the head and neck region respond well [12].

There are multiple studies supporting the efficacy of topical corticosteroids. Kwinter et al. reported response rates of 64 % in a study conducted on children who were treated with TCS alone [13]. Complete repigmentation rates are approximately 49.3 % [14].

The efficacy has been compared with other agents. When compared with topical calcineurin inhibitors, the response is equivocal to high [14, 15]. Repigmentation rates are however the same when compared with ultraviolet A (UVA) light phototherapy [16].

Even though TCS are very effective in the treatment of vitiligo, local side effects and topical steroid abuse limit the ultimate use of these agents. Skin atrophy, telangiectasia, hypertrichosis, acneiform eruptions, and striae caused by potent or very potent TCS are well known. Moreover, systemic absorption should be kept in mind while treating large areas of skin, thin skin and children with potent steroids. Lower potency TCS and newer class III TCS, like mometasone furoate and methylprednisolone aceponate, are devoid of these untoward side effects [11].

26.3 Topical Calcineurin Inhibitors (TCI)

Calcineurin, when activated, leads to transcription of IL-2 and TNF-α. Vitiliginous patches were found to have elevated levels of these cytokines. Inhibitors of calcineurin, like tacrolimus and pimecrolimus, are extremely effective in treating vitiligo, by increasing the proliferation of both melanoblasts and melanocytes [17]. This is particularly useful for new and actively spreading lesions on thin skin, as an alternative to TCS. Initially, twice-daily applications are recommended. If effective, the duration of use may be extended to 12 months [11]. The onset of action is earlier in comparison to TCS but the repigmentation is inferior. Occlusion may help in cases of recalcitrant lesions on the extremities [18]. Lesions on the head and neck are the most responsive, with the rates ranging from 63 to 89 % [19–21].

When combined with other agents, the response is even better. Topical tacrolimus combined with NB-UVB was reported to have repigmentation rates of greater than 50 % in 42 % of lesions in patients with chronic stable refractory vitiligo [22]. Similar results were also reported by Nordal et al. [23]. Also, combination with 308 nm excimer laser was reported to have a very high response rate of 100 % [24].

In controlled trials among the pediatric age group, efficiency of tacrolimus was compared with that of fluticasone, mometasone, and clobetasol, with a conclusion of similar efficiency of steroids and tacrolimus [25–28]. Moreover, tacrolimus in combination with oral prednisolone was effective in recent-onset vitiligo [29].

TCIs are safe for short-term or intermittent long-term use, side effects being erythema, pruritus, burning, irritation, and rarely hyperpigmentation and acne [30–33]. According to the FDA, topical tacrolimus should not be used in patients less than 2 years of age, and only 0.03 % tacrolimus is approved for patients aged 2–15 years [34]. Tacrolimus 0.1 % ointment with excimer laser is superior to placebo for UV-resistant areas. When used alone, the efficacy of tacrolimus 0.1 % ointment is similar to clobetasol propionate 0.05 % ointment. Pimecrolimus 1 % cream combined with narrow-band UVB is superior to placebo, especially for facial lesions [35].

26.4 Topical Vitamin D3 Analogs

Calcipotriene is an effective adjunct to topical corticosteroids in the treatment of vitiligo, on account of its immunomodulatory and proliferative effects on melanocytes. Even though advocated as a good add-on therapy, there are reports of repigmentation in children when used as a monotherapy [36, 37]. Combination with TCS provided the maximum benefit and was shown to be safe for both children and adults [1]. Moreover, there was increase in repigmentation rates, earlier-onset of repigmentation, and, most importantly, greater stability of repigmentation [38, 39].

Newman and Silverberg found that topical calcipotriene and betamethasone dipropionate is a promising combination to treat facial vitiligo [40]. Calcipotriene, however, is not effective when combined with NB-UVB [25, 41–43].

26.5 Photochemotherapy (Psoralens, Khellin, and L-Phenylalanine)

26.5.1 Psoralens

Photochemotherapy with topical 8-methoxypsoralen (8-MOP) can be used in patients with lesions covering less than 5 % body surface area and also in children less than 12 years of age (systemic PUVA is contraindicated). However, topical psoralens may lead to significant pruritus, erythema, edema, blisters, and skin necrosis even with minimum dosage. Thus, therapy with these agents mandates strict monitoring [1]. Application of 0.001 % 8-MOP or less, one to three times per week for 20–30 min, is recommended. The skin is then exposed to UVA radiation at 0.25–0.5 J/cm^2. The exposure time is increased by 15–30 s in subsequent sessions (maximum 10 min). This procedure has to be repeated until a dosage and exposure time are attained which produces erythema but not burning. Post-procedural advice is crucial to avoid untoward adverse effects. The patients should wash away the excess 8-MOP with soap and water immediately after the irradiation and apply UVA sunscreen to avoid additional environmental UVA exposure [44]. The advantage of topical PUVA is the need for fewer treatments and considerably smaller cumulative UVA doses, lower plasma levels, and reduced systemic and ocular phototoxicity [11].

26.5.2 Khellin

Khellin is a furanochrome extract of the plant *Ammi visnaga* (5,8-dimethoxy-2 methyl-4,5-furo-6,7 chromone). KUVA refers to khellin followed by UVA. It has a stimulatory effect on melanogenesis and melanocyte proliferation when combined with UVA light. Khellin can be topically applied in a moisturizing cream or Carbopol gel (3–5 %). Topical "KUVA-sun" is still used in sunny countries. It has been studied and found that topical khellin followed by UVA (KUVA) does not provide any significant benefit in patients with vitiligo [45, 46]. It is rather effective when given orally, but it has been abandoned.

26.5.3 Phenylalanine

Since phenylalanine is an essential amino acid responsible for initiation of melanogenesis, it is used as a photosensitizer for topical and/or oral supplementation of natural or artificial UVA light phototherapy in the management of vitiligo. The best responders are patients with less than 25 % body surface area involvement, with onset of disease before 21 years of age, and those having generalized and symmetrical lesions [47]. Lotti et al. reported a significant repigmentation in 29.3 % of patients applying topical L-phenylalanine as monotherapy [48]. The addition of topical L-phenylalanine to oral L-phenylalanine and light therapy makes it even more effective [49, 50].

26.6 Topical Depigmenting Agents

Topical agents like hydroquinone (HQ) and monobenzone induce melanocyte death, and these have been approved by the FDA for vitiligo [51]. It should be noted that depigmenting agents should be used in patients with extensive disfiguring vitiligo, and definitely when trial of conventional therapies have failed [11]. Unlike HQ, monobenzyl ether of hydroquinone (MBEH) always causes irreversible depigmentation [52]. A thin layer of MBEH 20 % cream is applied two to three times daily in a uniform manner and rubbed into the pigmented area. Since the depigmenting effect is significantly reduced on exposure to sunlight, prolonged exposure to sunlight is not permissible during treatment, or a sunscreen should be used. Depigmentation is achieved after 1–4 months. The drug should be withdrawn if there is no response after 4 months of treatment. However, if the desired degree of depigmentation is obtained, the drug should be continued in a maintenance dosage (twice weekly) [11].

The response rates range from 40 to 80 % [52]. Side effects include burning, itching, contact dermatitis, conjunctival melanosis, pingueculae, and corneal pigment deposition [1]. There are reports of development of resistance to treatment. To overcome this, prescribing MBEH with retinoic acid has been proposed [53].

26.7 Comparison of Various Topical Therapies

Clobetasol was shown to be superior in efficacy compared to pimecrolimus [54], but considering the adverse-effect profile of TCS, tacrolimus can be a better option [14]. Besides, the results with pimecrolimus is variable [55], thus re-establishing tacrolimus as a better option [21, 56]. However, pimecrolimus in combination with phototherapy is definitely a good option [57]. But, the combination of calcipotriol with TCS is the most favorable therapeutic modality with respect to the efficacy and safety profile, especially when applied on Indian skin [38].

26.8 Newer Drugs

26.8.1 Antioxidants

Recent advances in the etiopathogenesis of vitiligo suggest the role of reactive oxygen species (ROS) in the inhibition of melanogenesis. Therapy with antioxidants (topical and oral) leads to increased catalase activity and a decrease in ROS [58]. Combining oral and topical phenylalanine gives good results [59]. Moreover, Schallreuter et al. reported remarkable repigmentation on the face and hands of patients who were put on topical pseudocatalase with short-term UVB [60]. Sanclemente et al. concluded that topical catalase is as effective as 0.05 % betamethasone in vitiligo [61]. Side effects associated with the use of topical catalase/superoxide dismutase include transient erythema, pruritus, and peeling [61, 62].

26.8.2 Topical 5-Fluorouracil (5-FU)

Topical 5-FU has been studied for the treatment of vitiligo. It is hypothesized that direct overstimulation of melanocyte proliferation, inhibition of agents able to destroy melanocytes, and immunomodulation stabilizing the vitiligo disease could be responsible for the efficacy of 5-FU in vitiligo. However, topical application of 5-FU alone cannot induce any pigment spread in vitiligo patients; application on a dermabraded or ablated epidermis could cause a long-lasting and favorable pigment spread [7, 25, 63].

26.8.3 Piperine

Piperine and its analogs, PIP [5-(3,4-methylenedioxyphenyl)-2,4-pentadienoylpiperidine], tetrahydropiperine [THP, 5-(3,4-methylenedioxyphenyl)-pentanoylpiperidine], a cyclohexyl analog of piperine [CHP, 5-(3,4-methylenedioxyphenyl)-2,4-pentadienoylcyclohexylamine], and reduced CHP [rCHP, 5-(3,4-methylenedioxyphenyl)-2,4-pentanoylcyclohexylamine], have been reported to stimulate melanocyte replication in vitro and may be useful in treating vitiligo [8]. Treatments with these compounds and concomitant cutaneous exposure to ultraviolet (UV) radiation are better in efficacy than UV radiation alone [64].

26.8.4 Prostaglandin E2 (PGE2) Analogs

PGE2, by virtue of its growth-stimulatory effects, is capable of regulating the proliferation and maturation of melanocytes [65]. Kapoor et al. studied the efficacy and safety of topical PGE2 in the treatment of stable vitiligo (<5 % body surface area). Excellent response was seen in 55 % of patients. Side effects in the form of a transient burning sensation especially on the lips were reported in a few patients [66, 67].

26.8.5 Capsaicin and Curcumin

Treatment with these antioxidants inhibits caspase-induced apoptosis, increases the total antioxidant capacity of the body, decreases the generation of ROS and lipid peroxidation, and improves mitochondrial activity. Moreover, *C. melo* extracts have shown superoxide dismutase and catalase-like activities [68]. Thus, topical capsaicin and extracts of C. *melo* might protect against vitiligo progression [69]. However, well-designed randomized clinical trials are needed to support the use of these extracts for vitiligo because of conflicting reports regarding its effectiveness and efficacy [67, 70].

26.8.6 Camouflage

Keeping in mind the significant psychosocial trauma associated with vitiligo, camouflage has a considerable role in the management [71]. There is a wide choice of self-tanning agents; stains; dyes; whitening lotions; tinted cover creams; compact, liquid, and stick foundations; fixing powders; fixing sprays; cleansers; semipermanent and permanent tattoos; and dyes for pigmenting facial and scalp white hairs [11]. The results are even more gratifying in cases of vitiligo in children [72]. Dihydroxyacetone (DHA), one of the most effective camouflage agents, is an active ingredient of sunless tanners. DHA is an easy and convenient option for patients who want to camouflage their vitiligo, because the stain lasts up to 10 days. It reacts with proteins of the stratum corneum and forms brown chromophores called melanoidins, which temporarily impart a golden brown color to the skin [73]. The amount of tanning is proportional to the concentration of DHA used [74]. Thus, it becomes easy for the patient to choose the concentration of DHA that most closely matches their skin color [75, 76].

26.9 Conclusion

Success in the management of vitiligo depends on factors such as patient age, type of vitiligo, location, and extent of involvement. Treatment must also be tailored according to the individual requirements of the patients, to assure adherence. However, with the advent of surgical techniques, vitiligo is no longer considered a disease which cannot be cured, and topical therapies serve as an excellent adjunct to newer therapeutic modalities.

References

1. Felsten LM, Alikhan A, Petronic-Rosic V. Vitiligo: a comprehensive overview part II: treatment options and approach to treatment. J Am Acad Dermatol. 2011;65(3):493–514.
2. Birlea SA, Costin GE, Norris DA. Cellular and molecular mechanisms involved in the action of vitamin D analogs targeting vitiligo depigmentation. Curr Drug Targets. 2008;9(4):345–59.
3. Wu CS, Lan CC, Wang LF, Chen GS, Wu CS, Yu HS. Effects of psoralen plus ultraviolet A irradiation on cultured epidermal cells in vitro and patients with vitiligo in vivo. Br J Dermatol. 2007;156:122–9.
4. Falabella R, Barona MI. Update on skin repigmentation therapies in vitiligo. Pigm Cell Melanoma Res. 2008;22:42–65.
5. Shenoi SD, Prabhu S. Photochemotherapy (PUVA) in psoriasis and vitiligo. Indian J Dermatol Venereol Leprol. 2014;80:497–504.
6. Van doon Boorn JG, Melief CJ, Luiten RM. Monobenzone induced depigmentation: from enzymatic blockade to autoimmunity. Pigm Cell Melanoma Res. 2011;24:673–9.
7. Gauthier Y, Anbar T, Lepreux S, Cario-André M, Benzekri L. Possible mechanisms by which topical 5-fluorouracil and dermabrasion could induce pigment spread in vitiligo skin: an experimental study. ISRN Dermatol. 2013;2013:852497.
8. Faas L, Venkatasamy R, Hider RC, Young AR, Soumyanath A. In vivo evaluation of piperine and synthetic analogues asn potential treatments for vitiligo using a sparsely pigmented mouse model. Br J Dermatol. 2008;158:941–50.
9. Badri AM, Todd PM, Garioch JJ, Gudgeon JE, Stewart DG, Goudie RB. An immunohistological study of cutaneous lymphocytes in vitiligo. J Pathol. 1993;170:149–55.
10. van den Wijngaard R, Wankowicz-Kalinska A, Le Poole C, Tigges B, Westerhof W, Das P. Local immune response in skin of generalized vitiligo patients. Destruction of melanocytes is associated with the prominent presence of CLA+ T cells at the perilesional site. Lab Invest. 2000;80:1299–309.
11. Taieb A, Alomar A, Böhm M, Dell'anna ML, De Pase A, Eleftheriadou V, et al. Guidelines for the management of vitiligo: the European Dermatology Forum consensus. Br J Dermatol. 2013;168(1):5–19.
12. Cockayne SE, Messenger AG, Gawkrodger DJ. Vitiligo treated with topical corticosteroids: children with head and neck involvement respond well. J Am Acad Dermatol. 2002;46:964–5.
13. Kwinter J, Pelletier J, Khambalia A, Pope E. High-potency steroid use in children with vitiligo: a retrospective study. J Am Acad Dermatol. 2007;56:236–41.
14. Lepe V, Moncada B, Castanedo-Cazares JP, Torres-Alvarez MB, Ortiz CA, Torres-Rubalcava AB. A double-blind randomized trial of 0.1% tacrolimus vs 0.05% clobetasol for the treatment of childhood vitiligo. Arch Dermatol. 2003;139:581–5.
15. Coskun B, Saral Y, Turgut D. Topical 0.05% clobetasol propionate versus 1% pimecrolimus ointment in vitiligo. Eur J Dermatol. 2005;15:88–91.
16. Westerhof W, Nieuweboer-Krobotova L, Mulder PG, Glazenburg EJ. Left-right comparison study of the combination of fluticasone propionate and UV-A vs. either fluticasone propionate or UV-A alone for the long-term treatment of vitiligo. Arch Dermatol. 1999;135:1061–6.
17. Lan CC, Chen GS, Chiou MH, Wu CS, Chang CH, Yu HS. FK506 promotes melanocyte and melanoblast growth and creates a favourable milieu for cell migration via keratinocytes: possible mechanisms of how tacrolimus ointment induces repigmentation in patients with vitiligo. Br J Dermatol. 2005;153:498–505.
18. Hartmann A, Brocker EB, Hamm H. Repigmentation of pretibial vitiligo with calcineurin inhibitors under occlusion. J Deutschen Dermatologischen Gesellschaft. 2008;6:383–5.
19. Silverberg NB, Lin P, Travis L, Farley-Li J, Mancini AJ, Wagner AM, et al. Tacrolimus ointment promotes repigmentation of vitiligo in children: a review of 57 cases. J Am Acad Dermatol. 2004;51:760–6.

20. Grimes PE, Morris R, Avaniss-Aghajani E, Soriano T, Meraz M, Metzger A. Topical tacrolimus therapy for vitiligo: therapeutic responses and skin messenger RNA expression of proinflammatory cytokines. J Am Acad Dermatol. 2004;51:52–61.
21. Hartmann A, Brocker EB, Hamm H. Occlusive treatment enhances efficacy of tacrolimus 0.1% ointment in adult patients with vitiligo: results of a placebo-controlled 12-month prospective study. Acta Derm Venereol. 2008;88:474–9.
22. Fai D, Cassano N, Vena GA. Narrow-band UVB phototherapy combined with tacrolimus ointment in vitiligo: a review of 110 patients. J Eur Acad Dermatol Venereol. 2007;21:916–20.
23. Nordal E, Guleng G, Ro¨nnevig J. Treatment of vitiligo with narrowband-UVB (TL01) combined with tacrolimus ointment (0.1%) vs. placebo ointment, a randomized right/left double blind comparative study. J Eur Acad Dermatol Venereol. 2011;25:1440–3.
24. Passeron T, Ostovari N, Zakaria W, Fontas E, Larrouy JC, Lacour JP, et al. Topical tacrolimus and the 308-nm excimer laser: a synergistic combination for the treatment of vitiligo. Arch Dermatol. 2004;140:1065–9.
25. Korobko IV. Review of current clinical studies of vitiligo treatments. Dermatol Ther. 2012;25(S1):S17–27.
26. Kathuria S, Khaitan BK, Ramam M, Sharma VK. Segmental vitiligo: a randomized controlled trial to evaluate efficacy and safety of 0.1% tacrolimus ointment vs 0.05% fluticasone propionate cream. Indian J Dermatol Venereol Leprol. 2012;78:68–73.
27. Juan D, Qianxi X, Zhou C, Jianzhong Z. Clinical efficacy and safety of tacrolimus ointment in patients with vitiligo. J Dermatol. 2011;38:1092–4.
28. Ho N, Pope E, Weinstein M, Greenberg S, Webster C, Krafchik BR. A double-blind, randomized, placebo controlled trial of topical tacrolimus 0.1% vs. clobetasol propionate 0.05% in childhood vitiligo. Br J Dermatol. 2011;165:626–32.
29. Lee DY, Kim CR, Lee JH, Yang JM. Recent onset vitiligo treated with systemic corticosteroid and topical tacrolimus: need for early treatment in vitiligo. J Dermatol. 2010;37:1057–9.
30. Xu AE, Zhang DM, Wei XD, Huang B, Lu LJ. Efficacy and safety of tacrolimus cream 0.1% in the treatment of vitiligo. Int J Dermatol. 2009;48:86–90.
31. Mehrabi D, Pandya AG. A randomized, placebo-controlled, double-blind trial comparing narrowband UV-B plus 0.1% tacrolimus ointment with narrowband UV-B plus placebo in the treatment of generalized vitiligo. Arch Dermatol. 2006;142:927–9.
32. De D, Kanwar AJ. Tacrolimus-induced hyperpigmentation in a patch of vitiligo. Skinmed. 2008;7:93–4.
33. Bakos L, Bakos RM. Focal acne during topical tacrolimus therapy for vitiligo. Arch Dermatol. 2007;143:1223–4.
34. US Food and Drug Administration Web site. www.fda.gov. Accessed 1 Oct. 2015.
35. Wong R, Lin AN. Efficacy of topical calcineurin inhibitors in vitiligo. Int J Dermatol. 2013;52(4):491–6.
36. Parsad D, Saini R, Nagpal R. Calcipotriol in vitiligo: a preliminary study. Pediatr Dermatol. 1999;16:317–20.
37. Gargoom AM, Duweb GA, Elzorghany AH, Benghazil M, Bugrein OO. Calcipotriol in the treatment of childhood vitiligo. Int J Clin Pharmacol Res. 2004;24:11–4.
38. Kumaran MS, Kaur I, Kumar B. Effect of topical calcipotriol, betamethasone dipropionate and their combination in the treatment of localized vitiligo. J Eur Acad Dermatol Venereol. 2006;20:269–73.
39. Travis LB, Silverberg NB. Calcipotriene and corticosteroid combination therapy for vitiligo. Pediatr Dermatol. 2004;21:495–8.
40. Newman MD, Silverberg NB. Once-daily application of calcipotriene 0.005%-betamethasone dipropionate 0.064% ointment for repigmentation of facial vitiligo. Cutis. 2011;88:256–9.
41. Arca E, Tastan HB, Erbil AH, Sezer E, Koc E, Kurumlu Z. Narrow-band ultraviolet B as monotherapy and in combination with topical calcipotriol in the treatment of vitiligo. J Dermatol. 2006;33:338–43.

42. Hartmann A, Lurz C, Hamm H, Brocker EB, Hofmann UB. Narrow-band UVB311 nm vs. broad-band UVB therapy in combination with topical calcipotriol vs. placebo in vitiligo. Int J Dermatol. 2005;44:736–42.
43. Ada S, Sahin S, Boztepe G, Karaduman A, Kolemen F. No additional effect of topical calcipotriol on narrow-band UVB phototherapy in patients with generalized vitiligo. Photodermatol Photoimmunol Photomed. 2005;21:79–83.
44. Ortel B, Petronic-Rosic V, Calzavara-Pinton P. Phototherapeutic options for vitiligo. In: Krutmann J, Honigsmann H, Elmets CA, Bergstresser PR, editors. Dermatological phototherapy and photodiagnostic methods. Heidelberg: Springer; 2009. p. 151–83.
45. Orecchia G, Perfetti L. Photochemotherapy with topical khellin and sunlight in vitiligo. Dermatol. 1992;184:120–3.
46. Saraceno R, Nistico SP, Capriotti E, Chimenti S. Monochromatic excimer light 308 nm in monotherapy and combined with topical khellin 4% in the treatment of vitiligo: a controlled study. Dermatol Ther. 2009;22:391–4.
47. Greiner D, Ochsendorf FR, Milbradt R. Vitiligo therapy with phenylalanine/UV A. Catamnestic studies after five years [in German]. Hautarzt. 1994;45:460–3.
48. Lotti T, Buggiani G, Troiano M, Assad GB, Delescluse J, De Giorgi V, et al. Targeted and combination treatments for vitiligo. Comparative evaluation of different current modalities in 458 subjects. Dermatol Ther. 2008;21(S1):S20–6.
49. Camacho F, Mazuecos J. Treatment of vitiligo with oral and topical phenylalanine: 6 years of experience. Arch Dermatol. 1999;135:216–7.
50. Antoniou C, Schulpis H, Michas T, Katsambas A, Frajis N, Tsagaraki S, et al. Vitiligo therapy with oral and topical phenylalanine with UVA exposure. Int J Dermatol. 1989;28:545–7.
51. Hariharan V, Klarquist J, Reust MJ, Koshoffer A, McKee MD, Boissy RE, et al. Monobenzyl ether of hydroquinone and 4-tertiary butyl phenol activate markedly different physiological responses in melanocytes: relevance to skin depigmentation. J Invest Dermatol. 2010;130:211–20.
52. Njoo MD, Vodegel RM, Westerhof W. Depigmentation therapy in vitiligo universalis with topical 4-methoxyphenol and the Qswitched ruby laser. J Am Acad Dermatol. 2000;42:760–9.
53. Kasraee B, Fallahi MR, Ardekani GS, Ebrahimi S, Doroudchi G, Omrani GR, et al. Retinoic acid synergistically enhances the melanocytotoxic and depigmenting effects of monobenzylether of hydroquinone in black guinea pig skin. Exp Dermatol. 2006;15:509–14.
54. Eryilmaz A, Seckin D, Baba M. Pimecrolimus: a new choice in the treatment of vitiligo? J Eur Acad Dermatol Venereol. 2009;23:1327–49.
55. Dawid M, Veensalu M, Grassberger M, Wolff K. Efficacy and safety of pimecrolimus cream 1% in adult patients with vitiligo: results of a randomized, double-blind, vehicle-controlled study. J Dtsch Dermatol Ges. 2006;4:942–6.
56. Radakovic S, Breier-Maly J, Konschitzky R, et al. Response of vitiligo to once vs. twice-daily topical tacrolimus: a controlled prospective, randomized, observer-blinded trial. J Eur Acad Dermatol Venereol. 2009;23:951–3.
57. Esfandiarpour I, Ekhlasi A, Farajzadeh S, Shamsadini S. The efficacy of pimecrolimus 1% cream plus narrow-band ultraviolet B in the treatment of vitiligo: a double-blind, placebo-controlled clinical trial. J Dermatol Treat. 2009;20:14–8.
58. Dell'Anna ML, Mastrofrancesco A, Sala R, Venturini M, Ottaviani M, Vidolin AP, et al. Antioxidants and narrow band-UVB in the treatment of vitiligo: a double-blind placebo controlled trial. Clin Exp Dermatol. 2007;32:631–6.
59. Rojas-Urdaneta JE, Poleo-Romero AG. Evaluation of an antioxidant and mitochondria-stimulating cream formula on the skin of patients with stable common vitiligo [in Spanish]. Invest Clin. 2007;48:21–31.
60. Schallreuter KU, Wood JM, Lemke KR, Levenig C. Treatment of vitiligo with a topical application of pseudocatalase and calcium in combination with short-term UVB exposure: a case study on 33 patients. Dermatol. 1995;190:223–9.

61. Sanclemente G, Garcia JJ, Zuleta JJ, Diehl C, Correa C, Falabella R. A double-blind, randomized trial of 0.05% betamethasone vs. topical catalase/dismutase superoxide in vitiligo. J Eur Acad Dermatol Venereol. 2008;22:1359–64.
62. Tsiskarishvili N. Cuprum sulfate and vitix in the treatment of vitiligo in children [in Russian]. Georgian Med News. 2005;121:48–51.
63. Garg T, Chander R, Jain A. Combination of microdermabrasion and 5-fluorouracil to induce repigmentation in vitiligo: an observational study. Dermatol Surg. 2011;37:1763–6.
64. Soumyanath A, Venkatasamy R, Joshi M, et al. UV irradiation affects melanocyte stimulatory activity and protein binding of piperine. Photochem Photobiol. 2006;82:1541–8.
65. Parsad D, Pandhi R, Dogra S, Kumar B. Topical prostaglandin analog (PGE2) in vitiligo – a preliminary study. Int J Dermatol. 2002;41:942–5.
66. Kapoor R, Phiske MM, Jerajani HR. Evaluation of safety and efficacy of topical prostaglandin E2 in treatment of vitiligo. Br J Dermatol. 2009;160:861–3.
67. Lotti TM, Hercogová J, Schwartz RA, Tsampau D, Korobko I, Pietrzak A, et al. Treatments of vitiligo: what's new at the horizon. Dermatol Ther. 2012;25(S1):S32–40.
68. Yuksel EP, Aydin F, Senturk N, Canturk T, Turanli AY. Comparison of the efficacy of narrow band ultraviolet B and narrow band ultraviolet B plus topical catalase-superoxide dismutase treatment in vitiligo patients. Eur J Dermatol. 2009;19:341–4.
69. Becatti M, Prignano F, Fiorillo C, Pescitelli L, Nassi P, Lotti T, Taddei N. The involvement of Smac/DIABLO, p53, NF-kB, and MAPK pathways in apoptosis of keratinocytes from perilesional vitiligo skin: protective effects of curcumin and capsaicin. Antioxid Redox Signal. 2010;13(9):1309–21.
70. Schallreuter KU, Panske A, Chiuchiarelli G. Ineffective topical treatment of vitiligo with *Cucumismelo* extracts. Int J Dermatol. 2011;50:374–5.
71. Ongenae K, Dierckxsens L, Brochez L, van Geel N, Naeyaert JM. Quality of life and stigmatization profile in a cohort of vitiligo patients and effect of the use of camouflage. Dermatol. 2005;210:279–85.
72. Tedeschi A, Dall'Oglio F, Micali G, Schwartz RA, Janniger CK. Corrective camouflage in pediatric dermatology. Cutis. 2007;79:110–2.
73. Muizzuddin N, Marenus KD, Maes DH. Tonality of suntan vs sunless tanning with dihydroxyacetone. Skin Res Technol. 2000;6(4):199–204.
74. Draelos ZD. Self-tanning lotions: are they a healthy way to achieve a tan? Am J Clin Dermatol. 2002;3(5):317–8.
75. Hsu S. Camouflaging vitiligo with dihydroxyacetone. Dermatol Online J. 2008;14:23.
76. Rajatanavin N, Suwanachote S, Kulkollakarn S. Dihydroxyacetone: a safe camouflaging option in vitiligo. Int J Dermatol. 2008;47:402–6.

Chapter 27
Oral Medications in Vitiligo

Koushik Lahiri and Samujjala Deb

27.1 Introduction

The exact etiopathogenesis of vitiligo is yet to be determined, and hence there is a great dilemma regarding an effective modality of treatment for vitiligo. Treatment response is often variable. Thus, patients of vitiligo having skin of color suffer a negative impact on the quality of their lives [1–7].

Over the years, a number of studies have been carried out on different treatment modalities that may give the best outcomes. These help physicians decide on a course of treatment, supported by evidence-based medicine for different forms of vitiligo. The major studies published are from India [8], Saudi Arabia [9], America [10, 11], and Europe [12, 13].

In spite of much advancement in pharmacotherapy, treatment for vitiligo still remains a challenge for physicians. With the complex interplay of etiopathogenic factors, it still remains a mystery as to which treatment option will be best for different cases of vitiligo. The various modalities of treatment range from topical to systemic and from physical to surgical. The choice of treatment needs to be individualized based on the patients' age, extent of vitiligo, stability, side-effect profile, coexisting morbidity, and supporting evidence [10, 12, 14–19]. The various oral medications that have been used in vitiligo are discussed, together with some novel and alternative treatment modalities.

K. Lahiri (✉)
Apollo Gleneagles Hospitals, WIZDERM,
Greenwood Nook, Coral Isle-14 RB, 369/2 Purbachal, Kalikapur, EM Byepass,
Kolkata 700070, India
e-mail: doctorlahiri@gmail.com

S. Deb
St. John's Medical College & Hospital, Bangalore, Karnataka, India, 560034
e-mail: samujjala.deb@gmail.com

E.B. Handog, M.J. Enriquez-Macarayo (eds.), *Melasma and Vitiligo in Brown Skin*,
DOI 10.1007/978-81-322-3664-1_27

27.2 Systemic Corticosteroids

Oral corticosteroids are very effective in controlling actively spreading vitiligo when given in optimum doses and for appropriate indications. It mainly acts by suppressing of autoantibody production and inducing apoptosis of cytotoxic T cells. It halts the progression in rapidly progressing disease and also helps in repigmentation [20–23]. In the past, daily doses of corticosteroids were often used. In light of the untoward side effects like weight gain, diabetes mellitus, hirsutism, peptic ulcer, acneiform eruptions, and osteoporosis, low-dose pulse therapy regimens were tried which showed good response without the adverse effects [20].

27.2.1 Oral Pulse Therapy

This principle of administering systemic corticosteroids has shown a lot of promise in the treatment of unstable progressive vitiligo. In pulse therapy, intermittent large (suprapharmacologic) doses are administered to enhance the therapeutic effect and reduce the side effects of a particular drug. It was pioneered in India by Pasricha [22].

As an adjunct to phototherapy, Rath et al. observed that the highest repigmentation was seen when used in combination with narrowband ultraviolet B light (NBUVB) in comparison to broadband UVB (BBUVB) and psoralen with UVA phototherapy [24].

In one study, prednisolone was given in an oral dose of 2 mg/kg once weekly in 50 patients with extensive and rapidly spreading vitiligo; 93 % of patients showed cessation of disease progression with repigmentation in 88 % of cases, with side effects developing in only three patients [25].

27.2.1.1 Oral Minipulse (OMP) Therapy

Oral minipulse therapy is usually given using dexamethasone or betamethasone, 5 mg as a single oral dose, after having breakfast on any two consecutive days of the week. This regimen has similar therapeutic response without the potential adverse effects of daily corticosteroid therapy [26, 27].

The dosage can be increased to 7.5 mg in patients with inadequate response. In children the dose can be reduced to 2.5–3.5 mg per day for two consecutive days in a week after having a thorough discussion with parents and keeping the indications and side-effect profile in mind. The mini-pulse regimen can be used in patients with other concomitant diseases like hypertension and diabetes mellitus. It is best to avoid minipulse therapy in pregnant women.

Side effects are less in comparison to daily corticosteroid therapy but can be seen nevertheless. Most common are weight gain, acneiform eruptions, gastric discomfort, hiccups, headache, and bad taste in the mouth.

The treatment is usually continued till the appearance of new lesions is halted. The dose can then be progressively reduced over a span of 6–8 months. The usual protocol is to reduce the dose of betamethasone by 1 mg every 4–6 weeks. In another study, methylprednisolone was given as OMP in doses of 0.8 mg/day along with topical fluticasone in children for a duration of 6 months. The disease was arrested in 90 % cases with repigmentation seen in 65 % cases with minimal side effects [28].

Response is usually achieved within 1–3 months in most patients. Progression of the disease is halted, and many patients achieve partial to complete repigmentation. In some cases, repigmentation may not occur at all [26, 27].

In the study conducted by Radakovik et al., 10 mg of dexamethasone minipulse was given on two consecutive days per week for up to 24 weeks in 77 patients. In 88 % of patients, progression of disease activity was stopped following 18 weeks of treatment; 69 % of patients also showed side effects like weight gain, insomnia, agitation, hypertrichosis, and menstrual disturbances [27].

In cases with rapidly progressive vitiligo, phototherapy can be started following minipulse therapy. But there is limited data regarding the efficacy of phototherapy in vitiligo when given alongside steroid minipulse therapy.

27.2.2 Intravenous Pulse Therapy

In a study by Seiter et al., methylprednisolone was administered in a dose of 8 mg/kg for three consecutive days in a month in 14 patients with generalized vitiligo. Eighty-five percent of the patients showed cessation of disease progression with repigmentation in 71 % patients. But the patients who had static disease did not show any repigmentation. The therapy was well tolerated in all except by one patient who developed intermittent arterial hypertension [29].

In another study by Nagayata, five vitiligo patients were treated with 500 mg of intravenous methylprednisolone (half-dose steroid pulse) for three consecutive days, thrice every month. The patients were evaluated using a spectrophotometer. After completion of three such monthly cycles, three out of the five patients achieved arrest of disease progression with decrease of white contrast on spectrophotometric examination [30].

Lee et al. evaluated the safety and efficacy of intravenous methylprednisolone pulse in combination with phototherapy in generalized vitiligo. Thirty-six patients were treated with intravenous methylprednisolone, 500 mg on three consecutive days followed by twice weekly treatment with PUVA. 36.1 % patients in the study achieved greater than 50 % repigmentation [31].

27.3 Immunosuppressants and Biologics

Many immunosuppressive and biologic drugs have also been tried in the treatment of vitiligo. Immunosuppressants act by inhibiting the T-cell response toward the melanocytes. They may have an adjuvant role and help in reducing the dose of corticosteroids. Of the plethora of immunosuppressives, azathioprine, cyclophosphamide, cyclosporine, and methotrexate have been tried in vitiligo with varying results [32, 33].

There is still a lot of research and study needed to determine the therapeutic potential of immunosuppressants and biologics in the treatment of vitiligo. Till such data is available, it would be prudent to keep the adverse side effect profile of these drugs in mind when it comes to treating a patient with vitiligo.

27.3.1 Azathioprine

In the study by Radmaneesh et al., 60 patients with vitiligo were randomized to receive either azathioprine (0.6–0.76 mg/kg body weight) and oral PUVA or PUVA alone for 4 months. Following treatment after 4 months, 58.4 % patients achieved a mean total repigmentation in the azathioprine and oral PUVA group compared to 24.8 % in the oral PUVA group alone. Side effects seen were minimal in both the groups during the duration of the study [32]. In view of this finding, azathioprine may be given in rapidly progressing vitiligo where corticosteroids are contraindicated.

27.3.2 Cyclophosphamide

Cyclophosphamide was also tried in a study by Gokhale et al. in a group of 33 vitiligo patients. With 100 mg given daily, some repigmentation was seen in 29 patients with side effects being cytopenia, hair loss, and nausea [34]. Some studies have also shown the efficacy of cyclophosphamide along with oral minipulse of corticosteroids and methotrexate (7.5 mg weekly) in rapidly spreading vitiligo [22, 33].

27.3.3 Cyclosporine

Cyclosporine was tried in six patients in a dose of 6 mg/kg daily. Five patients showed little to no pigmentation after several months of therapy. Side effects seen were hypertension and renal dysfunction [35].

27.3.4 Antitumor Necrosis Factor-α (Anti-TNF-α)

An open-label pilot study was carried out by Rigopuolos on four patients with progressive non-segmental vitiligo to assess the therapeutic efficacy of etanercept. It was given weekly in a dose of 50 mg for 12 weeks followed by 25 mg weekly for another 4 weeks. The patients tolerated the drug well but there was no repigmentation [36].

In another case report, a patient with ankylosing spondylitis and progressive non-segmental vitiligo was treated with infliximab in doses of 350 mg intravenously at weeks 0, 2, and 6 and then on alternate weeks for a total span of 10 months. After 6 months, partial or complete repigmentation was seen in all or most spots with a halt in the progression of vitiligo [37]. But one point that needs to be kept in mind is that non-segmental vitiligo may itself be induced by anti-TNF-α agents [38].

27.4 Oral Psoralens

Since ancient time, UV light-based therapy has been used in the treatment of vitiligo. Psoralens are naturally occurring tricyclic furocoumarins in plants. In ancient India and Egypt, medical writings mention the use of *Ammi majus* [39] and *Psoralea corylifolia* plants [40] on whitish skin patches followed by exposure to sunlight. The active ingredients were later found out to be 8-methoxypsoralen, 5-methoxypsoralen, and 8-isoamyleneoxypsoralen [41].

In 1948, modern photochemotherapy was introduced by El-Mofty [42], who purified the topical and oral psoralens. When it was discovered that psoralens were maximally activated with UVA light of 360 mm wavelength [43, 44], fluorescent black lamps were used by investigators in combination with psoralens and the use of PUVA chemotherapy began [45]. PUVA is effective in causing repigmentation of vitiligo lesions as shown by many studies [43, 46].

The most commonly used psoralen is 8-methoxypsoralen (8-MOP). This is of plant origin but synthetic preparations are also available. TMP (4, 5, 8 trimethyl psoralen) is from a synthetic preparation which is less phototoxic after oral administration but is also less effective. 5-MOP is another naturally occurring psoralen in citrus fruits, celery, and parsley leaves. This is less erythmogenic by oral route and also does not lead to the development of intolerance reactions or adverse gastrointestinal effects. The time taken to achieve therapeutic levels in blood for psoralens varies with the type and amount of food [47].

The most common dosing schedule used is by giving 8-MOP at 0.4–0.6 mg/kg, after food intake, followed by exposure to sunlight after 2 h on alternate days in a week. Though 8-MOP and TMP can both be used, the latter is often utilized as it is less phototoxic [48]. The most suitable time for sun exposure is usually between 10:30 to 11:30 am and 3:30 to 4:30 pm, but these can be modified to suit the patients' schedule. It changes as per the geographic location of the subject, based on the latitude and longitude and also the position of the sun during that specific part of the year.

The duration of exposure is gradually increased from 5 to 15 min in a stepwise manner or till the appearance of mild erythema. The UVA doses range from 0.25 to 2 J/cm^2 initially with increments of 0.2–0.5 J/cm^2 every session, until erythema develops or a maximum dose is reached. A maximum of 6 J/cm^2 was cited by one study [27, 49–51]. In another study, the exposure was increased by 20 % instead of a fixed increase, with the end point remaining the same [52]. Therapy should be stopped if there is no response after 6 months or 50 treatments. Maximum number of treatments has been suggested to be a maximum of 150–200 sittings.

Studies comparing UVA-based therapy with narrowband phototherapy have shown that NB-UVB may be better in comparison to PUVA [53].

There are quite a few limitations associated with psoralen-based photochemotherapy. Oral administration of psoralens can lead to nausea and vomiting. The exposure to UVA needs to be done within 2 h of ingestion. The absorption of the drug is also variable depending on the type of food taken prior to the drug. Post therapy, photo-protection is needed for the skin and the eyes to prevent damage. Also UVA penetrates deeper in comparison to UVB; thus, incorrect administration can lead to painful blistering of the skin which can be severe enough to warrant a cessation of therapy. At the same time, there is poor color match and psoralens are only moderately effective in vitiligo [54].

Psoralen based therapy is also contraindicated in children less than 10 years of age for skin type 1 and less than 16 years for skin type 2. This is because of their increased susceptibility to ocular and cutaneous damage especially if they have concomitant risk factors for developing malignant melanoma [55]. No studies are available for patients of darker skin belonging to Fitzpatrick skin type IV, V, or IV.

Past history of non-melanoma skin cancer is not an absolute contraindication, but alternative therapies may be tried in patients with other important risk factors [55].

27.5 Khellin-Based Photochemotherapy

Another type of photochemotherapy using khellin as a photosensitizer has also been tried. Khellin (5, 8-dimethoxy-2-methyl-4,5-furo-6,7 chromone) is a furanchrome, derived as an extract from the plant *Ammi visnaga* and is used in conjunction with UVA phototherapy [7, 56, 57] This treatment is also known as KUVA. The main advantage of this regimen is the lack of phototoxicity. Thus, it can be used with natural sunlight even as a daily regimen. Its efficacy is limited because up to 30 % of patients can present with liver toxicity in the form of cytolysis. It is used at a dose of 100 mg orally given 2 h before treatment. Notwithstanding its usefulness, the efficacy and safety profile of oral khellin-based therapies in comparison to PUVA or other treatment modalities has not been studied extensively, and available data is limited.

27.6 Other Systemic Treatments in Vitiligo

27.6.1 Antioxidants

Keeping in mind the role of cellular oxidative stress in the progression of vitiligo, antioxidants have been tried in the treatment of vitiligo [58]. Pseudocatalase, vitamin E, vitamin C, ubiquinone, lipoic acid, *Polypodium leucotomos*, catalase/superoxide dismutase combination, and *Ginkgo biloba* are antioxidants that have been used alone or, more frequently, in combination with phototherapy [12].

Open trials have suggested that oral administration of single or multiple antioxidants stopped the progression of vitiligo and also promoted repigmentation [59].

Vitamin E has been reported to enhance recovery of skin lipid peroxidation following PUVA therapy according to few randomized clinical trials [60]. A study by Dell'Anna et al. has demonstrated a reduction in the requirement of UV dosages after administration of a mixture of α-lipoic acid, vitamin E, and vitamin C. It also helped to enhance repigmentation [61].

Polypodium leucotomos is a fern found in South America with a wide application in the treatment of diseases like vitiligo, melasma, psoriasis, and sunlight-induced damage. It has antioxidant, photosensitizing and immunomodulator actions that showed good results on concomitant administration with PUVA or UVB [62]. In a study by Middelkamp-Hup et al., 50 patients were enrolled in a double-blind randomized study wherein they received 250 mg of the extract thrice daily along with twice weekly treatment with NBUVB. After 25–26 weeks, 44 % of patients receiving the extract showed repigmentation in the head and neck area which was significantly more, in comparison to controls (27 % only); other areas like trunk, extremities, hands and feet had poorer response Repigmentation was higher in the patients who received NB-UVB along with leucotomos extract [62].

Another novel agent, *Gingko biloba*, is a traditional Chinese herb. It is a polyphenol compound having anti-inflammatory, immunomodulatory, and antioxidant properties and has shown promising results in the treatment of vitiligo. In a study by Parsad et al., 52 patients were enrolled in a randomized controlled study and were treated with either 40 mg of *Gingko biloba* extract or placebo thrice daily. After 6 months of therapy, 80 % of vitiligo patients had cessation of disease activity compared to 36.6 % of controls. Also 40 % of patients showed up to 75 % repigmentation compared to only 9 % of controls [63].

In another study by Szczurko et al., 12 patients were treated for 12 weeks with 120 mg extract, and all had arrest of disease progression [64]. The anti-inflammatory action of *Gingko biloba* leads to a reduction in the cyclooxygenase activity with a reduction in IL-8 and vascular endothelial growth factor in response to TNF-α [65]. The most common side effect seen was gastric discomfort [64]. An important side effect is coagulopathy; hence, this drug should be used with caution in patients on anticoagulants [66]. However, the number of patients enrolled in this study was limited. A definite consensus cannot be reached on the long-term safety profile and further studies are warranted [63–66].

27.7 Newer and Alternative Treatments in Vitiligo [67]

Vitiligo has been increasingly recognized as a disorder of autoimmune destruction of melanocytes [68–70]. Still, controversy exists regarding its true etiopathogenesis. A number of hypotheses have been put forward like immune dysregulation, neurogenic factors, catecholamine-mediated cytotoxicity, and oxidative stress [71, 72]. Over the years, a number of compounds have been experimentally tried in the treatment of vitiligo. Some have shown good results while others have had equivocal responses. In light of the enigmatic pathophysiology of vitiligo, research continues to discover newer and novel systemic treatment modalities for vitiligo.

27.7.1 L-Phenylalanine

L-Phenylalanine (l-Phe) is an essential amino acid and a precursor to tyrosine in the melanin biosynthetic pathway. It has been explored as a treatment option in vitiligo along with ultraviolet phototherapy. It has been hypothesized that metabolism and uptake of phenylalanine is defective in vitiligo [72, 73]. Phenylalanine appears to be beneficial in vitiligo, unrelated to its role in the melanin synthesis pathway.

It has also been hypothesized that l-Phe may interfere with the antibody production in vitiligo [74, 75].

In a study by Siddiqi et al., 149 patients of vitiligo were treated with l-Phe for 18 months. Patients were divided into three groups. Group I received l-Phe (100 mg/kg body weight) with UVA phototherapy twice weekly. Group II received l-Phe alone and group III did not receive any treatment. They found that 71.2 % of the patients in group I had repigmentation up to 77 % in comparison to no pigmentation seen in groups II and III [76].

In another study by Antoniou et al., patients received oral l-Phe and UVA phototherapy in one group and oral and topical l-Phe along with UVA phototherapy in another group. In both, 75 % repigmentation was seen [74].

In two other studies, 50 mg/kg of l-Phe was given to patients along with UVA phototherapy and repigmentation ranging from 85 to 95 % after 6–8 months [77, 78].

It can be thus concluded that l-Phe limits the antibody attack on melanocytes while UVA induces repigmentation. Thus l-Phe may be tried in vitiligo in conjunction with UVA phototherapy, and the evidence is supported by quite a few randomized clinical trials.

27.7.2 Vitamin B12 and Folic Acid

It has been seen that there is decreased serum levels of vitamin B12 and folic acid in vitiligo [79, 80].

An association between vitiligo and pernicious anemia has also been noticed [81, 82]. This has led researchers to study the role of vitamin B12 and folic acid supplementation in the management of vitiligo.

Montes et al. reported that among 15 vitiligo patients, 73.3 % had folic acid deficiency, 33.3 % had vitamin B12 deficiency, and 26.6 %6 had vitamin C deficiency. On daily supplementation, repigmentation was seen in all patients and a halt in the progression of disease in 80–100 % patients, over a span of 2 years [83]. In a study by Juhlin and Olsson of 100 vitiligo patients on oral supplementation with vitamin B12 and folic acid along with phototherapy with either sunlight or UVB, repigmentation was seen in 52.2 % cases with halt in progression of vitiligo over a span of 3–6 months [84].

On the contrary, in a randomized clinical trial by Tjioe et al., no significant difference was seen in 27 vitiligo patients on supplementation with vitamin B12 and folic acid (oral cobalamin 1000 ug sustained release and folic acid 5 mg, twice daily) along with UVB phototherapy [85].

Homocysteine levels have been found to be elevated in vitiligo patients and cause direct damage of melanocytes by oxidative stress [80]. It is likely that vitamin B12 and folic acid act by decreasing homocysteine levels in vitiligo [86].

Since vitamin B12 and folic acid are water soluble vitamins, they can be supplemented in vitiligo patients at a low cost and negligible side effect profile. But nevertheless, data supporting its therapeutic effect is limited and the only randomized trial did not show any difference in clinical efficacy on supplementing vitamin B12 and folic acid.

27.7.3 Zinc

Zinc acts by regulation of gene expression and also acts as a cofactor for superoxide dismutase. Adequate cellular levels of zinc are also needed to prevent cellular apoptosis. Decreased zinc levels activate caspase leading to cell death [87, 88]. In a study by Shameer et al., vitiligo patients were found to have 21.6 % lower level of serum zinc in comparison to controls [88]. Yaghoobi et al. carried out a randomized trial with 35 patients of vitiligo receiving topical corticosteroids with or without oral zinc sulfate supplementation in a dose of 220 mg, two capsules per day in teenager and adults, and 10 mg/kg of capsule or syrup for children. At 4 months, response to treatment was higher in the group receiving oral zinc supplementation [89].

Zinc supplementation has shown good results on concomitant treatment with topical corticosteroids, but further studies are needed. The only limiting adverse effect is gastrointestinal irritation with oral zinc therapy [89].

27.7.4 Minocycline

Minocycline is an antibiotic with anti-inflammatory and antioxidant property. In a study by Parsad et al., daily treatment with minocycline (100 mg once daily). After 4 weeks of treatment, minocycline was effective in halting the progression of vitiligo both during and after therapy [90]. Further research, however, is needed to elucidate the efficacy of minocycline therapy in vitiligo.

27.7.5 Vitamin D

Many studies have identified a possible correlation between low vitamin D levels and autoimmunity. A study done by Silverberg and Silverberg showed very low levels (<15 ng/ml) of 25-hydroxy vitamin D levels in patients with vitiligo vulgaris [91]. It has also been shown in a study by Sehrawat et al. that levels of 25-hydroxy vitamin D were found to increase significantly following increase in the cumulative dose of NBUVB [92]. A study conducted by Finamor et al. has showed that daily oral supplementation with 35,000 IU of vitamin D for 6 months showed significant repigmentation in 14 out of 16 vitiligo patients [93].

27.8 Conclusion

It is thus evident that despite of a plethora of systemic medications for vitiligo treatment, the dilemma regarding the best possible treatment modality persists. Patients often visit physicians after having tried both topical and oral medications for a long period of time with variable responses. Nevertheless, with a systematic and scientific approach, treatments with strong evidence supporting them can be prescribed to patients in order to stop the disease progression, enhance the process of repigmentation, and improve the quality of their lives [2–4, 8, 9, 11, 12].

Outside of the topical and systemic medications known for vitiligo, availability of surgical modalities is now an option for stable [94] as well as localized forms of vitiligo. Excellent results can be obtained when tried in appropriate patients as shown by Lahiri et al. in a number of studies [1, 19, 95, 96].

Patients must also be warned against the multitude of incorrect and harmful treatments which may worsen their disease. Extensive research continues toward finding a satisfactory treatment for vitiligo.

References

1. Lahiri K. Evolution and evaluation of autologous mini punch grafting in vitiligo. Indian J Dermatol. 2009;54:159–67.
2. Ongenae K, Van Geel N, Naeyaert JM. Evidence for an autoimmune pathogenesis of vitiligo. Pigment Cell Res. 2003;16(2):90–100.
3. Lotti T, Gori A, Zanieri F, Colucci R, Moretti S. Vitiligo: new and emerging treatments. Dermatol Ther. 2008;21(2):110–7.
4. Szczurko O, Boon HS. A systematic review of natural health product treatment for vitiligo. BMC Dermatol. 2008;8:2.
5. Handa S, Kaur I. Vitiligo: clinical findings in 1436 patients. J Dermatol. 1999;26:653–7.
6. Kent G, Al-abadie M. Factors affecting responses on dermatology life quality index among vitiligo sufferers. Clin Exp Dermatol. 1996;21:330–3.
7. Parsad D, Pandhi R, Dogra S, Kanwar AJ, Kumar B. Dermatology life quality index score in vitiligo and its impact on the treatment outcome. Br J Dermatol. 2003;148:373–4.

8. Parsad D, Gupta S. Standard guidelines of care for vitiligo surgery. Indian J Dermatol Venereol Leprol. 2008;74(S1):37–45.
9. Ismail SA, Sayed DS, Abdelghani LN. Vitiligo management strategy in Jeddah, Saudi Arabia as reported by dermatologists and experienced by patients. J Dermatol Treat. 2014;25:205–11.
10. Felsten LM, Alikhan A, Petronic-Rosic V. Vitiligo: a comprehensive overview part II: treatment options and approach to treatment. J Am Acad Dermatol. 2011;65(3):493–514.
11. Felsten LM, Alikhan A, Petronic-Rosic V. Vitiligo: a comprehensive overview: part I. Introduction, epidemiology, quality of life, diagnosis, differential diagnosis, associations, histopathology, etiology, and work-up. J Am Acad Dermatol. 2011;65(3):473–91.
12. Taieb A, Alomar A, Bohm M, Dell'anna ML, De Pase A, Eleftheriadou V, et al. Guidelines for the management of vitiligo: the European Dermatology Forum consensus. Br J Dermatol. 2013;168(1):5–19.
13. Ezzedine K, Lim HW, Suzuki T, Katayama I, Hamzavi I, Lan CC, et al. Revised classification/nomenclature of vitiligo and related issues: the Vitiligo Global Issues Consensus Conference. Pigm Cell Melanoma Res. 2012;25(3):E1–13.
14. Lotti T. Vitiligo: problems and solutions. Int J Immunopath Pharmacol Dermatol. 2002;13:325–8.
15. Taieb A, Piccardo M. Clinical practice: vitiligo. N Engl J Med. 2009;360:160–9.
16. Buggiani G, Tsampau D, Hercogovà J, Rossi R, Brazzini B, Lotti T. Clinical efficacy of a novel topical formulation for vitiligo: compared evaluation of different treatment modalities in 149 patients. Dermatol Ther. 2012;25(5):472–6.
17. Kathuria S, Khaitan BK, Ramam M, Sharma VK. Segmental vitiligo: a randomized controlled trial to evaluate efficacy and safety of 0.1% tacrolimus ointment vs 0.05% fluticasone propionate cream. Indian J Dermatol Venereol Leprol. 2012;78(1):68–73.
18. Lahiri K. Stability in vitiligo? What's that? J Cutan Aesthet Surg. 2009;2(1):38–40.
19. Lahiri K, Malakar S. The concept of stability of vitiligo: a reappraisal. Indian J Dermatol. 2012;57:83–9.
20. Brosthoff H, Brosthoff J. Vitiligo and steroids. Lancet. 1978;2:688.
21. Thomas PS. Prednisolone causing amelioration of both vitiligo and chronic active hepatitis. Br J Hosp Med. 1978;38:464.
22. Pasricha JS, Seetharam KA, Dashore A. Evaluation of five different regimens for the treatment of vitiligo. Indian J Dermatol Venereol Leprol. 1989;55:18–21.
23. Gupta R. Causes of vitiligo. In: Gupta R, editor. Leucoderma (vitiligo). 1st ed. New Delhi: Atlantic Publishers and Distributors; 2007. p. 20–40.
24. Rath N, Kar HK, Sabhnani S. An open labeled, comparative clinical study on efficacy and tolerability of oral minipulse of steroid (OMP) alone, OMP with PUVA and broad/narrowband UVB phototherapy in progressive vitiligo. Indian J Dermatol Venereol Leprol. 2008;74:357–60.
25. Gupta RR. Modified oral mini pulse steroid therapy in unstable vitiligo: a novel once a week regimen. Presented at 29th Annual Conference of IADVL; 2001. Unpublished.
26. Imran M. Childhood vitiligo: response to methylprednisolone OMP therapy and topical fluticasone preparation. Indian J Dermatol. 2010;54:124–7.
27. Pasricha JS, Khaitan BK. Oral minipulse therapy with betamethasone in vitiligo patients having extensive or fast spreading disease. Int J Dermatol. 2001;44:814–7.
28. Radakovik Fijan S, Furnissn-Friedl AM, Tanew A, Honigsman H. Oral dexamethasone pulse treatment for vitiligo. J Am Acad Dermatol. 2001;44:814–7.
29. Seiter S, Ugurel S, Tilgen W, Reinhold U. Use of high-dose methylprednisolone pulse therapy in patients with progressive and stable vitiligo. Int J Dermatol. 2000;39:624–7.
30. Nagata Y, Tanemura A, Ono E, Tanaka A, Kato K, Yamada M, Katayama I. Preliminary colorimetric assessment of progressive nonsegmental vitiligo under short-term intravenous methylprednisolone pulse therapy. J Cosm Dermatol Sci Appl. 2014;4:135–40.
31. Lee Y, Seo YJ, Lee JH, Park JK. High-dose prednisolone and psoralen ultraviolet a combination therapy in 36 patients with vitiligo. Clin Exp Dermatol. 2007;32:499–501.

32. Radmaneesh M, Saedi K. The efficacy of combined PUVA and low dose azathioprine for early and enhanced repigmentation in vitiligo patients. J Dermatol Treat. 2006;17:151–3.
33. Sandra A, Pai S, Shenoi SD. Unstable vitiligo responding to methotrexate. Indian J Dermatol Venereol Leprol. 1998;64:309.
34. Gokhale BB. Cyclophosphamide and vitiligo. Int J Dermatol. 1979;18:92.
35. Gupta AK, Ellis CN, Nickoloff BJ, Nickoloff BJ, Goldfarb MT, Ho VC, et al. Oral cyclosporine in the treatment of inflammatory and noninflammatory dermatoses. A clinical and immunopathologic analysis. Arch Dermatol. 1990;126:339–50.
36. Rigopoulos D, Gregorious S, Larios G, Larios G, Moustou E, Belayeva-Karatza E, Kalogeromitros D. Etanercept in the treatment of vitiligo. Dermatol. 2007;215:84–5.
37. Smith DI, Heffernan MP. Vitiligo after the resolution of psoriatic plaques during treatment with adalimumab. J Am Acad Dermatol. 2008;58:S50–1.
38. Ramı'rez-Herna'ndez M, Marras C, Martı'nez-Escribano JA. Infliximab- induced vitiligo. Dermatol. 2005;210:79–80.
39. McKenna WB. Ammi majus Linn in the treatment of vitiligo. Scott Med J. 1957;2:69–70.
40. Benedetto AV. The psoralens. A historical perspective. Cutis. 1977;20:469–71.
41. Fowlks WL. The chemistry of the psoralens. J Invest Dermatol. 1959;32:249–54.
42. El Mofty AM. A preliminary clinical report on the treatment of leucoderma with Ammi majus Linn. J Egypt Med Assoc. 1948;31:651–65.
43. Pathak MA, Fellman JH. Activating and fluorescent wave-lengths of furocoumarins: psoralens. Nature. 1960;185:382–3.
44. Buck HW, Magnus IA, Porter AD. The action spectrum of 8-methoxypsoralen for erythema in human skin: preliminary studies with a monochromator. Br J Dermatol. 1960;72:249–55.
45. Fulton Jr JE, Leyden J, Papa C. Treatment of vitiligo with topical methoxsalen and blacklite. Arch Dermatol. 1969;100:224–9.
46. Bouattour H, Chaabouni M. Comparative analytical study of the effects of psoralens in vitiligo (findings in 70 patients) (author's transl). Ann Dermatol Venereol. 1978;105:507–10.
47. Sharma VK, Jerajani HR, Srinivas HR, Kanwar AJ, Premalatha S, Sengupta SR, et al. Guidelines for medical management of vitiligo. In: Sharma VK, editor. IADVL therapeutic guidelines: guidelines for vitiligo, Stevens Johnson Syndrome-Toxic Epidermal Necrolysis and psoriasis. 1st ed. New Delhi: IADVL; 2009. p. 1–72.
48. Morison WL, Baugham RD, Day RM, Forbes PD, Hoenigsmann H, Krueger GG, et al. Consensus workshop on the toxic effects of long-term PUVA therapy. Arch Dermatol. 1998;134:595–8.
49. Grimes PE, Minus HR, Chakrabarti SG, Enterline J, Halder R, Gough JE, et al. Determination of optimal topical photochemotherapy for vitiligo. J Am Acad Dermatol. 1982;7:771–8.
50. El Mofty M, Mostafa W, Esmat S, Youssef R, Azzam O, Hunter N, et al. Narrow band ultraviolet B 311 nm in the treatment of vitiligo: two right-left comparison studies. Photodermatol Photoimmunol Photomed. 2006;22:6–11.
51. Bhatnagar A, Kanwar AJ, Parsad D, De D. Comparison of systemic PUVA and NB-UVB in the treatment of vitiligo: an open prospective study. J Eur Acad Dermatol Venereol. 2007;21:638–42.
52. Westerhof W, Nieuweboer-Krobotova L. Treatment of vitiligo with UV-B radiation vs topical psoralen plus UV-A. Arch Dermatol. 1997;133:1525–8.
53. Yones SS, Palmer RA, Garibaldinos TM, Hawk JL. Randomized double-blind trial of treatment of vitiligo: efficacy of psoralen–UV-A therapy vs narrowband–UV-B therapy. Arch Dermatol. 2007;143:578–84.
54. Kwok YK, Anstey AV, Hawk JL. Psoralen photochemotherapy (PUVA) is only moderately effective in widespread vitiligo: a 10-year retrospective study. Clin Exp Dermatol. 2002;27:104–10.
55. British Photodermatology Group. An appraisal guideline for PUVA. Br J Dermatol. 1994;130:246–55.

56. Ortel B, Tanew A, Honigsmann H. Treatment of vitiligo with khellin and ultraviolet A. J Am Acad Dermatol. 1988;18:693–701.
57. Orecchia G, Perfetti L. Photochemotherapy with topical khellin and sunlight in vitiligo. Dermatol. 1992;184:120–3.
58. Dell'Anna ML, Picardo M. A review and a new hypothesis for non-immunological pathogenetic mechanisms in vitiligo. Pigm Cell Res. 2006;19:406–11.
59. Picardo M, Dell'Anna ML. Vitamins and antioxidants: topical and systemic. In: Picardo M, Taieb A, editors. Vitiligo. Berlin: Springer; 2010. p. 369–74.
60. Akyol M, Celik VK, Ozcelik S, Polat M, Marufihah M, Atalay A. The effects of vitamin E on the skin lipid peroxidation and the clinical improvement in vitiligo patients treated with PUVA. Eur J Dermatol. 2002;12:24–6.
61. Dell'Anna ML, Mastrofrancesco A, Sala R, Venturini M, Ottaviani M, Vidolin AP, et al. Antioxidants and narrow band-UVB in the treatment of vitiligo: a double-blind placebo controlled trial. Clin Exp Dermatol. 2007;32:631–6.
62. Middelkamp-Hup MA, Bos JD, Riuz-Diaz F, Gonzalez S, Westerhof W. Treatment of vitiligo vulgaris with narrow band UVB and oral Polypodium leucotomos extract: a randomized double-blind placebo controlled study. J Eur Acad Dermatol Venereol. 2007;21:942–50.
63. Parsad D, Pandhi R, Juneja A. Effectiveness of oral Ginkgo biloba in treating limited, slowly spreading vitiligo. Clin Exp Dermatol. 2002;28:285–7.
64. Szczurko O, Shear N, Taddio A, Boon H. Ginkgo biloba for the treatment of vitiligo vulgaris: an open label pilot clinical trial. BMC Complement Altern Med. 2011;11:21.
65. Trompezinski S, Bonneville M, Pernet I, Denis A, Schmitt D, Viac J. Gingko biloba extract reduces VEGF and CXCL-8/IL-8 levels in keratinocytes with cumulative effect with epigallocatechin-3-gallate. Arch Dermatol Res. 2010;302(3):183–9.
66. Bent S, Goldberg H, Padula A, Avins AL. Spontaneous bleeding associated with Ginkgo biloba: a case report and systematic review of the literature: a case report and systematic review of the literature. J Gen Intern Med. 2005;20(7):657–61.
67. Cohen BE, Elbuluk N, Mu EW, Orlow SJ. Alternative systemic treatments for vitiligo: a review. Am J Clin Dermatol. 2015;16(6):463–74.
68. Harris JE, Harris TH, Weninger W, Wherry EJ, Hunter CA, Turka LA. A mouse model of vitiligo with focused epidermal depigmentation requires IFN-gamma for autoreactive CD8(+) T-cell accumulation in the skin. J Invest Dermatol. 2012;132(7):1869–76.
69. Spritz RA. Recent progress in the genetics of generalized vitiligo. J Genet Genomics. 2011;38(7):271–8.
70. Spritz RA. Shared genetic relationships underlying generalized vitiligo and autoimmune thyroid disease. Thyroid. 2010;20(7):745–54.
71. Egli F, Walter R. Images in clinical medicine. Vitiligo and pernicious anemia. N Engl J Med. 2004;350(26):2698.
72. Schallreuter KU, Chavan B, Rokos H, Hibberts N, Panske A, Wood JM. Decreased phenylalanine uptake and turnover in patients with vitiligo. Mol Genet Metab. 2005;86(S1):S27–33.
73. Schallreuter KU, Zschiesche M, Moore J, Panske A, Hibberts NA, Herrmann FH, et al. In vivo evidence for compromised phenylalanine metabolism in vitiligo. Biochem Biophys Res Commun. 1998;243(2):395–9.
74. Antoniou C, Schulpis H, Michas T, Katsambas A, Frajis N, Tsagaraki S, et al. Vitiligo therapy with oral and topical phenylalanine with UVA exposure. Int J Dermatol. 1989;28(8):545–7.
75. Ryan WL, Carver MJ. Inhibition of antibody synthesis by L-phenylalanine. Science. 1964;143(3605):479–80.
76. Siddiqui AH, Stolk LM, Bhaggoe R, Hu R, Schutgens RB, Westerhof W. L-phenylalanine and UVA irradiation in the treatment of vitiligo. Dermatol. 1994;188(3):215–8.
77. Cormane RH, Siddiqui AH, Westerhof W, Schutgens RB. Phenylalanine and UVA light for the treatment of vitiligo. Arch Dermatol Res. 1985;277(2):126–30.
78. Thiele B, Steigleder GK. Repigmentation treatment of vitiligo with L-phenylalanine and UVA irradiation [in German]. Z Hautkr. 1987;62(7):519–23.

79. Karadag AS, Tutal E, Ertugrul DT, Akin KO, Bilgili SG. Serum holotranscobalamine, vitamin B12, folic acid and homocysteine levels in patients with vitiligo. Clin Exp Dermatol. 2012;37(1):62–4.
80. Shaker OG, El-Tahlawi SM. Is there a relationship between homocysteine and vitiligo? A pilot study. Br J Dermatol. 2008;159(3):720–4.
81. Howitz J, Schwartz M. Vitiligo, achlorhydria, and pernicious anemia. Lancet. 1971;1(7713):1331–4.
82. Sabry HHSJ, Hashim HM. Serum levels of homocysteine, vitamin B12, and folic acid in vitiligo. Egypt J Dermatol Venereol. 2014;34:65–9.
83. Montes LF, Diaz ML, Lajous J, Garcia NJ. Folic acid and vitamin B12 in vitiligo: a nutritional approach. Cutis. 1992;50(1):39–42.
84. Juhlin L, Olsson MJ. Improvement of vitiligo after oral treatment with vitamin B12 and folic acid and the importance of sun exposure. Acta Derm Venereol. 1997;77(6):460–2.
85. Tjioe M, Gerritsen MJ, Juhlin L, van de Kerkhof PC. Treatment of vitiligo vulgaris with narrow band UVB (311 nm) for one year and the effect of addition of folic acid and vitamin B12. Acta Derm Venereol. 2002;82(5):369–72.
86. Singh S, Singh U, Pandey SS. Increased level of serum homocysteine in vitiligo. J Clin Lab Anal. 2011;25(2):110–2.
87. Shameer P, Prasad PV, Kaviarasan PK. Serum zinc level in vitiligo: a case control study. Indian J Dermatol Venereol Leprol. 2005;71(3):206–7.
88. Bagherani N, Yaghoobi R, Omidian M. Hypothesis: zinc can be effective in treatment of vitiligo. Indian J Dermatol. 2011;56(5):480–4.
89. Yaghoobi R, Omidian M, Bagherani N. Comparison of therapeutic efficacy of topical corticosteroid and oral zinc sulfate-topical corticosteroid combination in the treatment of vitiligo patients: a clinical trial. BMC Dermatol. 2011;11:7.
90. Parsad D, Kanwar AJ. Oral minocycline in the treatment of vitiligo—a preliminary study. Dermatol Ther. 2010;23:305–7.
91. Silverberg JI, Silverberg AI, Malka E, Silverberg NB. A pilot study assessing the role of 25 hydroxy vitamin D levels in patients with vitiligo vulgaris. J Am Acad Dermatol. 2010;62(6):937–41.
92. Sehrawat M, Arora TC, Chauhan A, Kar HK, Poonia A, Jairath V. Correlation of vitamin D levels with pigmentation in vitiligo patients treated with NBUVB therapy. ISRN Dermatol. 2014;3:1–6.
93. Finamor DC, Sinigaglia-Coimbra R, Neves LC, Gutierrez M, Silva JJ, Torres LD, et al. A pilot study assessing the effect of prolonged administration of high daily doses of vitamin D on the clinical course of vitiligo and psoriasis. Dermato Endocrinol. 2013;5:222–34.
94. Batchelor JM, Tan W, Tour S, Yong A, Montgomery AA, Thomas KS. Validation of the vitiligo noticeability scale: a patient-reported outcome measure of vitiligo treatment success. Br J Dermatol. 2016;174(2):386–94.
95. Lahiri K. Punch grafting in vitiligo. Indian J Dermatol Venereol Leprol. 1998;64:310–1.
96. Lahiri K, Malakar S, Sarma N, Banerjee U. Inducing repigmentation by regrafting and phototherapy (311 nm) in punch grafting failure cases of lip vitiligo: a pilot study. Indian J Dermatol Venereol Leprol. 2004;70:156–8.

Chapter 28
Vitiligo Management: Procedural Options

Swetalina Pradhan and Somesh Gupta

28.1 Introduction

Vitiligo is an idiopathic acquired pigmentary disorder characterized by solitary or multiple depigmented macules that may arise in a localized, segmental, or generalized distribution [1]. Though not life-threatening, it adds a huge negative psychological and social impact on patients [2, 3]. The treatment of vitiligo has been challenging, and medical therapies are considered as the primary mode of treatment. However, some cases are refractory to medical treatment, and as such, surgical interventions can be used alone or in conjunction with medical management.

28.2 Principles of Surgery

The basic objective of surgical treatment should be to achieve complete and permanent cosmetically acceptable repigmentation toward the color of the surrounding normal skin in the shortest possible time with minimal or no side effects. The basic principle is to introduce active melanocytes to the lesion sites which will then establish and function as epidermal melanin units. Transfer of active melanocytes can be done either through tissue grafts or cellular grafts.

S. Pradhan
All India Institute of Medical Sciences, Bhubaneswar, India

S. Gupta (✉)
All India Institute of Medical Sciences, New Delhi, India
e-mail: someshgupta@hotmail.com

E.B. Handog, M.J. Enriquez-Macarayo (eds.), *Melasma and Vitiligo in Brown Skin*,
DOI 10.1007/978-81-322-3664-1_28

Table 28.1 Assessment of vitiligo stability

	Parameters for assessing stability of vitiligo	Consensus recommendation of IADVL[a] taskforce on stability [5]
History of progression	The absence of new lesions	No new lesions
Extension of old lesions	No extension of old lesions	No progression of existing lesions
Koebner phenomenon	The absence of Koebner phenomenon either based on history or by checking for experimentally induced vitiligo	The absence of Koebner phenomenon during the past 1 year
Spontaneous repigmentation		Should be considered as a favorable sign for the transplantation procedure
Minigrafting test or test grafting	The original test was proposed by Falabella et al. to select patients with stable vitiligo who may respond to melanocyte transplantation [4]. The test is considered positive if unequivocal repigmentation took place beyond 1 mm from the border of the implanted graft over a period of 3 months	May be considered whenever there is a doubt about the stability, or the patient is unable to give a clear history on stability

[a]Indian Association of Dermatologists, Venereologists, and Leprologists

Table 28.2 Patient selection criteria for vitiligo surgery

1.	Patients not responding to medical treatment
2.	Patients with stable lesions of vitiligo vulgaris, localized or segmental vitiligo lesions, though it may be done for all types of vitiligo (including segmental, generalized, and acro-facial types) Test graft should be always used to confirm the stability of vitiligo in case of a doubt or inconclusive history
3.	Patients with realistic expectations and who are psychologically stable

28.2.1 Criteria of Vitiligo Stability

Stability is the most important parameter before instituting any surgical treatment for vitiligo. The outcome of surgery is good in stable lesions, whereas unstable lesions respond poorly (Table 28.1).

28.2.2 Patient Selection Criteria (Table 28.2)

28.2.2.1 Patient Age

No current guidelines exist regarding the age group selection for vitiligo surgery. Children may be difficult candidates. The procedure generally performed under local anesthesia may be not tolerated by this younger age group. On the other hand, surgery done under general anesthesia poses unacceptable risk. Moreover, progress of the vitiligo is hard to predict in children. Hence, it has been suggested that surgical procedures should not be performed in children. However, in various studies, it has been found that results of the transplantation procedures yielded better results in younger individuals than in older ones [6, 7]. Thus no consensus exists in this aspect, and physicians should exercise their judgment after taking all aspects of the individual patient into consideration.

28.2.3 Pre-procedure Preparation

28.2.3.1 Preoperative Counseling and Informed Consent [5]

The nature of the disease, procedure, expected outcome, and possible complications after the procedure must be explained to the patient. The need for concomitant medical therapy should be emphasized. Patients should understand that proper results may take time to appear (few months to more than a year). They should be provided with adequate opportunity to seek information through brochures, computer presentations, and one-on-one discussions.

The consent form should specifically state the limitations of the procedure, possible future disease progression, and whether more procedures will be needed for optimal outcome. A detailed consent form describing the procedure and possible complications should be signed by the patient.

28.2.3.2 Preoperative Investigations (Based on the Procedure)

Complete blood counts, coagulation profile platelet count, blood sugar, screening for hepatitis B, VDRL, HIV (ELISA), routine urinalysis, serum creatinine, blood urea nitrogen, SGOT, SGPT (if large areas are going to be phenolized), and ECG may be needed in elderly patients.

28.2.3.3 Anesthesia [5]

The recipient site is locally anesthetized by infiltration of 2 % lidocaine HCl (Xylocaine), the pain of which can be reduced by prior application of topical combination anesthetic lidocaine 2.5 %/prilocaine 2.5 % (EMLA® cream) under occlusion for 1–2 h. Adrenaline should not be used on the recipient site as it makes the judgment difficult regarding the adequacy of the denudation to the required depth. Tumescent anesthesia and nerve blocks may be used in larger areas. If grafting is planned for extensive areas, general anesthesia may be needed in a hospital setting Recent studies suggest that adequate anaesthetsia can be achieved in a significant

Table 28.3 Grafts used for vitiligo surgery

Tissue grafts	Cellular grafts
Punch grafting/minigraft	Autologous, non-cultured epidermal cell suspension
Suction blister grafting/epidermal grafting	Autologous, cultured melanocyte transplantation
Split-thickness skin grafting	Autologous, cultured epithelial grafts
Modified grafting techniques Mesh grafting Flip-top grafting Hair follicle grafting	

proportion of patients by using topical anaesthesia alone, provided adequate amount of EMLA cream is applied under effective occlusion for sufficient duration.

28.3 Methods of Surgical Modalities

Surgical modalities for vitiligo have been broadly classified into two types: tissue grafts and cellular grafts (Table 28.3). Special methods of treatment used in selected situation are tattooing and therapeutic wounding.

28.3.1 *Tissue Grafts*

28.3.1.1 Autologous Minipunch Grafting (PG)

Among the surgical modalities for vitiligo, minipunch grafting is the easiest, fastest, least aggressive, and minimally expensive.

A. Evolution

Norman Orentreich in 1972 first reported autograft repigmentation in humans and treated a black woman with long-standing leukoderma. Orentriech deployed nine, 1 and 2 mm diameter, normal skin autografts and observed the "pigment spread phenomenon" and reported a maximum of 1 mm pigment spread from both the 1 and 2 mm grafts [8]. Falabella treated vitiligo and secondary leukoderma by minigraft technique. He used minigrafts of size 1–1.2 mm in diameter from donor site and grafted them onto chambers of the same size at the recipient site spacing them 3 to 4 mm apart and further secured them using Monsel's solution and pressure dressing [9, 10]. Because of similar size, the grafts did not snugly fit into the recipient chambers which led to circular peri-graft scarring. Hence, Loewenthal's method of using donor grafts larger than the recipient chambers was used by Falabella leading to better fixation of the grafts and lesser textural alterations. The procedure proved to be a highly effective modality in various studies [11–15].

B. Test grafting
Test grafting is done to confirm the stability of the disease before attempting repigmentation of the entire area. Few grafts (1–1.2 mm) are placed in the center of the depigmented lesion to be scrutinized. Dressing is done by adhesive tape (Micropore®) and kept for a couple of weeks. After removal of the tape, the area is exposed to sunlight for 15 min daily, for a period of 3 months. No treatment is given during this test period. All test sites are visualized under Wood's light. The test is considered positive if unequivocal repigmentation takes place beyond 1 mm from the border of the implanted grafts. Apart from stability, it also gives a fair idea about the perigraft pigment spread which will guide to maintain adequate distance to be kept between the recipient chambers in future attempts. Over the years, this test has been acknowledged as a powerful tool for detecting stability of vitiligo and thereby anticipating success of the surgery in terms of repigmentation.

C. Instruments
The instruments required are cylindrical skin biopsy punches (1.2 to 1.5mm), "S"-shaped scissors, ring forceps, iris scissors, Adson's toothed forceps, and a sterile petri dish/bowl.

D. Procedure

- Recipient area
  The recipient area is prepared first. Lignocaine 2 %, with or without adrenaline, is infiltrated as a local anesthetic. To minimize the chance of developing any perigraft halo, the initial recipient chambers are made on or very close to the border of the lesion. The punched out chambers are spaced according to the result of test grafting or at a gap of 5–10 mm from each other.
- Donor area
  The donor area is either the upper lateral portion of the thigh or the gluteal area. Punch impressions are made very close to each other so that a maximum number of grafts can be taken from a small area. In one sitting, up to 200 grafts can be harvested and grafted (average, 25–60). The remaining (extra) grafts can be stored in a refrigerator (on a shelf, not in the freezer) for reuse (to replace rejected grafts up to 24–48 h later).
- Same-sized punches are used for both the donor and recipient areas.
- The grafts are placed directly from the donor area to the recipient area which speeds up the procedure and lessens the chance of infection. The needle of the syringe or tip of the scissors can be used for the proper placement of grafts so that the graft edges are not folded and tissue is not placed upside down.
- Hemostasis is achieved by applying firm pressure with a saline-soaked gauze piece over the area.
- The recipient area is dressed with the three layers of paraffin-embedded, non-adherent sterile gauze (Jelonet®), sterile Surgipad®, and bio-occlusive Micropore® from inside to out.
- For the donor area, only Surgipad® and Micropore® are used.

E. Post-procedure instructions

- The recipient area may be immobilized, if necessary.
- For special areas like the lips, the patients are advised to be on a liquid diet for the first 24 h, preferably with a straw, and are allowed a normal diet after this period.
- To find out any dislodgment of grafts, dressings may be opened after 24 h, and if any are found, they need to be replaced.
- Finally, dressings are removed after 4–7 days [12, 13, 16].
- Antibiotics and anti-inflammatory drugs are administered for 8–10 days.
- PUVA/PUVASOL or NB-UVB for 3–6 months is done to enhance repigmentation [12, 13, 17–19].

F. Mechanism of pigmentation after grafting
The graft of the donor area functions independently of the recipient area. It produces active melanin, and the melanocytes from the infundibulum of hair follicles present in the graft spread centrifugally to the basal cell layer and thereby recolonize the epidermis of recipient area with active and functional melanocytes leading to perigraft pigmentation [8, 10, 20].

G. Complications [21] (Table 28.4)

H. Advantages and disadvantages (Table 28.5)

Table 28.4 PG complications: recipient and donor sites

Recipient site	Donor site
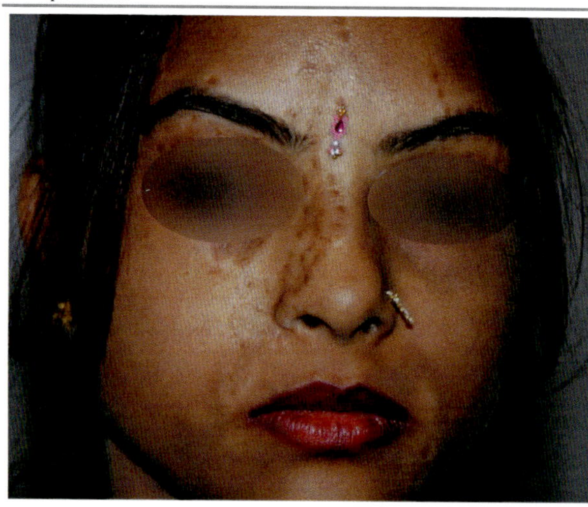 **Fig. 28.1** After minigrafting, good repigmentation evident but cobblestoning seen Cobblestoning (Fig. 28.1) Polka dot Variegated appearance and color mismatch Static graft (no pigment spread) Depigmentation of graft Perigraft halo Graft dislodgment/rejection Hypertrophic scar and keloid formation Target-like pigmentation [22]	Keloid Hypertrophic scar Superficial scar Depigmentation/spread of disease Contact dermatitis to adhesive tapes

Table 28.5 PG: advantages and disadvantages

Advantages	Disadvantages
Simple, safe, and inexpensive office procedure Needs no special training for a dermatologist. High success rate and excellent cosmetic results Large lesions and any site except the angle of the mouth can be treated Areas of residual vitiligo between grafts or rejected can be regrafted Specifically suitable for the areola Perhaps the only suitable method for the palm	Commonly associated with side effects Perfect color match does not occur Phototherapy is required after grafting to achieve pigmentation

28.3.1.2 Suction Blister Grafting/Epidermal Grafting (SBEG)

Suction blister epidermal grafting is an established technique for the treatment of recalcitrant and stable vitiligo. The pigmented epidermis is harvested from the donor site by using suction to raise a blister which is then transferred to the vitiliginous area.

A. Evolution
   Falabella, in 1971, first used epidermal sheets to treat vitiligo by in vivo separation of the viable epidermis [23]. However, various modified techniques have been used for producing the blister, including the use of syringes, three-way connectors, surgical glue, and modified BFY dermis– epidermis separator, making the procedure simple with improved results [24–27].
B. Instruments
   Required are the following instruments: disposable syringes (10, 20, and 50 cc), three-way cannulas, dermabrader (manual or electrical), iris scissors, non-toothed forceps, artery forceps, sterile glass slides, and surgical glue (N-butyl-2-cyanoacrylate). If available, lasers (CO_2 or Er:YAG) may be used.
C. Procedure

   - Donor Area
     Preferred sites include the medial aspect of the forearm, the medial/lateral aspect of the upper arm, and the medial or posterior aspect of the upper thigh. After surgical cleansing, a topical local anesthetic is applied to the area as the procedure is painful; alternatively, 1 % lidocaine (Xylocaine) can be injected as a field block.
   - Raising of the Blister
     Blisters may be raised using syringes, suction pump, suction cups, or a negative pressure cutaneous suction chamber system [24, 28, 29]. The most commonly used is the syringe suction. The bases of syringes sized 10 and 20 ml, coated with petroleum jelly (Vaseline), are applied on the donor site. Approximately 20–30 ml of air is aspirated using a 50 ml syringe and a three-way cannula. The three-way cannula is locked, and the 50 cc syringe is disconnected. This maintains constant negative pressure within the 10 or 20 cc syringe. It usually takes 1.5–3 h for the development of blisters. The best

result is a single unilocular nonhemorrhagic blister. In case of smaller blisters, one can either increase the negative pressure in the syringe by another 5 ml or intradermally inject saline into the blister to expand it [18].

- Blister deroofing
  The roofs of the blisters are gently cut using iris scissors. The graft is then placed on a glass slide with the dermal side facing upward. The graft is then cleaned and spread to its maximum size and kept moist with normal saline. The donor site is then cleaned and bandaged using nonadherent dressing such as chlorhexidine gauze.
- Recipient site
  The recipient area is surgically cleaned using methylated spirit and povidone iodine and then anesthetized using plain lignocaine 1 %. The area is then dermabraded using a manual or motorized dermabrader, a microdermabrader, or a CO_2 laser till minute pinpoint bleeding spots are visible. Gupta et al. used hypodermic needle as a dermabrading device for the smaller recipient area preparation before suction blister grafting [30]. Dermabrasion should extend for 1–2 mm beyond the border of the vitiliginous area. Hemostasis is achieved by pressure, and the area is covered with saline-soaked gauze pieces. Cryoblistering or suction blistering has also been used for the preparation of the recipient site [31].
- Transfer of grafts
  The grafts are then placed such that the dermal side of the graft is now in contact with the dermabraded area. A gap of 0.5 cm can be left between two grafts because there is a pigment spread.
- Graft fixation
  With sterile moist gauze, firm pressure is given over the graft to remove any serous collection underneath. This helps in graft adherence. The recipient area is dressed with double layer framycetin tulle moist gauze, followed by sterile gauze and Elastocrepe bandage. Alternately, surgical glue (N-butyl-2-cyanoacrylate) can be applied along the edges of the grafts for fixation. Donor area is dressed with dry sterile pads.

D. Post-procedure instructions

- The dressing over the donor and recipient sites is removed after 24 h and 7 days, respectively. The patient is advised to keep the area immobile. Usually, the grafts fall off in 1–2 weeks.
- Oral or topical Psoralen-UVA or PUVASOL can be started from the day of removal of dressing to facilitate repigmentation.

E. Principle of suction blister epidermal grafting
In suction blister grafting, the cleavage occurs between the basal cells and the basal lamina of the basement membrane zone. Hence, only the epidermal portion of the donor area is grafted. So the graft generally acquires the characteristics of the recipient site rather than the donor site, resulting in a better color match and cosmetic outcome [32]. The melanocyte transfer takes place within 48–72 h from the graft to the recipient site.

Table 28.6 SBEG complications: donor and recipient sites

Donor site	Recipient site
Ecchymosis	Hyperpigmentation
Hematoma	Incomplete pigmentation
Pigmentary changes	Perigraft halo
Secondary infection	Graft rejection
	Allergic contact dermatitis

F. Complications (Table 28.6)
G. Advantages and disadvantages (Table 28.7)

28.3.1.3 Split-Thickness Skin Grafting (STSG)

Split-thickness skin grafting involves transfer of epidermis and often the uppermost part of superficial dermis into the dermabraded patch of vitiligo, thereby achieving the transfer of melanocytes and keratinocytes from donor graft to the recipient area [8]. The thickness of the graft ranges from 0.1 to 0.7 mm [35].

A. Evolution
   In 1964, Behl was the first to report the use of thin Thiersch's skin grafts to treat vitiligo [36]. Since then, various modifications of the same procedure like ultrathin epidermal sheets or ultrathin split-thickness grafting (less than 0.08–0.15 mm) have been tried for the treatment of vitiligo [37–40].
B. Instruments
   These include dermabrader (manual or electrical), skin grafting equipment, graft spreading rods/spatula, non-traumatizing ring forceps, iris scissors, surgical glue-Cyanoacrylate adhesive (N-butyl-2-cyanoacrylate), and a sterile petri dish/bowl.
C. Procedure

   - Donor area
     Preferred sites include the gluteal area and anterolateral aspect of the thigh, abdomen, and arms [37, 41]. After shaving off the hairs and proper cleansing with povidone iodine and 70% ethanol, the area is anesthetized with 1% lidocaine (Xylocaine) without adrenaline. The area is then stretched, and a thin, even split-thickness graft is harvested, using either a sterile razor blade mounted on a Kocher's forceps or a blade-holding instrument. Alternatively, a hand dermatome, Humby's knife, Silver's knife, or an air-driven power dermatome may be used for harvesting the grafts [42–44]. The grafts thus obtained are transferred to a petri dish containing normal saline. The donor area is dressed with nonadherent dressing.
   - Recipient area
     After proper cleansing with povidone iodine and 70% ethanol, the area is abraded using a dermabrader, until pinpoint hemorrhages are seen uniformly all over the lesion. The area is then cleaned with normal sterile saline and covered with a gauze piece soaked in normal saline. The grafts obtained are then placed upside down on the sterile glass slides. The slide is placed on the

Table 28.7 SBEG: advantages and disadvantages

Advantages	Disadvantages
Safe, easy, and inexpensive method	Time-consuming
Very good success rates (Fig. 28.2 a–e)	Painful procedure
Repigmentation is faster	Larger areas require multiple sittings
Very good color match	Improper handling may lead to tearing of the graft
Best method for lips, eyelids, and areola [33, 34]	Wrong placement of graft leads to failure of repigmentation
	Not suitable for palms and soles
	Color mismatch (Fig. 28.3 a, b)

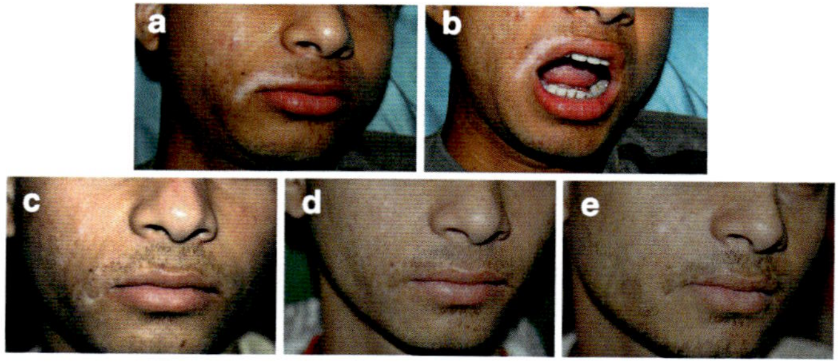

Fig 28.2 (**a**, **b**) Segmental Vitiligo - before suction blister epidermal grafting; (**c–e**) Post-procedure - good repigmentation of both vitiligo skin and leukotrichia

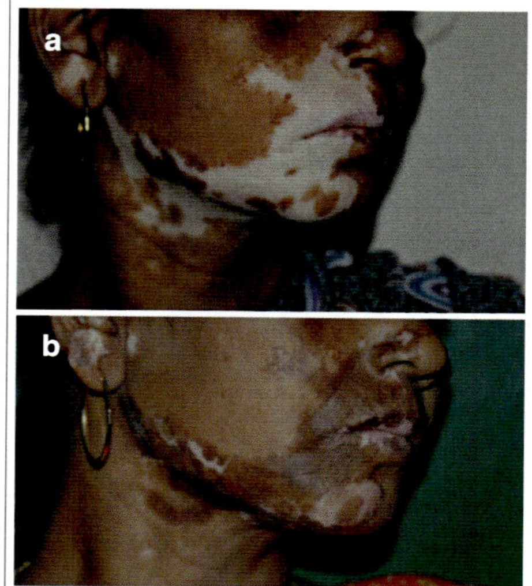

Fig 28.3 (**a**) Segmental Vitiligo - before suction blister epidermal grafting (**b**) after the procedure, note color mismatch

recipient area and pressed against the skin. Any blood or exudates between the graft and recipient area are evacuated by firm pressure over the graft with the help of wet gauze, without displacing the graft. The graft is immobilized by using surgical adhesive, octyl-2-cyanoacrylate and pressure dressing. The adhesive gives excellent results to secure the graft and also has antimicrobial properties against Staphylococci, *Pseudomonas*, and *E. coli* [45]. The recipient site can also be prepared using a pulsed Erbium-YAG laser or ultrapulse CO_2 laser [46].

D. Post-procedure instructions

- Patients are advised to avoid excessive movement of the grafted area and to follow up after 1 week for a change of dressing. Donor site dressing is also changed after 1 week.
- Prophylactic oral antibiotics are given for 1 week to prevent postoperative infection.
- If there is perigraft depigmentation or achromic fissures, NB-UVB is required postoperatively for complete repigmentation.

E. Principle of split-thickness skin grafting
Three biological changes occur following skin grafting [41].

- Graft take adherence
This stage is comprised of two phases. The first phase occurs within 72 h of the placement of the graft. Fibrin bonding occurs between the graft and recipient area leading to graft adherence. The second phase begins with the onset of vascular anastomosis and fibrovascular growth.
- Graft revascularization
The graft and host vessels get connected with the formation of new vascular channels.
- Contracture
The contraction of the elastin fibers leads to the contracture of the graft after harvesting, and a similar phenomenon also occurs at the recipient site. The above two factors contribute to achromic fissures and perigraft halo which follows the grafting. Overlapping of the graft edges at the recipient site can prevent these complications.

F. Complications (Tables 28.8 and 28.9)
G. Advantages and disadvantages

28.3.1.4 Modifications of Techniques at Special Sites [32]

A. Eyelids
The thinnest graft should be selected for the upper eyelid. For small area, suction blister graft is ideal. Thin or ultrathin split-thickness skin grafts give good results if the entire eyelid is involved. Strict immobilization for the first 72 h is essential for graft uptake.

Table 28.8 STSG complications: recipient and donor sites

Recipient site	Donor site
Graft rejection Textural abnormalities like "curling" or "branching," resulting in peripheral beading at the graft edge or a "stuck on tire patch" appearance Hyperpigmentation Perigraft halo Hypertrophy Milia Secondary infection Reactivation of vitiligo	Post inflammatory hyperpigmentation Scarring Recurrence or Koebnerization

Table 28.9 STSG: advantages and disadvantages

Advantages	Disadvantages
Pigmentation can instantly cover larger areas over a short period of time Difficult areas such as eyelids, inner canthus of eyes, areola, nipples, and genitals can be treated readily Pigmentation achieved is uniform [47] Repigmentation of leukotrichia is also possible [48, 49] Less time-consuming as compared to other procedures	Prolonged hyperpigmentation particularly on the exposed areas in dark-skinned patients Superficial scarring and chances of vitiligo at the donor site Larger area requires multiple sitting Requires surgical skill for graft harvesting Tips, palms, soles, and mucous membranes are difficult to treat by this method Scarring and contracture at the recipient area [50] Risk of malignant transformation in keratinized grafts applied in the oral mucosa [51]

B. Lips
   Suction blister grafts for small areas and thin split-thickness skin grafts for larger areas give a good cosmetic outcome on the lips.
C. Areola
   The entire areola should be grafted in order to maintain a uniform color.
D. Acral areas
   Minipunch grafting is most suitable for the fingers, toes, palms, and soles. Suction blister grafting or thin split-thickness skin grafting is suitable for the dorsal sites.
E. Genitals
   The history of genital herpes should be always ruled out before attempting surgical treatment. Long-term prophylaxis with acyclovir should be given in proven and doubtful cases and the prognosis clearly explained. Suction blister grafts, thin split-thickness skin grafts, minipunch grafts, and non-cultured melanocyte suspensions can be tried, depending on the size of the vitiligo patch and expertise of the surgeon [52].
F. Hairy areas
   The hair should be plucked out instead of shaving before grafting to delay hair regrowth and thereby preventing lifting up of the graft. Alternatively, a chemical depilatory may be used.

28.3.1.5 Mesh Grafting (MG)

Mesh grafting is a technique where the graft is expanded by making slits in it such that it appears like a mesh [53].

A. Instruments
   These include a Padgett or Duvals dermatome, an ampligreffe or Discard-A-pad, and a dermabrader.
B. Procedure
   - Donor site
     Under general anesthesia, a 0.01 mm thickness graft is obtained from the anterolateral aspect of the thigh, using a Padgett dermatome. The grafts, with the dermis facing upward, are transferred to an ampligreffe, specifically placed on its slightly inclined metal plate. With one end of the graft inserted between the spiral barrels of the ampligreffe, the latter's handle is then rotated. There occurs the formation of a diamond-shaped mesh when the graft passes between the two barrels of the ampligreffe. The resultant mesh is of four times the size of the original graft.
   - Recipient site
     After the recipient site is cleaned and dermabraded, the graft is transferred and bandaged with saline-soaked dressing or framycetin (Sofratulle®). The donor site is also dressed using aseptic precautions.
C. Post-procedure instructions
   - The dressing at the recipient site is removed after a week.
   - Phototherapy is started immediately or after a week.
D. Advantages and disadvantages (Table 28.10)

28.3.1.6 Flip-Top Pigment Transplantation

Flip-top technique is a method devised by McGovern and colleagues in which the graft is placed between a flap of the epidermis and dermis at the recipient site [54].

A. Instruments: sterile blade and surgical glue
B. Procedure

Table 28.10 MG: advantages and disadvantages

Advantages	Disadvantages
Larger areas can be covered due to graft expansion Rapid harvesting of the graft Allows coverage of areas with variable contours No risk of scarring at recipient site	Risk of scarring at the donor site Thick graft might lead to beading at the margin Cosmetic results are inferior as compared to other methods

- Donor area
  After cleaning, a thin split-thickness graft is harvested from either the medial aspect of the upper arm or lateral aspect of the thigh, by using a sterile blade. The grafts are kept moist in saline-soaked gauzes.
- Recipient area
  The recipient site is cleaned. A flap of the epidermis is raised using a sterile blade. One end of the epidermis is left in contact with the dermis, and the flap is turned to expose the dermis. The graft is placed with its dermal side in contact with the dermis of the recipient site. The flap is put back in position to cover the graft. Cyanoacrylate glue is used to secure the graft and the flap. Both the donor and recipient areas are dressed.

C. Post-procedure instructions

- The dressing is removed after a week.
- Phototherapy is started after removal of dressing.

D. Advantages and disadvantages (Table 28.11)

28.3.1.7 Hair Follicle Grafting

Repigmentation of vitiligo occurs from hair follicle melanocytes. Hence, hair follicle transplantation over a vitiligo patch leads to repigmentation of the patch, especially in hair-bearing areas with leukotrichia [55, 56].

A. Procedure

- Donor area
  The occipital area of the scalp is the preferred site. The hairs are trimmed to 1–2 mm length. Field block anesthesia is given with 2 % lidocaine. A 0.8 mm punch with Folligraft® is used to obtain follicular units. The hair suspension thus obtained is preserved in a sectioned petri dish filled with normal saline.
- Recipient site
  The recipient vitiligo patch is anesthetized with topical anesthetic cream followed by a small amount of injected local anesthesia (2 % lidocaine). The prepared hair follicles are transplanted uniformly over the incision site created with a scalpel. The recipient site is dressed.

Table 28.11 Flip-top pigment transplantation: advantages and disadvantages

Advantages	Disadvantages
Flap of epidermis acts as a biological dressing Less chances of secondary infection and falling of graft Inexpensive Easy to perform Quick method	Requires skill to harvest a thin graft There is beading at the margins

B. Post-procedure instructions

- After a week, the dressing is removed and checked for graft uptake.
- Phototherapy is started after removal of the dressing.

C. Principle of hair follicle grafting
This procedure is based on the concept of the existence of undifferentiated stem cells in the hair follicle, which forms a good source of melanocytes for repigmentation [55]. Hair melanocytes have a remarkable synthetic capacity, and a relatively small number of melanocytes can potentially produce sufficient melanin for pigmentation [57]. After a few weeks of grafting, the melanocytes spread to surrounding depigmented epidermis, and the skin appears repigmented.

D. Advantages and disadvantages (Table 28.12)

Table 28.12 Hair follicle grafting: advantages and disadvantages

Advantages	Disadvantages
Scarless surgery Good technique for management of leukotrichia Vitiligo in hairy and non-glabrous areas No cobblestoning Good color match	Requiring expertise and time

28.3.2 *Cellular Grafts*

Tissue grafting techniques in vitiligo, though easy to perform and give appreciable results, have various deficiencies in the form of cobblestoning, pigment mismatch, stuck-on appearance, inadequate pigment cover, and patient discomfort. There has always been an inclination toward the use of advanced technology in the treatment of each and every condition. Replenishing melanocytes selectively in vitiliginous macules by autologous melanocytes is one such promising treatment. Two types of techniques are used: autologous melanocyte-rich cell suspension (non-cultured) technique and the cultured melanocyte technique. Both are based on the principle of seeding melanocytes (i.e., introduction of melanocytes from the normal skin into a region of the depigmented skin).

28.3.2.1 Non-cultured Epidermal Cellular Grafting

A. Evolution
In 1992, Gauthier and Surleve-Bazeille described the technique in which a donor sample was obtained from the scalp by superficial shaving using a dermatome with a razor blade and then treated with trypsin 0.25 % for 18 h

for dermal–epidermal separation [58]. Subsequently, epidermal cells were extracted, and a cellular suspension was prepared. This suspension was inoculated into blisters raised with liquid nitrogen at the recipient area. In 1998, Olsson and colleagues used the gluteal skin as donor sample and reduced trypsinization time to 50 min. The cellular suspension was directly applied onto a dermabraded vitiligo lesion [59]. Since then, many advances have been made in the procedure, along with preparation of the recipient area. De-epithelialization of the graft recipient area bed can be achieved by cryotherapy, induction of suction blisters or dermabrasion using a high-speed dermabrader, and laser abrasion. Similarly, the use of special culture media has been replaced by phosphate-buffered saline (PBS) or saline solution without xenobiotics (e.g., bovine serum or pituitary extract or other foreign proteins).

B. Instruments
These include skin grafting knife/Silver's knife, dermabraders (manual metallic or electrical), incubator, centrifuge, laminar flow bench, petri dishes, iris scissors, jeweler's forceps, ring forceps, spatula, and test tube marking pen.

C. Procedure

- Donor area
  The medial aspect of the thigh or the lateral aspect of the gluteal region is selected as the donor site. About one-tenth the size of the recipient area is selected for harvesting the graft. A very superficial sample of the skin is obtained using Silver's skin grafting knife after anesthetizing the area. The superficial wound is then dressed with liquid paraffin dressing and sterile gauze pad.
- Trypsinization and cell separation in laboratory
  The skin graft is immediately transferred to 6 ml of 0.25 % trypsin-EDTA solution in a petri dish and is incubated at 37 °C for 50 min.
- Removal of excess trypsin
  The grafts are then transferred into a petri dish containing 8 ml of melanocyte nourishment medium [i.e., Dulbecco's Modified Eagle Medium/F12 (DMEM)] which acts as a diluting agent to wean off the trypsin action. All the subsequent steps are performed in a laminar airflow bench under strict aseptic conditions. The epidermis is further separated from the dermis with forceps. The epidermis is further broken into smaller pieces in a petri dish and washed with the DMEM/F12 medium and finally transferred to a test tube also containing DMEM/F12.
- Centrifugation

The test tube is then centrifuged for 6 min at 3000 rpm. The supernatant is discarded, and the pellet at the bottom is suspended in a 1 ml insulin syringe.

- Recipient area
  After surgical cleaning and anesthesia, the vitiliginous area is dermabraded until pinpoint bleeding is seen. The cell suspension is applied evenly on the denuded area and spread uniformly with spatula. The area is then covered with a collagen dressing which is again covered with sterile liquid paraffin and gauze pieces. The patient is made to lie down for 30 min (elevation of body part, if required, i.e., foot) and then allowed to leave with the instructions to avoid vigorous activities and to carry out only restricted movements for next 7 days.

D. Post-procedure instructions

- Oral antibiotics and analgesics are given for 5 days.
- The dressings are removed after 1 week in most cases.
- The patients are followed up at 1, 3, and 6 months after the procedure for assessing repigmentation.
- Phototherapy can be initiated after 3 weeks.

E. Complications (Table 28.13)
F. Advantages and disadvantages (Table 28.14)

Table 28.13 Non-cultured epidermal cellular grafting complications: donor and recipient sites

Donor area	Recipient area
Scarring Infection Koebnerization Milia	Infection

Table 28.14 Non-cultured epidermal cellular grafting: advantages and disadvantages

Advantages	Disadvantages
Tenfold large areas can be treated at a time Excellent cosmetic results Excellent texture and color matching No stuck-on look No cobblestoning	Expensive procedure Requires special setup Needs expertise

G. Modifications of the procedure

- The use of hyaluronic acid
  Hyaluronic acid can be added to the suspension to increase viscosity and thereby preventing running away of the suspension [60].
- In vivo technique for preparation of cell suspension
  This is a novel technique suggested by Gupta et al. in which cell separation and harvesting are performed inside sterile blisters induced by suction on the patient's thigh and injecting the solution containing 1 ml of 0.25 % trypsin 0.002 % EDTA solution into the blister. The body heat serves as the incubator at a temperature of around 37°C. This technique has the advantage of being simple, easy to learn, inexpensive, and requiring only minimal processing and handling of the tissue outside the body [61].
- Noncultured hair follicle outer root sheath cell suspension (Fig. 28.4a–d)
  In this technique, the clee suspension is prepared from outer root sheath cells of extracted hair follicles. Hair follicle contains more numerous and larger melanocytes as compared to epidermis.
- Mechanical separation of epidermal cells instead of enzymatic separation
  Epidermal scrapings (till the level of the papillary dermis) are applied directly onto the dermabraded recipient area [62]. However, questions regarding the homogeneity of the repigmentation remain to be investigated.

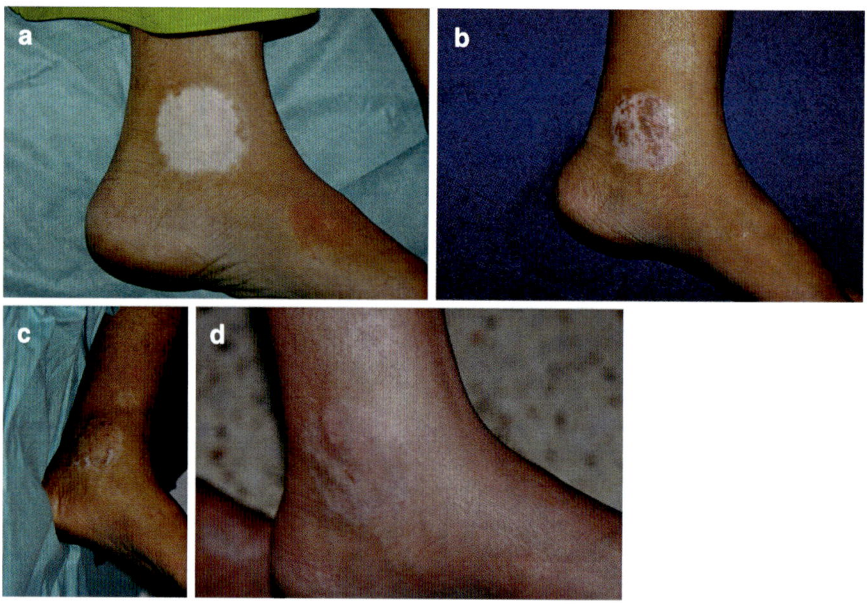

Fig. 28.4 (**a**) Acral Vitiligo - before hair follicular outer root sheath cell suspension. (**b–d**) After the procedure - good repigmentation evident

28.3.2.2 Cultured Melanocyte Transplantation (CMT)

Autologous melanocyte culture is an effective surgical mode of treatment in stable and recalcitrant lesions of vitiligo in which large areas of the skin can be covered with a smaller donor skin. Cultured melanocytes have a donor to recipient area ratio of around 1:100, and hence a very small donor graft is adequate to cover a very large area.

A. Evolution

Eisinger and Marko in 1980 successfully cultured melanocytes from the newborn foreskins and adult skin [63]. In 1987, cultured melanocytes were used to treat leukoderma. Lerner et al. successfully treated a patient of piebaldism with the use of cultured melanocytes [64]. The procedure of obtaining cultured melanocytes and the preparation of recipient area for the melanocyte transplantation have undergone several modifications in the last few decades.

B. Procedure

- The initial steps are similar to the ones used for autologous, non-cultured melanocyte plus keratinocyte grafting till the formation of a cell suspension pellet.
- The cell suspension is cultured in tissue culture flasks along with 05 ml of M2 medium [F12 medium supplemented with bFGF (20 ng/ml), isobutyl methylxanthine (0.1 mm), cholera toxin (10 ng/ml), glutamine 2 mm, and 10 % fetal bovine serum (serum-free tetradecanoylphorbol acetate)]. The culture is maintained at 37 °C in 95 % air and 5 % CO_2 atm (using anaerobic gas chargers) in an incubator for a total of 21 days. The tissue culture fluid was replaced on a daily basis.
- Cell viability is assessed by trypan blue exclusion assay, which is based on uptake of trypan blue dye by nonviable cells as a result of disintegration of the cellular membrane. The density of melanocytes is counted under a microscope using a Neubauer's chamber. A density of 1000–2000 melanocytes/mm^2 is achieved before transplantation.
- The cultured grafts are transferred to a petri dish containing 8 ml of DMEM media and then centrifuged at 3000 rpm for 6 min.
- The cell suspension pellet is obtained, and the subsequent steps of cellular transplantation to the recipient area are similar to the non-cultured epidermal cell suspension method.

C. Post-procedure instructions

- The patient is asked to give rest to the operated area and to limit mobility at the site.
- The dressing at both donor and recipient sites is removed on the seventh day.
- The patients are called after 1, 3, and 6 months to assess the extent of repigmentation.

D. Advantages and disadvantages (Table 28.15)

Table 28.15 CMT: advantages and disadvantages

Advantages	Disadvantages
Very small donor graft is adequate to cover a very large area The cells can be cryopreserved for future use	Lack of complete standardization Expensive laboratory equipment Technical complexity

E. Modifications of the procedure

- Amniotic Membrane as a Scaffold for Melanocyte Transplantation
  In a study by Redondo et al., cultured epidermal melanocytes were replated onto the basement membrane (BM) side of the amniotic membrane and were allowed to grow for another 3–4 days [65]. The amniotic membranes were then placed on the dermabraded recipient site with the BM side down. Excellent repigmentation was achieved in all patients along with repigmentation of the marginal area.
  The amniotic membranes have anti-inflammatory and antimicrobial properties with lack of antigenicity, facilitating the reepithelialization of the skin and reducing scarring.
- Hyaluronic Acid Micropore Sheets as Scaffold [66]
  The cultured melanocytes and keratinocytes are transferred onto a 10×10 cm-sized sheet of hyaluronic acid, and the cells are allowed to proliferate and form a keratinizing stratified epithelium. This sheet is then transferred to dermabraded recipient sites, and repopulation of the areas occurs via passage of cells through the micropores.
- Autologous Cultured Epithelial Graft (CEG)
  There has been limited data on these methods [66]. The melanocytes and keratinocytes can be cultured together by this technique, and hence it is useful in vitiligo patients who are refractory to all other known therapies [66]. No major complications have been reported in various studies, but this technique is expensive and requires sophisticated laboratory and trained personnel.

28.3.3 Other Methods

28.3.3.1 Micropigmentation

Tattooing or micropigmentation is defined as uniform implantation of minute inert pigment granules into the dermis so as to artistically create a permanent cosmetic camouflage [67, 68].

A. Instruments

- Electrically driven tattooing machine and tattoo pigments
- The pigment to be used for micropigmentation should be nontoxic and nonirritating, with a particle size of about 6 μm, insoluble, light and tissue stable, and inert to immunologic destruction.

- Various chemical substances and their colors of pigmentation are as follows:
  - White: titanium dioxide
  - Red: cinnabar, mercuric sulfate (cadmium sulfide added to make red brighter)
  - Black: iron oxide
  - Yellow: cadmium sulfide
  - Camel yellow: iron oxide
  - Light brown: iron oxide
  - Dark brown: iron oxide

B. Procedure

- Pigment preparation is done by mixing various pigment powders to achieve the desired shade. One to two drops of a wetting agent such as normal saline, water, or 80 % alcohol are added to make a pigment paste.
- A thick layer of pigment paste is applied to the site under local anesthesia lignocaine 2 %. The site to be tattooed is stretched with the thumb and index finger while the tattooing machine, held in the pen-holding manner, makes repeated vertical movements of needles up and down on the surface of the skin. Tattooing is done in the entire area in an overlapping manner. Pressure is exerted with the thumb and index finger to maintain hemostasis.

C. Post-procedure instructions

- Prophylactic antibiotics and anti-inflammatory drugs may be given postoperatively.
- Follow-up at 4–6 weeks and 6 months may require touch-up tattooing for the areas of pigment shed off.

D. Principles of Micropigmentation
The pigment particles are implanted intradermally between the superficial and middle dermis; these particles get permanently fixed, both intracellularly and extracellularly, within dermal mononuclear cells and collagen fibers, respectively. Over the years, a small amount of this pigment may migrate to the regional lymph nodes with resultant fading.

E. Complications (Table 28.16)

F. Advantages and disadvantages (Table 28.17)

Table 28.16 Complications

Ecchymosis Crusting Edema Reactivation of herpes simplex virus infection Secondary bacterial infection Contact allergy to pigments	Tattoo may act as foci of localized dermatoses in diseases associated with Koebnerization Rarely precipitation of cutaneous malignant melanoma, basal cell carcinoma, and reticulohistiocytoma

Table 28.17 Tattooing: advantages and disadvantages

Advantages	Disadvantages
Results are immediate Chances of rejection are less Inexpensive, safe, and simple office procedure Needs no hospitalization or expertise Can be done on any anatomical site Can be easily repeated if required	Mismatched color Change in shade from brown to slate bluish black Loss of pigment (pigment extrusion) Leaching (pigment fading)

28.3.3.2 Therapeutic Wounding

It is a therapeutic modality where superficial wounding of the epidermis is done for small and stable patches of vitiligo to achieve repigmentation.

A. Evolution
This procedure for the vitiliginous skin is performed without subsequent grafting. Various modalities like dermabrasion, CO_2 laser and Er:YAG laser ablation, cryosurgery, needling, and spot chemical peeling with 88 % phenol solution or trichloroacetic acid 30–50 % have been used for wounding the vitiligo patch and inducing repigmentation [69–75].
B. Mechanism of repigmentation
Following therapeutic wounding, there occurs inflammation followed by reepithelialization from the remnants of dermal appendages like sebaceous glands, hair follicles, and sweat glands [69, 70, 74]. Various cytokines, such as leukotrienes C4 and D4, TGF-α, interleukin-1, and endothelin-1 liberated during inflammatory and healing phase, stimulate the follicular and perilesional melanocytes and induce perifollicular and perilesional pigmentation [69, 70, 74, 76–78].

Superficial Dermabrasion (Spot or Regional)

A. Procedure

- It is performed under local or general anesthesia.
- Multiple, parallel, side-to-side, and above-downward strokes with an electric dermabrader or to-and-fro, longitudinal, and horizontal, crisscross strokes with a manual metallic abrader are made from one border to another border of the vitiligo patch, till punctuate bleeding points appear. The complete lesion is evenly dermabraded extending 1 cm beyond the vitiliginous area (feathering).

B. Post-procedure instruction

- Topical PUVA or PUVASOL therapy is advised for the next 3–6 months after the lesion has healed.

C. Complications

- Postoperative hypo- or hyperpigmentation, erythema, secondary infection, and scarring

D. Advantages and disadvantages (Table 28.18)

Table 28.18 Superficial dermabrasion: advantages and disadvantages

Advantages	Disadvantages
Inexpensive	Can be used for cosmetically unimportant area
Safe and simple office procedure	25 % (ideally up to 50 %) of the black hair required
Quick results	Multiple sittings required for larger regions

CO_2 Laser Ablation (Spot or Regional)

A. Procedure

- After anesthesia, small adjacent areas are uniformly ablated using the free-hand method with the laser in the continuous mode. There occurs immediate bubbling of the epidermis (which turns grayish white).
- After removal of the epidermis, healthy erythematous to pinkish dermis is seen.
- The wound is then dressed with an antibiotic ointment.

B. Post-procedure instruction

- Topical PUVA or PUVASOL therapy is advised for the next 3–6 months after the lesion has healed.

C. Complications

- Persistent erythema, pigmentary changes, and scarring

D. Advantages and disadvantages (Table 28.19)

Table 28.19 CO_2 laser ablation: advantages and disadvantages

Advantages	Disadvantages
Simple freehand technique	At least 25 % of black hair required
No bleeding	Expensive equipment

Liquid Nitrogen Cryosurgery

A. Procedure

- This is done by therapeutically wounding the hairy vitiligo area by freezing it with liquid nitrogen (−196°C) for 10–20 s through a single freeze–thaw cycle. Within a few minutes, a violet color appears at the periphery and moves centrally. A hemorrhagic blister forms on the surface which turns into an eschar, lasting for a few days or weeks.

B. Complications (Table 28.20)

Table 28.20 Liquid nitrogen cryosurgery complications: immediate and delayed

Immediate	Delayed
Pain Headache (for lesions on the forehead, temples, or scalp) Edema Hemorrhage Blister formation Syncope	Hemorrhage Postoperative infection Granulation tissue formation Pseudoepitheliomatous hyperplasia Hyperpigmentation Milia Hypertrophic scars Arthralgia

Needling

A. Procedure

- Multiple, superficial, tiny puncture wounds spaced 1 mm apart are made at the junctional hyperpigmented border with a sterile #26 injection needle at an angle of 30–45° with the tip of the needle pointing toward the depigmented zone. Hemostasis is achieved with pressure. A scab may form by the second to fourth day and falls off by the eighth to tenth day.

B. Post-procedure instruction

- Treatment with topical PUVA/PUVASOL is continued.

Chemical Wounding with 50 % TCA or 88 % Phenol

A. Procedure

- Eighty-eight percent phenol is applied using a cotton-tipped applicator with uniform smooth strokes until there is ivory white uniform frosting. Feathering is done by gently painting the phenol from the periphery of the lesion into the surrounding normal skin.
- No neutralization is required for phenol; however, ice cold water is needed for neutralization if TCA is used, once frosting is observed.

B. Post-procedure instruction

- PUVA/PUVASOL therapy is started after 15 days and continued till there is coalition of perifollicular and perilesional pigmentation.

C. Complications

- Immediate burning sensation and discomfort, hyperpigmentation, and superficial scarring

D. Advantages and disadvantages (Table 28.21)

Table 28.21 Chemical wounding: advantages and disadvantages

Advantages	Disadvantages
Safe, simple, and inexpensive	Multiple sittings required
No specialized training, equipment, or local anesthesia	At least 25 % black hair needed

Donor Dermabrasion to Obtain Melanocytes and Keratinocytes

Described by Dilip Kachawa, this unique method involves dermabrasion of the donor area. The dermabraded epidermis is collected and applied directly onto the similarly dermabraded recipient area. In this method, the donor area needed for collecting grafting material is approximately one-third of recipient area [79].

28.3.3.3 Body Hair Transplantation in Vitiligo

Chouhan et al. reported successful repigmentation of vitiligo with leukotrichia after body hair transplantation [79].

A. Procedure

- Donor hairs are collected using the follicular unit extraction (FUE) method with 0.8 mm punch under local anesthesia. Follicular units are simultaneously transplanted in the directions of existing hairs using a 19 g needle in the depigmented macules with 5 mm gap between the follicles.

B. Post-procedure instruction

- Phototherapy is restarted in the recipient area a week after the procedure.

28.3.3.4 Smashed Skin Grafting or Smash Grafting

Smashed skin grafting is a variant of the split-thickness skin graft with a slight modification [80]. In this method, the split-thickness graft obtained undergoes a process of "smashing" before being applied onto the donor site.

A. Procedure

- The amount of donor tissue removed is only one-tenth of the recipient area. The tissue is "smashed" or simply cut into very minute pieces using a sterile curved suture-cutting scissor to make a fine homogenous donor material. The final tissue thus obtained after thorough smashing looks just like a paste consisting of minute particles of the skin.

- The smash graft is then applied to the recipient area. The recipient site is then left open for 15–30 min for the exudates to dry up a little bit. The recipient area is dressed using a nonadherent material, and the patient is advised to keep the area immobile.

B. Post-procedure instruction

- Topical PUVA/PUVASOL is started after 2 weeks.

C. Advantages

- Need simple instruments
- Cost-effective to the patient
- Minimal residual changes at the donor and recipient sites
- Unlike suction blister and thin split-thickness graft, smash graft can be applied without any epidermal or dermal side consideration.
- Easy to master with training and expertise

28.4 Conclusion

Proper patient selection and establishment of stability on vitiligo lesions are very vital in considering surgical modalities as a form of management for refractory vitiligo cases. With all the surgical options available and presented in the chapter, the decision as to what surgical procedure to carry out for a particular candidate will then depend on what is best for the patient and the expertise of the dermatologist–surgeon.

References

1. Goldinger SM, Dummer R, Schmid P, Burg G, Seifert B, Lauchli S. Combination of 308-nm xenon chloride excimer laser and topical calcipotriol in vitiligo. J Eur Acad Dermatol Venereol. 2007;21(4):504–8.
2. Mohanty S, Kumar A, Dhawan J, Sreenivas V, Gupta S. Noncultured extracted hair follicle outer root sheath cell suspension for transplantation in vitiligo. Br J Dermatol. 2011;164(6):1241–6.
3. Rusfianti M, Wirohadidjodjo YW. Dermatosurgical techniques for repigmentation of vitiligo. Int J Dermatol. 2006;45:411–7.
4. Falabella R, Arrunategui A, Barona MI, Alzate A. The minigrafting test for vitiligo: detection of stable lesions for melanocyte transplantation. J Am Acad Dermatol. 1995;32:228–32.
5. Prasad D, Gupta S. Standard guidelines of care for vitiligo surgery. Ind J Dermatol Venereol Leprol. 2008;74:37–45.
6. Gupta S, Kumar B. Epidermal grafting in vitiligo: influence of age, site of lesion, and type of disease on outcome. J Am Acad Dermatol. 2003;49:99–104.
7. Gupta S, Kumar B. Epidermal grafting for vitiligo in adolescents. Pediatr Dermatol. 2002;19:159–62.

8. Orentriech N, Selmanwitz VJ. Autograft repigmentation of leucoderma. Arch Dermatol. 1972;105:784–6.
9. Falabella R. Repigmentation of stable leukoderma by autologous minigrafting. J Dermatol Surg Oncol. 1986;12:172–9.
10. Falabella R. Treatment of localized vitiligo by autologous minigrafting. Arch Dermatol. 1988;124:1649–55.
11. Savant SS. Autologous miniature punch grafting in stable vitiligo. Indian J Dermatol Venereol Leprol. 1992;58:310–4.
12. Lahiri K, Sengupta SR. Treatment of stable and recalcitrant depigmented skin conditions by autologous punch grafting. Indian J Dermatol Venereol Leprol. 1997;63:11–4.
13. Malakar S, Dhar S. Treatment of stable and recalcitrant vitiligo by autologous miniature punch grafting: a prospective study of 1,000 patients. Dermatol. 1999;198:133–9.
14. Feetham HJ, Chan JL, Pandya AG. Characterization of clinical response in patients with vitiligo undergoing autologous epidermal punch grafting. Dermatol Surg. 2011;38:14–9.
15. Malakar S, Lahiri K. Punch grafting for lip leukoderma. Dermatol. 2004;208:125–8.
16. Falabella R. Repigmentation of segmental vitiligo by autologous minigrafting. J Am Acad Dermatol. 1983;9:514–21.
17. Skouge JW, Morison WL, Diwan RV, Rotter S. Autografting and PUVA: a combination therapy for vitiligo. Dermatol Surg Oncol. 1992;18:357–60.
18. Hann SK, Im S, Bong HW, Park YK. Treatment of stable vitiligo with autologous epidermal grafting and PUVA. J Am Acad Dermatol. 1995;32:943–8.
19. Lahiri K, Malakar S, Sarma N, Banerjee U. Repigmentation of vitiligo with punch grafting and narrow-band UV-B (311 nm) a prospective study. Int J Dermatol. 2005;45:649–55.
20. Ortonne JP, Schmitt D, Thivolet J. PUVA induced repigmentation of vitiligo, scanning electron microscopy of hair follicles. J Invest Dermatol. 1980;74(1):40–2.
21. Lahiri K. Evolution and evaluation of autologous mini punch grafting in vitiligo. Ind J Dermatol. 2009;54:159–67.
22. Bisen N, Bhat RM, Lahiri K, Kambil SM. Target-like pigmentation after minipunch grafting in stable vitiligo. Ind J Dermatol. 2014;59:355–6.
23. Falabella R. Epidermal grafting: an original technique and its application in achromic and granulating areas. Arch Dermatol. 1971;104:592–600.
24. Gupta S, Shroff S, Gupta S. Modified technique of suction blistering for epidermal grafting in vitiligo. Int J Dermatol. 1999;38:306–9.
25. Gupta S. Double syringe blistering by adding a three-way connector. J Dermatol Treat. 2001;12:219.
26. Kim HV, Yun SK. Suction device for epidermal grafting in vitiligo: employing a syringe and a manometer to provide an adequate negative pressure. J Dermatol Surg. 2001; 26:702–4.
27. Li J, Fu WW, Zheng ZZ, Zhang QQ, Xu Y, Fang L. Suction blister epidermal grafting using a modified suction method in the treatment of stable vitiligo: a retrospective study. Dermatol Surg. 2011;37:999–1006.
28. Burm JS. Simple suction device for autologous epidermal grafting. Plast Reconstr Surg. 2000;106:1225–6.
29. Alexis AF, Wilson DC, Todhunter JA, Stiller MJ. Reassessment of the suction blister model of wound healing: introduction of a new high pressure device. Int J Dermatol. 1999; 38:613–7.
30. Gupta S, Gupta S, Kumar A. The hypodermic needle as a dermabrading device for recipient area preparation for skin grafting in vitiligo. J Am Acad Dermatol. 2015;72:e105–6.
31. Lee DY. The use of suction blisters for recipient site in epidermal grafting: the implications for vitiligo. J Eur Acad Dermatol Venereol. 2009;23:241–2.
32. Khunger N, Kathuria SD, Ramesh V. Tissue grafts in vitiligo surgery – past, present, and future. Indian J Dermatol. 2009;54(2):150–8.
33. Gupta S, Sandhu K, Kanwar A, Kumar B. Melanocyte transfer via epidermal grafts for vitiligo of labial mucosa. Dermatol Surg. 2004;30:45–8.

34. Nanda S, Relhan V, Grover C, Reddy BS. Suction blister epidermal grafting for management of eyelid vitiligo: special considerations. Dermatol Surg. 2006;32:387–91.
35. Robinson JK. Surgery of the skin: procedural dermatology. 3rd ed. Philadelphia: Elsevier Mosby; 2015.
36. Behl PN. Treatment of vitiligo with homologous thin Thiersch skin grafts. Curr Med Pract. 1964;8:218–21.
37. Kahn AM, Cohen MJ. Vitiligo: treatment by dermabrasion and epithelial sheet grafting. J Am Acad Dermatol. 1995;33:646–8.
38. Kahn AM, Cohen MJ. Repigmentation in vitiligo patients. Melanocyte transfer via ultra-thin grafts. Dermatol Surg. 1998;24:365–7.
39. Olsson MJ, Juhlin L. Epidermal sheet grafts for repigmentation of vitiligo and piebaldism, with a review of surgical techniques. Acta Derm Venereol. 1997;77:463–6.
40. Behl PN, Azad O, Kak R. Autologous thin Thiersch's grafts in vitiligo: experience of 8000 cases, 50,000 grafts (1959–98) with modified technique in 198 cases in the year 1997–98. Ind J Dermatol Venereol Leprol. 1999;65:117–21.
41. Khunger N. Thin split-thickness skin grafts for vitiligo. In: Gupta S, Narang T, Olsson MJ, Ortonne JP, editors. Surgical management of vitiligo. Malden/Oxford: Blackwell Publishing Ltd; 2007. p. 108–14.
42. McGregor IA, McGregor AD. Free skin grafts. In: McGregor IA, McGregor AD, editors. Fundamental techniques of plastic surgery. 9th ed. Edinburg: Churchill Livingstone; 1995. p. 35–9.
43. Ozdemir M, Cetinkale O, Woff R, Wolf R, Kotoyan A, Mat C, et al. Comparison of two surgical approaches for treating vitiligo: a preliminary study. Int J Dermatol. 2002;41:135–8.
44. Olsson M, Juhlin L. Long-term follow-up of leukoderma patients treated with transplants of autologous cultured melanocytes, ultrathin epidermal sheets and basal cell layer suspension. Br J Dermatol. 2002;47:893–904.
45. Torium DM, O'Grody K, Desai D, Bagal A. Cyanoacrylate adhesive. Plast Reconstr Surg. 1998;102:2209–19.
46. Kahn AM, Ostad A, Moy RL. Grafting following short pulse CO_2 laser de-epithelialization. Dermatol Surg. 1996;22:965–7.
47. Khandpur S, Sharma VK, Manchanda Y. Comparison of minipunch grafting versus split-skin grafting in chronic stable vitiligo. Dermatol Surg. 2005;31:436–41.
48. Agrawal K, Agrawal A. Vitiligo: surgical repigmentation of leukotrichia. Dermatol Surg. 1995;21:711–5.
49. Bose SK. Is there any treatment of leukotrichia in stable vitiligo? J Dermatol. 1997;24:615–7.
50. Rhee PH, Friedman CD, Ridge JA, Kusiak J. The use of processed allograft dermal matrix for intraoral resurfacing: an alternative to split-thickness skin grafts. Arch Otolaryngol Head Neck Surg. 1998;124:1201–4.
51. Sa'do B, Nakamura N, Higuchi Y, Zeki S, Harada H, Tashiro H. Squamous cell carcinoma of the oral cavity derived from a skin graft: a case report. Head Neck. 1994;16(1):79–82.
52. Mulekar SV, Al Issa A, Al Eisa A, Asaad M. Genital vitiligo treated by autologous, noncultured melanocyte-keratinocyte cell transplantation. Dermatol Surg. 2005;31:1737–40.
53. Srinivas CR, Rai R, Uday Kumar P. Meshed split skin graft for extensive vitiligo. Ind J Dermatol Venereol Leprol. 2004;70:165–7.
54. McGovern TW, Bolognia J, Leffell DL. Flip-top pigment transplantation. Arch Dermatol. 1999;135:1305–7.
55. Aziz Jalali M, Jafari B, Isfahani M, Nilforoushzadeh MA. Treatment of segmental vitiligo with normal-hair follicle autograft. Med J Islam Repub Iran. 2013;27:210–4.
56. Malakar S, Dhar S. Repigmentation of vitiligo patches by transplantation of hair follicles. Int J Dermatol. 1999;38:237–8.

57. Slominski A, Wortsman J, Plonka PM, Schallreuter KU, Paus R, Tobin DJ. Hair follicle pigmentation. J Invest Dermatol. 2005;124(1):13–21.
58. Gauthier Y, Surleve-Bazeille JE. Autologous grafting with non-cultured melanocytes: a simplified method for treatment of depigmented lesions. J Am Acad Dermatol. 1992;26:191–4.
59. Olsson MJ, Juhlin L. Melanocyte transplantation in vitiligo. Lancet. 1992;340:981.
60. van Geel N, Ongenae K, De Mil M, Naeyaert JM. Modified technique of autologous non cultured epidermal cell transplantation for repigmenting vitiligo: a pilot study. Dermatol Surg. 2001;27:873–6.
61. Gupta S, Sahni K, Tembhre MK, Mathur S, Sharma VK. A novel point-of-care in vivo technique for preparation of epidermal cell suspension for transplantation in vitiligo. J Am Acad Dermatol. 2015;72:e65–6.
62. Kachhawa D, Kalla G. Keratinocyte-melanocyte graft technique followed by PUVA therapy for stable vitiligo. Indian J Dermatol Venereol Leprol. 2008;74:622–4.
63. Eisinger M, Marko O. Selective proliferation of normal human melanocytes in vitro in the presence of phorbol ester and cholera toxin. Proc Natl Acad Sci U S A. 1982;79:2018–22.
64. Lerner AB, Halaban R, Klaus SN, Moellmann GE. Transplantation of human melanocytes. J Invest Dermatol. 1987;89:219–24.
65. Redondo P, Giménez de Azcarate A, Marqués L, Garcia-Guzman M, Andreu E, Prosper F. Amniotic membrane as a scaffold for melanocyte transplantation in patients with stable vitiligo. Dermatol Res Pract. 2011;5:321–39.
66. Andreassi L, Pianigiani E, Andreassi A, Taddeucci P, Biagioli M. A new model of epidermal culture for the surgical treatment of vitiligo. Int J Dermatol. 1998;37:595–8.
67. Savant SS. Tattooing. In: Savant SS, Shah RA, Gore D, editors. Textbook & atlas of dermatosurgery and cosmetology. Mumbai: AS CAD Publishers; 1998. p. 222–6.
68. Roberts TA, Ryan SA. Tattooing and high-risk behavior in adolescents. Pediatr. 2002;110:1058–63.
69. Savant SS. Therapeutic spot and regional dermabrasion in stable vitiligo. Ind J Dermatol Venereol Leprol. 1996;62:139–45.
70. Savant SS. Therapeutic spot dermabrasion. Study of 197 sites in 11 skin conditions. Ind J Dermatol Surg. 1999;1:6–15.
71. Savant SS. Therapeutic wounding. In: Savant SS, editor. Textbook and atlas of dermatosurgery and cosmetology. 2nd ed. Mumbai: ASCAD; 2005. p. 370–7.
72. Savant SS. Cryosurgery with liquid nitrogen in stable vitiligo. Ind J Dermatol Venereol Leprol. 1999;65:246–7.
73. Ahmad TJ, Rashid T, Rani Z. Needling: an adjunct to narrowband ultraviolet B therapy in localized fixed vitiligo. J Pak Asso Dermatol. 2008;18:149–53.
74. Savant SS, Shenoy S. Chemical peeling with phenol for the treatment of stable vitiligo and alopecia areata. Indian J Dermatol Venereol Leprol. 1999;65:93–8.
75. Savant SS. Surgical therapy of vitiligo: current status. Ind J Dermatol Venereol Leprol. 2005;71:307–10.
76. Morelli JG, Yohn JJ, Lyons MB, Murphy RC, Norris DA. Leukotrienes C4 and D4 as potent mitogens for cultured human neonatal melanocytes. J Invest Dermatol. 1989;93(6):719–22.
77. Morelli JG, Kincannon J, Yohn JJ, Zekman T, Weston WL, Norris DA. Leukotriene C4 and TGF-alpha are stimulators of human melanocyte migration in vitro. J Invest Dermatol. 1992;98(3):290–5.
78. Yohn JJ, Morelli JG, Walchak SJ, Rundell KB, Norris DA, Zamora MR. Cultured human keratinocytes synthesize and secrete endothelin-I. J Invest Dermatol. 1993;100(1):23–6.
79. Chouhan K, Kumar K, Kanwar AJ. Body hair transplantation in vitiligo. J Cutan Aesthet Surg. 2013;6(2):111–2.
80. Krishnan A, Kar S. Smashed skin grafting or smash grafting – a novel method of vitiligo surgery. Int J Dermatol. 2012;51(10):1242–7.

Chapter 29
Phototherapy in Vitiligo

Molly C. Powers and Henry W. Lim

29.1 Introduction

Dating back many centuries, heliotherapy, or sunlight for therapeutic uses, has been used to treat a variety of skin conditions. Over 3500 years ago in Egypt, individuals would ingest a boiled extract from a weed growing in the Nile Delta and then expose themselves to the sunlight for the treatment of vitiligo. In India, this similar practice continued with the Atharva-Veda "healers." These healers would supply *Psoralea corylifolia* seeds and advise patients with "leukoderma" to ingest them followed by sun exposure [1, 2]. These practices represent the earliest forms of photochemotherapy or PUVA.

In the late nineteenth century, the continued health benefits of sunlight in several medical conditions were discovered. In 1877, Downes and Blunt demonstrated the bactericidal properties of sunlight on bacillus anthrax [1–4]. Three years later, Palm of Edinburgh reported the therapeutic role of the sun in treating rickets [4]. In 1896, dermatologist Niels Ryberg Finsen reported the successful treatment of lupus vulgaris in a personal friend with artificial light, also known as the "Finsen lamp" [1, 2]. The "Finsen lamp" used light generated from carbon arcs with a common glass lens initially, then later used a fused quartz lens to allow separation of visible light and ultraviolet rays. The "Finsen lamp" was used to treat over 800 patients with lupus vulgaris. During that time period, without the availability of antibiotics and anti-inflammatory medications, this was a tremendous breakthrough in medicine. Finsen was awarded the Nobel Prize in Medicine in 1903 – the only dermatologist to ever be awarded one [1, 2, 5–8].

The modern era of phototherapy began in 1947 after the identification of 8-methoxypsoralen (8-MOP) and 5-methoxypsoralen (5-MOP) from the *Ammi*

M.C. Powers • H.W. Lim, MD (✉)
Department of Dermatology, Henry Ford Hospital – New Center One,
3031 West Grand Blvd, Suite 800, Detroit, MI 48202, USA
e-mail: hlim1@hfhs.org

E.B. Handog, M.J. Enriquez-Macarayo (eds.), *Melasma and Vitiligo in Brown Skin*,
DOI 10.1007/978-81-322-3664-1_29

majus plant [9, 10]. While it is recognized that the use of psoralen with ultraviolet A (UVA) is a form of photochemotherapy, in this chapter, for simplicity, the term "phototherapy" will be used to cover all forms of UV-based therapy.

The first use of oral psoralen in contemporary medicine was performed in 1967 with 8-MOP with ultraviolet light for the treatment of psoriasis [11]. In 1972, Mortazawi used topical 8-MOP with blacklight UVA tubes in a total body radiation unit for the treatment of psoriasis; however the output from the lightbulbs was insufficient to yield adequate response [12]. Later a team of dermatologists, photophysicists, and electrical engineers collaborated to develop high-intensity UVA fluorescent tubes, which, as reported by Parrish et al. in 1974, was successfully used for the treatment of psoriasis in combination with oral 8-MOP, a treatment now commonly known as "PUVA" or psoralen + UVA [13]. Since its introduction, PUVA became a widely used treatment for many dermatoses including psoriasis, vitiligo, mycosis fungoides, and atopic dermatitis.

In 1981, Parrish and Jaenicke reported that the most efficient action spectrum for the treatment of psoriasis is between 296 and 313 nm, ultimately leading to the development of narrowband ultraviolet B (NB-UVB) lightbulbs with a peak emission in 311–313 nm [14]. NB-UVB phototherapy is currently the most widely used form of phototherapy worldwide.

29.2 Impact of Vitiligo

Vitiligo results in significant highly visible disfigurement, and the effects on overall well-being, especially psychosocial, must not be overlooked. As the most visible organ, the skin reflects not only information about our physical health but also participates in social communications to others. Vitiligo has been found to evoke negative emotions including shame, embarrassment, anxiety, depression, and other insecurities, which may ultimately lead to significant influences on personal and social life, daily functioning, and psychological status [15–18].

Vitiligo has important significance in individuals with skin of color. For example, in the Indian population, the depigmented patches are not only more visible in comparison to individuals with lighter skin but also associated with an enormous stigma. Many Indian cultures view vitiligo as a serious disease, which may lead to ostracism, social restrictions, difficulties in employment, and may be considered as a barrier to marriage [19].

29.3 Phototherapy in Vitiligo

29.3.1 Narrowband Ultraviolet B Therapy (NB-UVB)

Although the precise pathogenesis of vitiligo has not been fully elucidated, the role of autoimmunity is the most favored hypothesis. NB-UVB treatment in vitiligo is thought to be twofold. It induces localized immunosuppression, which can therefore downregulate the autoimmune process [20–22]. UVB irradiation leads to increased levels of IL-10, which are associated with the local induction of antigen-specific T-cell tolerance. This increase in IL-10 also causes an increase in the T regulatory cells (Tregs), which in turn helps to suppress self-reactive antigens [20]. Furthermore, NB-UVB has proven to elicit a more optimal level of Th17 and Treg cells in the vitiliginous skin, again, allowing for increased tolerance of self-antigens [22, 23]. Not only does NB-UVB help to promote a favorable balance of Th17 and Treg cells, it has also been implicated in inducing apoptosis in T lymphocytes in psoriatic plaques [24].

The ultimate goal of phototherapy is to repigment the vitiliginous skin. There are several proposed mechanisms for NB-UVB's role in repigmentation. Firstly, it has been discovered that the melanocytes within the hair follicles appear to be immunologically privileged and are typically spared in the vitiliginous skin [20]. For this reason, the proliferation and migration of these melanocytes are essential for repigmentation [25]. NB-UVB results in phosphorylation of focal adhesion kinase and MMP-2, leading to increased migration of melanocytes from the hair follicles and uninvolved perilesional skin. This phenomenon may help to explain why the sites lacking hair follicles, such as the fingertips and mucosal surfaces, are difficult to repigment [26–29]. In addition, NB-UVB results in the increased production of melanogenic growth factors from keratinocytes [30]. These growth factors include basic fibroblastic growth factor (bFGF) and endothelin-1, ultimately leading to the proliferation of melanocytes [26, 27, 30, 31]. Lastly, NB-UVB results in increased expression of tyrosinase, the key enzyme in melanogenesis [25].

There are two ways to initiate NB-UVB phototherapy. Some treatment centers recommend initiating at a fixed dose, considering all vitiliginous areas as the equivalent of skin phototype I. This is the method used at our center (Henry Ford Medical Center, Detroit, Michigan, USA). The approximate MED for skin phototype I is 400 mJ/cm^2. We then initiate treatment at 70 % of the MED, which is 280 mJ/cm^2 [32]. In other centers, the constitutional skin type of the patient's unaffected skin is used as a basis of determining the initial dose. In this method, either MED of the unaffected skin is determined, and treatment started at 70 % of MED, or alternately, skin type protocol is used.

With either of these two methods, treatment dose is increased by 5–15 % with each session. Treatment is done 2–3× a week to a maximum of 1 J/cm^2 to the face and 3 J/cm^2 to the body, if tolerated. During the repigmentation phase, treatment should not be less than twice weekly; treatments completed once a week would not allow for appropriate increase in dose and therefore should not be utilized.

In those patients who are responsive, repigmentation should be evident within 20–30 treatments. Phototherapy is usually continued for a total of 40–60 treatments. Once the response has plateaued, frequency is tapered to twice weekly for 4 weeks, once weekly for 4 weeks, and then discontinued.

29.3.2 Psoralen Plus Ultraviolet A (PUVA)

Photochemotherapy, or psoralen plus ultraviolet A (PUVA), consists of taking a photosensitizer followed by irradiation with UVA. In the United States (US) and in many parts of the world, 8-MOP is used; in Europe, 5-MOP is also available [1, 2, 5, 33, 34]. An additional photosensitizer, 4-, 5-, 8-trimethyl psoralen (TMP, trioxsalen), is a synthetic compound that was also used in PUVA therapy, frequently in combination with sunlight. However, it is no longer available in the USA and in many parts of the world [35]. Methoxsalen conjugates and forms covalent bonds with DNA upon photoactivation, leading to monofunctional and bifunctional adducts [35–37]. This has apoptotic, antiproliferative, anti-angiogenic, and immunosuppressive effects [38].

There are similar cutaneous immunosuppressive properties between PUVA and NB-UVB; however, the proposed mechanisms to stimulate pigmentation differ. With PUVA therapy, the psoralens help to stimulate melanogenesis through their photoconjugation to the DNA in melanocytes leading to further mitosis and proliferation [39]. It produces increased melanin synthesis in melanocytes, with subsequent increase of melanosome transfer to keratinocytes. Lastly, there is a stimulation of cAMP, which leads to activation and synthesis of tyrosinase in melanocytes [39, 40].

Prior to or shortly after starting PUVA therapy, a baseline ophthalmology examination should be obtained, and then yearly thereafter. Similar to NB-UVB phototherapy, PUVA is administered two to three times weekly. Treatments should be spaced 48 h apart as the peak erythema following PUVA exposure occurs at 48 h. 8-MOP is given at 0.4–0.5, up to 0.6 mg/kg for recalcitrant cases, with a maximum of 70 mg per treatment. The photosensitizer should be taken one hour prior to UVA exposure with a light, nonfatty meal as fatty foods can limit the absorption. Ideally, the patient should take the photosensitizer on an empty stomach; however, this often leads to gastrointestinal (GI) disturbances. Consistency of the meal (timing and type of food) is important to ensure consistency in the GI absorption of 8-MOP as food can substantially impact the peak blood levels [41]. On the day of treatment, it is important that the patient practice photoprotection, including the use of UV-protective glasses when outdoor, once the patient has ingested the psoralen.

We recommend the initial starting dose of UVA to be 0.25–0.5 J/cm^2, increasing by 0.25–0.5 J/cm^2 until mild, symptomatic erythema is observed in vitiligo lesions. Since the limiting skin type is the vitiligo lesions, the equivalent of skin type I, a maximum of 8 J/cm^2 is recommended.

Similar to NB-UVB, patients should show evidence of response after 20–30 treatments. Protocol for tapering and discontinuation of treatment is similar to that of NB-UVB.

29.3.3 Psoralen and Solar Exposure (PUVAsol)

PUVAsol is the use of topical or systemic psoralen derivatives in combination with natural sunlight. It is commonly used in regions where there is adequate sunlight and/or insufficient access to artificial ultraviolet lamps. Individuals apply or ingest the indicated psoralen (often TMP) then expose themselves to sunlight, initially of short duration, then titrating upward to achieve adequate erythema [42, 43]. This has been shown to be effective in both localized and generalized vitiligo as demonstrated by Handa et al. [44].

Nonetheless, there are several limitations of this therapy. Most importantly, there is no standardization in the total dose received from sun exposure. Due to variations in solar intensity pertaining to climate alterations, it is very difficult to maintain consistency in the dose of ultraviolet radiation. PUVAsol has been shown to lead to more frequent and severe adverse phototoxic events. For these reasons, it has been almost completely replaced by NB-UVB phototherapy.

29.3.4 Targeted Phototherapy: Excimer Laser and Lamp

Targeted phototherapy comprised of the use of both the excimer laser and the excimer lamp. Both produce radiation at 308 nm. Excimer laser and excimer lamp are believed to have similar mechanism to NB-UVB, including immunosuppression and pro-pigmentary properties. Excimer laser produces a pulsing (200 Hz), coherent radiation at a 308 nm wavelength and is based on a self-contained system of xenon chloride (XeCl) gases [45]. It allows for the targeted delivery of higher fluences to affected lesions. The excimer lamp produces an almost continuous, incoherent radiation with a monochromatic spectrum of between 295 and 315 nm with peak absorption of 308 nm [46, 47]. Excimer laser/lamp is ideal for individuals with a smaller body surface area (BSA) affected by vitiligo, by selectively treating the vitiliginous areas and sparing the uninvolved skin. This allows for decreased side effects, such as tanning of the uninvolved skin (except for tanning of immediate adjacent area); it also allows for decreased dose of total cumulative radiation delivered.

At our center, excimer laser is used. For initiation, we start at 150 mJ/cm^2 and increasing by 5–15 % per session up to a maximum of 1 J/cm^2 for the face and 3 J/cm^2 for the body.

29.3.5 Home Phototherapy

In-office phototherapy is often inconvenient for patients. It may require multiple co-pays, increased driving time, and therefore expenses, lost wages, and any combination of the aforementioned [48]. Therefore, for patients who are known to be responsive to phototherapy and requiring maintenance therapy or for patients who otherwise have no access to a phototherapy center, home phototherapy is an appropriate option.

There are several models available, most of which allow exposure of the entire body surface. Koek et al. found that home phototherapy, as compared with outpatient NB-UVB for psoriasis, leads to similar safety and efficacy, lower burden of treatment, and increased patient satisfaction [49]. There are fewer studies on the use of home phototherapy in vitiligo; however, Tien Guan et al. compared home-based phototherapy with Daavlin Dermapal system thrice weekly and institution-based excimer lamp twice weekly for 6 months. Results showed better efficacy in the home-based phototherapy group with 72 % and 50 % achieving good and excellent repigmentation, respectively, in contrast to only 54 and 26 % in the institution-based group. However, these results were not statistically significant. The authors believed that the better efficacy shown was due to the superior compliance in the home-based group with 92 % of the home-based phototherapy group remaining adherent to treatment regimen as opposed to 70 % in the excimer group [50]. Clearly, more studies need to be done on the efficacy of home phototherapy in vitiligo.

Another form of home phototherapy is the handheld NB-UVB devices. These devices are portable, lightweight, and suitable for the treatment of small areas of the affected skin. Handheld NB-UVB devices have been used in the treatment of scalp psoriasis and were found to be effective, well tolerated, safe, and easy to use [51, 52]. However, the efficacy of these handheld devices in vitiligo has not been well established.

29.4 Adjuvants in Phototherapy

Two of the most important factors to consider in the treatment of vitiligo are the body surface area involved and the stability of the disease. Stability of the disease is defined by Njoo et al., using the vitiligo disease activity score (VIDA). Briefly, if there are new or progressing lesions in the preceding 6 weeks, the score is +4; in the preceding 6–12 weeks, yields score of +3; in the preceding 3–6 months, yields score of +2; and in the preceding 6–12 months, yields score of +1. The disease has been defined as stable if there is no activity in the past 12 months [53].

The use of systemic medications in unstable vitiligo should be considered. In order to stabilize the disease, the use of systemic corticosteroids can be employed. Kim et al. used monotherapy with low-dose prednisolone at 0.3 mg/kg for months 1 and 2, 0.15 mg/kg/day for month 3, and 0.075 mg/kg/day for the fourth and final month; this resulted in 87.7 % arrested progression and 70.4 % repigmentation of vitiligo [54]. In a study conducted by Parsad et al., it was demonstrated that monotherapy with 100 mg minocycline daily was effective in stopping the progression of vitiligo in 29 of 32 patients with slowly progressive vitiligo [55]. Singh et al. later demonstrated similar efficacy of monotherapy with dexamethasone (2.5 mg/day on two consecutive days a week) and minocycline (100 mg/day) in decreasing the progression of the disease [56].

Figure 29.1 demonstrates a phototherapy treatment algorithm of vitiligo pertaining to body surface area (BSA) affected and the disease stability. Adjuvants that have been used for phototherapy are summarized in Table 29.1.

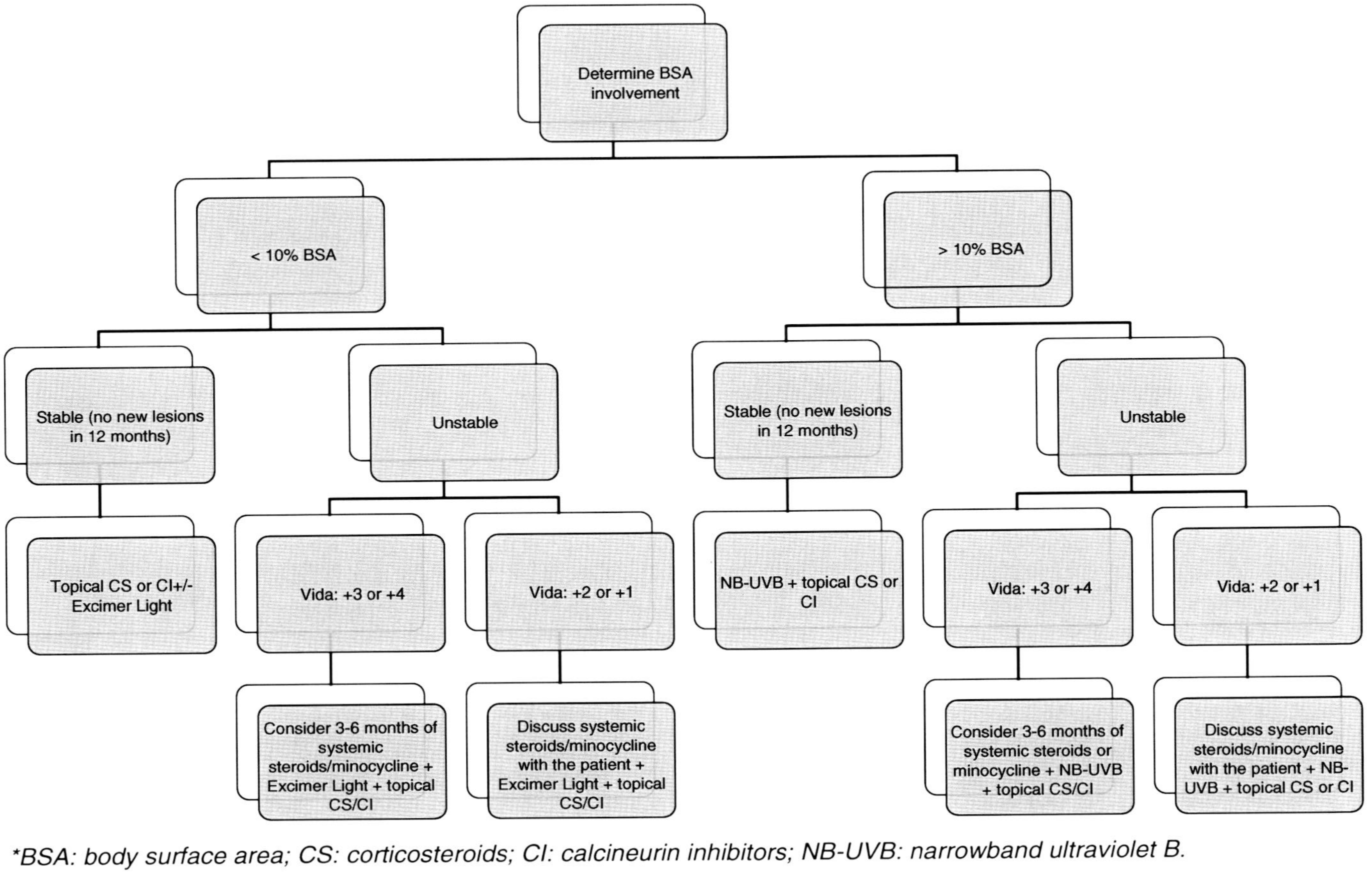

Fig. 29.1 Phototherapy algorithm. *BSA* body surface area, *CS* corticosteroids, *CI* calcineurin inhibitors, *NB-UVB* narrowband ultraviolet B

Table 29.1 Combinations in phototherapy

Author (year)	*N*	Type of trial	Therapy combined with light	Results
NB-UVB combination therapy				
Middelkamp-Hup et al. (2007)	49	RCT	Polypodium leucotomos	Patients attending more than 80 % of required NB-UVB sessions showed increased repigmentation in the head and neck area in the P. leucotomos group vs. placebo (50 vs. 19 %, $P<0.002$)
Lim et al. (2014)	55	Randomized multicenter trial	Afamelanotide	In the combination therapy group, repigmentation was 48.64 %(95 %CI, 39.49–57.80 %) at day 168 vs. 33.26 % (95 %CI, 24.18–42.33 %) in the NB–UVB monotherapy group
Dell'Anna (2007)	28	RCT	Antioxidant (contained alpha-lipoic acid, vitamins C and E, polyunsaturated fatty acids and cysteine monohydrate)	47 % of patients in the NB-UVB + antioxidant had >75 % repigmentation compared to NB-UVB + placebo ($P<0.05$)
Leone et al. (2006)	32	RCT	Vit D analogues (tacalcitol)	Combination therapy of NB-UVB + tacalcitol yielded significantly higher repigmentation than NB-UVB alone ($p<0.005$)
Arca et al. (2006)	37	Randomized, non-placebo controlled trial (blinding not disclosed)	Vit D Analogues (calcipotriol)	NB-UVB + calcipotriol yielded 46 % of subjects with >50 % repigmentation with NB-UVB alone yielding 42 % (not significant)
Bakis-Petsoglou et al. (2009)	32	RCT	Pseudocatalase cream	No statistically significant difference in repigmentation between NB-UVB + placebo cream and NB-UVB + pseudocatalase cream after 24 weeks

(continued)

Table 29.1 (continued)

Author (year)	*N*	Type of trial	Therapy combined with light	Results
Excimer (laser or lamp) combination therapy				
Kawalek et al. (2004)	24 (vitiligo patches); 8 patients	RCT	Excimer laser ± tacrolimus	50 % of the lesions treated with excimer + tacrolimus achieved >75 % repigmentation compared to 20 % in the excimer treatment group alone. ($P<0.05$)
Passeron et al. (2004)	14	RCT	Excimer laser ± tacrolimus	70 % of the excimer/ tacrolimus group achieved >75 % repigmentation compared with 20 % of excimer monotherapy lesions; UV resistant areas showed statistically significant repigmentation with combination than laser monotherapy ($P<0.002$); however, no statistical difference was shown in UV-resistant areas ($P=0.61$)
Lu-yan et al. (2006)	35	RCT	Excimer lamp ± vit D analogues	Topical tacalcitol with excimer yielded (25.7 %) of patients with >75 % repigmentation compared to excimer with placebo vehicle ($P<0.05$)
Goldinger et al. (2007)	9	Prospective right/left comparative, single-blinded study	Excimer laser with calcipotriol	After 24 treatments, in 8/9 patients, both sites (with and without calcipotriol) showed pigmentation with no statistically significant difference
Bae et al. (2015)	159	Retrospective chart review	Excimer laser with tacrolimus and short-term corticosteroids for segmental vitiligo	50.3 % of the 159 patients with segmental vitiligo achieved >75 % repigmentation using combinations excimer laser, topical tacrolimus, and short-term systemic corticosteroids

Selection of studies based on large randomized trials when possible

29.5 Comparisons

29.5.1 NB-UVB Versus PUVA

Westerhof and Nieuweboer were the first to report the use of NB-UVB for the treatment of vitiligo in 1997. They compared the use of NB-UVB and topical PUVA each administered twice weekly for 4 months. They reported that 67 % of NB-UVB patients developed repigmentation as compared with 46 % of topical PUVA patients [57]. Several subsequent studies by Parsad et al., Bhatnagar et al., and Yones et al. all demonstrated NB-UVB's superior efficacy on repigmentation compared to PUVA [58–60]. Currently, NB-UVB is used as first-line treatment for patients with widespread vitiligo, not only for its greater clinical efficacy over PUVA but also for the elimination of systemic psoralen-related side effects, the better color match, the superior safety in children, and the relative lack of long-term photocarcinogenesis risk.

29.5.2 NB-UVB Versus Excimer Laser/Lamp

The first head-to-head study comparing NB-UVB with excimer laser was conducted by Hong et al. using a split-body study. It was discovered that twice weekly, excimer laser produced more rapid and profound repigmentation than NB-UVB after 10, 15, and 20 treatments each [61]. Casacci et al. conducted another split-body study with twice-weekly dosing of both NB-UVB and excimer lamp for 6 months. The patients receiving excimer lamp treatment achieved faster repigmentation [62]. However, a more recent prospective intra-patient, placebo-controlled, randomized trial conducted by Verhaeghe et al. showed a higher percentage of lesions treated with localized 311 nm NB-UVB achieving 50 % repigmentation as compared with sites treated with 308 nm excimer lamp after 24 sessions [63]. In conclusion, while there are several more studies demonstrating the clinical superiority of excimer laser and excimer lamp to NB-UVB, larger-scale studies need to be conducted to evaluate this further.

29.5.3 Excimer Lamp Versus Excimer Laser

A single-center, randomized comparative study by Le Duff et al. compared the efficacy of the excimer laser versus the excimer lamp in the treatment of vitiligo. No statistically significant difference between the two excimer devices was demonstrated. They did note that the lamp takes longer to deliver the same dose as the laser. It also produces more erythema, believed to be due to longer treatment time [64]. Similarly, in 2005, Köllner et al. found no statistically significant difference in the treatment of psoriasis with excimer laser, excimer lamp, and NB-UVB for 10 weeks of treatment [65].

29.6 Limitations and Side Effects

Major limitations with phototherapy include the accessibility of phototherapy treatment centers and the time and effort necessary for patients to receive the treatment. Insurance coverage and treatment cost are other factors that need to be considered. While home phototherapy units do make it more convenient for the patients, they are primarily used as maintenance treatment.

Short-term adverse events for NB-UVB and excimer laser/lamp include UV erythema and possible keratitis/conjunctivitis [66]. While there have been no long-term studies on the use of NB-UVB for vitiligo, Hearn et al. evaluated over 3800 psoriatic patients previously treated with NB-UVB and found no increased incidence in skin cancers (both nonmelanoma and melanoma) in patients treated with NB-UVB alone; however, there was a small increase in the incidence of basal cell carcinoma among patients treated with both NB-UVB and PUVA [67]. No long-term side effects of excimer therapy have been described; however, in view of short duration of treatment and the small number of treatment sessions, it is highly unlikely that photoaging and photocarcinogenesis would occur secondary to excimer therapy.

The side effects of PUVA are well known. Acute side effects include psoralen-induced nausea and less commonly, vomiting, acute phototoxicity, melanonychia, and distal onycholysis. Chronic side effects include lentigines, photoaging, squamous cell carcinoma, basal cell carcinoma, and melanoma [35, 66]. With the replacement of PUVA with NB-UVB for the treatment of vitiligo and with the relatively shorter duration of treatment course, this is no longer a clinically significant issue for vitiligo.

29.6.1 Vitiligo and Skin Cancer

The incidence of skin cancer among vitiligo patients has yielded contradictory results. In 2002, Shallreuter et al. reported no increased risk for sun-induced skin cancers or sun-induced skin damage by biopsy [68]. Hexsel et al. later reported a small increase in the incidence of nonmelanoma skin cancers in vitiligo patients; however, the results were not statistically significant [69]. There is further research to suggest that individuals with vitiligo, including those with prior phototherapy treatment (including NB-UVB and PUVA), have an overall decreased risk in the incidence of both melanoma and nonmelanoma skin cancers as reported by Teuling et al. and Paradisi et al. [70, 71]. Conversely, Nijsten et al. demonstrated that psoriatic patients who underwent PUVA therapy had an increased incidence of nonmelanoma skin cancer, even decades after PUVA treatment [72]. Additional studies need to be conducted for further evaluation.

29.7 Conclusion

Phototherapy is an essential and important treatment for individuals with vitiligo. Individuals with greater than 10% BSA would be candidates for NB-UVB with topical corticosteroids or calcineurin inhibitors. Individuals with less than 10% BSA should be considered for either excimer lamp or laser to the affected areas. The addition of systemic medications including dexamethasone or minocycline may be considered for unstable vitiligo.

References

1. Hönigsmann H. History of phototherapy in dermatology. Photochem Photobiol Sci. 2013;12:16.
2. McDonagh A. Phototherapy: from ancient Egypt to the new millennium. J Perinatol. 2001;21:S7–12.
3. Saleeby CW. Sunlight and health. 3rd ed. London: Nisbet & Co; 1923–1926.
4. Palm TA. The geographic distribution and etiology of rickets. Practitioner. 1890;45:270–9.
5. Roelandts R. The history of phototherapy: something new under the sun? J Am Acad Dermatol. 2002;46:926–30.
6. Finsen NR. Om Lysets Indvirkninger paa Huden [On the effects of light on the skin]. Hospitalstidende. 1893;36:721–8.
7. Finsen NR. Om Anvendelse i Medicinen af koncentrerede kemiske Lysstraaler. [On the application in medicine of concentrated chemical rays of light]. Copenhagen: Gyldendalske Boghandels Forlag; 1896. p. 5–52.
8. Grzybowski A, Pietrzak K. From patient to discoverer—Niels Ryberg Finsen (1860–1904)—the founder of phototherapy in dermatology. Clin Dermatol. 2012;30(4):451–5.
9. Fahmy IR, Abu-Shady H, Schönberg A. Crystalline principle from Ammi majus L. Nature. 1947;160(4066):468.
10. Fahmy IR, Abu-Shady H. *Ammi majus* Linn: the isolation and properties of ammoidin, ammidin and majudin, and their effect in the treatment of leukoderma. Q J Pharm Pharmacol. 1948;21(4):499–503.
11. Oddoze L, Témime, Marchand JP, Benne M. L'association "meladipine" per os et ravons U.V. dans le rtaitement du psoriasis. [Combined oral meladinine and ultraviolet rays in the treatment of psoriasis]. Bull Soc Fr Dermatol Syphiligr. 1967;74(5):609–10.
12. Mortazawi SM. Meladinine and UVA in vitiligo, psoriasis, parapsoriasis and acne vulgaris. Dermatol Monatsschr. 1972;158:908–9.
13. Parrish JA, Parrish TB, Fitzpatrick TB, Tanenbaum L, Pathak MA. Photochemotherapy of psoriasis with oral methoxsalen and longwave ultraviolet light. N Engl J Med. 1974;291(23):1207–11.
14. Parrish JA, Jaenicke KF. Action spectrum for phototherapy of psoriasis. J Invest Dermatol. 1981;76(5):359–62.
15. Jayaprakasam A, Darvay A, Osborne G, McGibbon D. Comparison of assessments of severity and quality of life in cutaneous disease. Clin Exp Dermatol. 2002;27:306–8.

16. Harlow D, Poyner T, Finlay AY, Dykes PJ. Impaired quality of life of adults with skin disease in primary care. Br J Dermatol. 2002;143:979–82.
17. Halioua B, Beumont MG, Lunel F. Quality of life in dermatology. Int J Dermatol. 2000;39:801–6.
18. Jowett S, Ryan T. Skin disease and handicap: an analysis of the impact of skin conditions. Soc Sci Med. 1985;20:425–9.
19. Pahwa P, Mehta M, Khaitan BK, Sharma VK, Ramam M. The psychosocial impact of vitiligo in Indian patients. Ind J Dermatol Venereol Leprol. 2013;79(5):679–85.
20. Fitzpatrick TB. Mechanisms of phototherapy in vitiligo. Arch Dermatol. 1997;133:1591–2.
21. Moftah NH, El-Barbary RA, Ismail MA, Ali NA. Effect of narrow band-ultraviolet B on $CD4^+$ $CD25^{high}$ $FoxP3^+$T-lymphocytes in the peripheral blood of vitiligo patients. Photodermatol Photoimmunol Photomed. 2014;30(5):254–61.
22. Hegazy RA, Fawzy MM, Gawdat HI, Samir N, Rashed LA. T helper 17 and Tregs: a novel proposed mechanism for NB-UVB in vitiligo. Exp Dermatol. 2014;23(4):283–6.
23. Ponsonby AL, Lucas RM, van der Mei IA. UVR, vitamin D and three autoimmune diseases–multiple sclerosis, type 1 diabetes, rheumatoid arthritis. Photochem Photobiol. 2005;81:1267–75.
24. Ozawa M, Ferenczi K, Kikuchi T, Cardinale I, Austin LM, Coven TR, et al. 312-nanometer ultraviolet B light (narrow-band UVB) induces apoptosis of T cells within psoriatic lesions. J Exp Med. 1999;189:711–8.
25. Cui J, Shen LY, Wang GC. Role of hair follicles in the repigmentation of vitiligo. J Invest Dermatol. 1991;97:410–6.
26. Wu CS, Yu CL, Wu CS, Lan CCE, Yu HS. Narrow-band ultraviolet-B stimulates proliferation and migration of cultured melanocytes. Exp Dermatol. 2004;13(12):755–63.
27. Dong D, Jiang M, Xu X, Guan M, Wu J, Chen Q, Xiang L. The effects of NB-UVB on the hair follicle-derived neural crest stem cells differentiating into melanocyte lineage in vitro. J Dermatol Sci. 2012;66(1):20–8.
28. Morelli JG, Kincannon J, Yohn JJ, Zekman T, Weston WL, Norris DA. Leukotriene C4 and TGF-alpha are stimulator of human melanocyte migration in vitro. J Invest Dermatol. 1992;98:290–5.
29. Horikama T, Norris DA, Johnson TW, Zekman T, Dunscomb N, Bennion SD, et al. DOPA-negative melanocytes in the outer root sheath of human hair follicles express premelanosomal antigens but not a melanosomal antigen or the melanosome-associated glycoproteins tyrosinase TRP-1, and TRP-2. J Invest Dermatol. 1996;106:28–35.
30. Hirobe T. Role of keratinocyte-derived factors involved in regulating the proliferation and differentiation of mammalian epidermal melanocytes. Pigment Cell Res. 2005;18:2–12.
31. Halaban R, Langdon R, Birchall N, Cuono C, Baird A, Scott G, et al. Basic fibroblast growth factor from human keratinocytes is a natural mitogen for melanocytes. J Cell Biol. 1988;107(4):1611–9.
32. Scherschun L, Kim JJ, Lim HW. Narrow-band ultraviolet B is a useful and well-tolerated treatment for vitiligo. J Am Acad Dermatol. 2001;44(6):999–1003.
33. Grimes PE. Vitiligo. An overview of therapeutic approaches. Dermatol Clin. 1993;11:325–38.
34. Taneja A. Treatment of vitiligo. J Dermatol Treat. 2002;13:19–25.
35. Gupta AK, Anderson TF. Psoralen photochemotherapy. J Am Acad Dermatol. 1987;17:703–34.
36. Canton M, Caffieri S, Dall'Acqua F, Di Lisa F. PUVA-induced apoptosis involves mitochondrial dysfunction caused by the opening of the permeability transition pore. FEBS Lett. 2002;522:168–72.
37. Averbeck D. Recent advances in psoralen phototoxicity mechanism. Photochem Photobiol. 1989;50:859–82.
38. Ceoviæ R, Pasiæ A, Lipozenciæ J, JakiæRazumoviæ J, Szirovicza L, Kostoviæ K. Antiproliferative, antiangiogenic and apoptotic effect of photochemotherapy (PUVA) in psoriasis patients. Coll Antropol. 2007;31:5516.

39. Abdel-Naser MB, Hann SK, Bystryn JC. Oral psoralen with UV-A therapy releases circulating growth factor(s) that stimulates cell proliferation. Arch Dermatol. 1997;133:1530–3.
40. Wu CS, Lan CC, Wang LF, Chen GS, Wu CS, Yu HS. Effects of psoralen plus ultraviolet A irradiation on cultured epidermal cells in vitro and patients with vitiligo in vivo. Br J Dermatol. 2007;156:122–9.
41. Chakrabarti SG, Grimes PE, Minus HR, Kenney Jr JA, Pradhan TK. Determination of trimethylpsoralen in blood, ophthalmic fluids, and skin. J Invest Dermatol. 1982;79:374.
42. Theodoridis A, Tsambaos D, Sivenas C, Capetanakis J. Oral trimethylpsoralen in the treatment of vitiligo. Acta Derm Venereol. 1976;56:253–6.
43. Parsad D, Saini R, Verma N. Combination of PUVAsol and topical calcipotriol in vitiligo. Dermatol. 1998;197:167–70.
44. Handa S, Pandhi R, Kaur I. Vitiligo: a retrospective comparative analysis of treatment modalities in 500 patients. J Dermatol. 2001;28:461–6.
45. Baltás E, Csoma Z, Iynácz F, Dobzy A, Keměny L. Treatment of vitiligo with the 308 nm xenon chloride excimer laser. Arch Dermatol. 2002;138:1619–20.
46. Shi Q, Li K, Fu J, Wang Y, Ma C, Li Q, et al. Comparison of the 308-nm excimer laser with the 308-nm excimer lamp in the treatment of vitiligo – a randomized bilateral comparison study. Photodermatol Photoimmunol Photomed. 2013;29(1):27–33.
47. Park KK, Liao W, Murase JE. A review of monochromatic excimer light in vitiligo. Br J Dermatol. 2012;167(3):468–78.
48. Yentzer BA, Gustafson CJ, Feldman SR. Explicit and implicit copayments for phototherapy: examining the cost of commuting. Dermatol Online J. 2013;19(6):18563.
49. Koek MB, Buskens E, van Weelden H, Steegmans PH, Bruijnzeel-Koomen CA, Sigurdsson V. Home versus outpatient ultraviolet B phototherapy for mild to severe psoriasis: pragmatic multicentre randomised controlled non-inferiority trial (PLUTO study). BMJ. 2009;338:b1542.
50. Tien Guan ST, Theng C, Chang A. Randomized, parallel group trial comparing home-based phototherapy with institution-based 308 excimer lamp for the treatment of focal vitiligo vulgaris. J Am Acad Dermatol. 2015;72(4):733–5.
51. Dotterud LK, Braun R. UV-B comb versus betamethasone solution in scalp psoriasis. Tidsskr Nor Laegeforen. 2000;120(16):1858–9.
52. Caccialanza M, Piccinno R, Cappio M, Rozza M, Mainardi L. Phototherapy of psoriasis of the scalp. Results in 21 patients treated with a special portable ultraviolet rays lamp. Giornale Italiano Dermatologia Venereologia. 1989;124(11–12):61–5.
53. Njoo MD, Das PK, Bos JD, Westerhof W. Association of the Köebner phenomenon with disease activity and therapeutic responsiveness in vitiligo vulgaris. Arch Dermatol. 1999;135:407–13.
54. Kim SM, Lee HS, Hann SK. The efficacy of low dose oral corticosteroids in the treatment of vitiligo patients. Int J Dermatol. 1999;38:546–50.
55. Parsad D, Kanwar A. Oral minocycline in the treatment of vitiligo – a preliminary study. Dermatol Ther. 2010;23(3):305–7.
56. Singh A, Kanwar AJ, Parsad D, Mahajan R. Randomized controlled study to evaluate the effectiveness of dexamethasone oral minipulse therapy versus oral minocycline in patients with active vitiligo vulgaris. Ind J Dermatol Venereol Leprol. 2014;80:29–35.
57. Westerhof W, Nieuweboer-Krobotova L. Treatment of vitiligo with UV-B radiation vs topical psoralen plus UV-A. Arch Dermatol. 1997;133(12):1525–8.
58. Parsad D, Kanwar AJ, Kumar B. Psoralen-ultraviolet A vs. narrow-band ultraviolet B phototherapy for the treatment of vitiligo. J Eur Acad Dermatol Venereol. 2006;20(2):175–7.
59. Bhatnagar A, Kanwar AJ, Parsad D, De D. Comparison of systemic PUVA and NB-UVB in the treatment of vitiligo: an open prospective study. J Eur Acad Dermatol Venereol. 2007;21:638–42.
60. Yones SS, Palmer RA, Garibaldinos TM, Hawk JLM. Randomized double-blind trial of treatment of vitiligo: efficacy of psoralen—UV-a therapy vs. narrowband—UV-B therapy. Arch Dermatol. 2007;143:578–84.

61. Hong SB, Park HH, Lee MH. Short term effects of 308 nm xenon chloride excimer laser and narrow band ultraviolet B in the treatment of vitiligo: a comparative study. J Korean Med Sci. 2005;20:273–8.
62. Casacci M, Thomas P, Pacifico A, Bonnevalle A, Paro Vidolin A, Leone G. Comparison between 308-nm monochromatic excimer light and narrowband UVB phototherapy (311–313 nm) in the treatment of vitiligo – a multicentre controlled study. J Eur Acad Dermatol Venereol. 2007;21:956–63.
63. Verhaeghe E, Lodewick E, van Geel N, Lambert J. Intrapatient comparison of 308-nm monochromatic excimer light and localized narrow-band UVB phototherapy in the treatment of vitiligo: a randomized controlled trial. Dermatol. 2011;223(4):343–8.
64. Le Duff F, Fontas E, Giacchero D, Sillard L, Lacour JP, Ortonne JP, Passeron T. 308-nm excimer lamp vs. 308-nm excimer laser for treating vitiligo: a randomized study. Br J Dermatol. 2010;163(1):188–92.
65. Köllner K, Wimmershoff MB, Hintz C, Landthaler M, Hohenleutner U. Comparison of the 308-nm excimer laser and a 308-excimer lamp with 311-nm narrowband ultraviolet B in the treatment of psoriasis. Br J Dermatol. 2005;152(4):750–4.
66. DePry J, Brescoll J, Szczotka-Flynn L, Rambhatla P, Lim HW, Cooper K. Phototherapy-related ophthalmologic disorders. Clin Dermatol. 2015;33(2):247–55.
67. Hearn RMR, Kerr AC, Rahim KF, Ferguson J, Dawe RS. Incidence of skin cancers in 3867 patients treated with narrow-band ultraviolet B phototherapy. Br J Dermatol. 2008;159:931–5.
68. Shallreuter KU, Tobin DJ, Panske A. Decreased photodamage and low incidence of non-melanoma skin cancer in 136 sun-exposed Caucasian patients with vitiligo. Dermatol. 2002;204(3):194–201.
69. Hexsel CL, Eide MJ, Johnson CC, Krajenta R, Jacobsen G, Hamzavi I, Lim HW. Incidence of nonmelanoma skin cancer in a cohort of patients with vitiligo. J Am Acad Dermatol. 2009;60(6):929–33.
70. Teulings GE, Overkamp M, Ceylan E, Nieuweboer-Krobotova L, Bos JD, Nijsten T, et al. Decreased risk of melanoma and nonmelanoma skin cancer in patients with vitiligo: a survey among 1307 patients and their partners. Br J Dermatol. 2013;168(1):162–71.
71. Paradisi A, Tabolli S, Didona B, Sobrino L, Russo N, Abeni D. Markedly reduced incidence of melanoma and nonmelanoma skin cancer in a noncurrent cohort of 10,040 patients with vitiligo. J Am Acad Dermatol. 2014;71(6):1110–6.
72. Nijsten TE, Stern RS. The increased risk of skin cancer is persistent after discontinuation of psoralen + ultraviolet A: a cohort study. J Invest Dermatol. 2003;121(2):252–8.

Chapter 30
Vitiligo and Quality of Life

Marcia Ramos-e-Silva, Felipe Cupertino de Andrade, and João Paulo Niemeyer-Corbellini

30.1 Definition

The World Health Organization (WHO) defined quality of life (QoL) as "the perception of the individual regarding his position in life, the context of cultural and value systems in which he lives, and in relation to his objectives, expectations, rules and references" [1]. QoL is a multidimensional term determined not only by health aspects. Multiple nonmedical aspects shape its relevance (i.e., socioeconomic situation and degree of independence; professional career, personality, and psychological state; social relations and relations with the environment; happiness, ambition, beliefs, expectations, and religious experience) [2].

30.2 History

The QoL theme has already been raised by philosophers along the entire human history. In the IV century BC, Socrates stated that the most important is not life itself but its quality. Since 1948, when the WHO defined health as being not only the absence of disease and sickness but also the presence of physical, mental, and social well-being, aspects related to QoL had been growing in relevance in the assistance and investigation of health issues. The first clinical publications incorporating the term QoL appeared in the 1960s of the past century, and the last quarter of that century saw a dramatic increase regarding interest in QoL [3].

M. Ramos-e-Silva, MD, PhD (✉) • F.C. de Andrade • J.P. Niemeyer-Corbellini
Sector of Dermatology and Post-Graduation Course, University Hospital and School of Medicine, Federal University of Rio de Janeiro, Rio de Janeiro, Brazil
e-mail: ramos.e.silva@dermato.med.br

E.B. Handog, M.J. Enriquez-Macarayo (eds.), *Melasma and Vitiligo in Brown Skin*,
DOI 10.1007/978-81-322-3664-1_30

30.2.1 Quality of Life in Dermatology

Skin diseases have always caused an adverse effect on the life of patients. However, only in the last 20 years has this effect begun to be measured consistently through QoL studies [4]. There is a great interest in the evaluation of QoL in dermatological afflictions, given that these diseases usually have a significant impact in social relations, in the psychological state of mind, and in daily activities [2]. Since expectations regarding health and the ability to cope with limitations and incapacities can affect an individual's perception and satisfaction, two individuals with the same clinical health state may have different impacts regarding their QoL [5].

30.2.2 Quality of Life in Vitiligo

Since vitiligo does not cause physical deficiency, it is often considered only a cosmetic problem. However, alterations caused by this disease can affect the emotional and psychological well-being of the patient and entail important repercussions in his life. Additionally, vitiligo is a chronic disease with unpredictable natural course turning it into a burden on the QoL of the patients. The disease, which usually has its onset at a time in life where people begin to consolidate their individuality and sexual identity, can have a great impact on the self-image, self-esteem, and interpersonal relations. Actually, it has been reported that people with vitiligo have a negative self-image of their body with low corporal self-esteem. Furthermore, they may suffer stigmatization making them ashamed of their body and damaging their social life [6]. It seems inadequate therefore that to describe the severity of the disease, merely physical indicators are used (i.e., affected body surface area (BSA) or the number of body locations affected). Only 9 % of the studies that evaluate the efficacy of the treatment apply QoL as one of their references [7]. The evaluation of QoL requires specific instruments for its assessment in order to provide a detailed image of the individual impact caused by the disease.

30.3 Instruments for Evaluation of QoL in Dermatoses in General

In order to measure QoL, it is necessary to understand the factors that influence it. Despite existence of several definitions for QoL, the majority of the researchers agree that the factors involved can be classified into two main groups: objective and subjective. The subjective factors include the self-evaluation of the physical condition, mental condition, and social and interpersonal relations; on the other hand, objective factors are those related to medical and psychological diagnoses, results from laboratory exams and socioeconomic status [8].

30.3.1 Dermatology Life Quality Index (DLQI)

DLQI was developed by Finlay and Kahn in 1994. It was the first questionnaire specifically destined for QoL in dermatology. Of simple construction and with easy routine application, it has already been used in over 272 studies in 32 countries, being available in 55 languages. The questionnaire assesses the events that occurred in the foregoing week, allowing an easy recollection by the patients and can thus be used in comparative studies. The DLQI comprises ten questions addressing six different domains (symptoms, daily activities, leisure, work or school, personal relations, and treatment), and its score varies from zero (least impact in the QoL) to 30 (highest impact in QoL) [9].

30.3.2 Children's Dermatology Life Quality Index (CDLQI)

CDLQI was developed in 1995 based on the impact of dermatoses on children's QoL. It presents a similar score structure as DLQI and is recommended to be used for children over 7 years of age [10]. Subsequently, in 2003, an illustrated version of the CDLQI was created, faster and easier to fill out, being preferred by parents and children [11].

30.3.3 Skindex

Skindex is a useful instrument to measure QoL in patients with different cutaneous diseases. In its initial structure, it comprised 61 items divided in eight dimensions (cognitive effects, social effects, depression, fear, embarrassment, irritation, physical discomfort, and physical limitations) [12]. This is an extensive questionnaire with questions addressing the past 4 weeks, with excellent validity and reliability. Afterward, it was reduced to 29 items, originating the Skindex-29 [13], and later shortened again to 16 items, becoming Skindex-16 [14].

30.4 Specific Instruments for the Evaluation of QoL in Vitiligo

Recently, some authors have proposed the creation and validation of scales regarding the QoL evaluation, specifically aimed at vitiligo.

30.4.1 Vitiligo Quality of Life Scale (VitiQoL)

VitiQoL is a scale with 15 items that incorporates the majority of information from preexistent questionnaires specifically aimed at vitiligo and its impact in the foregoing week, with good reliability [15].

30.4.2 Vitiligo Life Quality Index (VLQI)

VLQI is a form with 25 questions regarding vitiligo, adapted from existent questionnaires and with new additional questions aimed at specific dermatoses such as the Psoriasis Quality of Life Scale (PSORIQoL), Acne Quality of Life Scale (AQOLS), and Atopic Dermatitis Quality of Life Scale (QoLiAD), presenting converging results with DLQI when tested simultaneously [16].

30.4.3 Vitiligo Impact Scale-22 (VIS-22)

VIS-22 presents with 22 specific questions regarding the disease, adapted from the VIS scale [17], which consisted of 27 questions, but had its number reduced with the purpose to bring greater balance to the evaluation [18].

30.5 QoL in Vitiligo Patients

Vitiligo patients, on the average, present a moderate DLQI score (ranging from 4.4 to 17.1), comparable to other dermatoses as psoriasis and atopic dermatitis. Additionally, DLQI is correlated to the extension of the affected BSA. Individuals with over 25 % affected BSA present difficulty in the performance of daily tasks (i.e., shopping, gardening, or choosing clothes) and difficulties in socializing (i.e., taking part in sport activities or begin and maintain affective and sexual relations) [19].

Through application and interpretation of Skindex-29, the main complaints referred by the patients can be highlighted. These include worries that the disease may worsen (60 %), a sentiment of anger, embarrassment, depressive feelings, affected social life, and shame. Emotional problems are more frequent in women. Individuals with age over 40 have more difficulty to maintain personal relations and social conviviality. The extension of the involvement and lesions in exposed areas has a strong impact in the daily functionality [6].

Treatment of vitiligo is required not only for cosmetic reasons but also for the promotion of the patient's well-being. This was evident with the improvement in the DLQI after therapy intervention, regardless of the effectiveness of the repigmentation

[20]. The regular use of corrective makeup also promotes an improvement in the QoL, with occurrence of a reduction in the DLQI score after a month of use in exposed lesion areas, showing a benefit of the cosmetic camouflage [21]. Group therapy with patients affected by vitiligo or persons who are accustomed to the disease is also effective in improvement of the QoL. This was shown to reduce the disease stigma [22].

Regarding younger age groups, the CDLQI score is lower in children from age 7–14 years, without impairment to the QoL. In adolescents between 15 and 17 years, CDLQI is significantly higher. There is no difference in scores among sexes. Facial lesions are the most disturbing for the patients and parents, followed by the lower limbs; the latter, however, shows no impairment to QoL [23]. Patients who have some parent with the disease have even lower scores, with mothers and best friends being relevant sources of emotional support [24]. Nevertheless, 40% of patients who underwent negative experiences in childhood, mainly provocations and bullying, present a reduction in QoL during their adult life [25].

30.6 QoL in Patients with Higher Phototypes

Patients with higher phototypes seem to present greater emotional and functional impairment and therefore, a worse QoL [26]. By observing the average DLQI found in several countries (Estonia: 4.7, UK: 4.8, Belgium: 4.9, Japan: 5.9, Germany: 7.0, Iran: 7.1–8.2, China: 8.4, India: 10.7, and Saudi Arabia: 14.7 and 17.1), the highest scores were associated to populations with higher skin phototypes [27]. However, patients from Tanzania obtained a DLQI score of 7.2, higher than the European population but lower than in countries as China, India, and Saudi Arabia [28]. This may have occurred due to the socioeconomic bias of the patients taking part in the study. As there are also religious and cultural biases in countries as India and the Middle East, more studies are required for a better assessment of the impact of phototypes in the QoL of vitiligo patients.

30.7 Conclusion

The chronic nature of vitiligo, the long-term treatment, the lack of a uniform and effective therapy, and the unpredictable course of the disease are demoralizing and discouraging factors for the patients. Many health professionals still consider vitiligo as a cosmetic health problem, failing to include in their assessment the psychological and sociological components which are closely linked to the illness, and therefore, underestimate the relevance of treatment for those patients.

Keeping in mind the maintenance of the quality of life can also have an influence on the choice of the treatment in the clinical routine and, consequently, on the patient's willingness to be treated. By employing the measures of the quality of life in the clinical practice ensures that the treatment is focused on the patient and not on his illness. Talking to the patients is necessary, asking how they feel about their condition, discussing the impact of vitiligo on their daily routine, and learning how to cope with it. An empathic approach is important, given the high psychological and social morbidity.

The first step therefore, regarding the improvement of the quality of life, is to establish a good relation between the doctor and the patient for motivation of the therapy, especially in unsuccessful phases.

References

1. Both H, Essink-Bot ML, Busschbach J, Nijsten T. Critical review of generic and dermatology-specific health-related quality of life instruments. J Invest Dermatol. 2007;127(12):2726–39.
2. Halioua B, Beumont MG, Lunel F. Quality of life in dermatology. Int J Dermatol. 2000;39(11):801–6.
3. McKenna SP, Doward LC. The needs-based approach to quality of life assessment. Value Health. 2004;7(S1):S1–3.
4. Finlay AY. Quality of life measurement in dermatology: a practical guide. Br J Dermatol. 1997;136(3):305–14.
5. Testa MA, Simonson DC. Assessment of quality-of-life outcomes. N Engl J Med. 1996;334(13):835–40.
6. Sampogna F, Raskovic D, Guerra L, Pedicelli C, Tabolli S, Leoni L, et al. Identification of categories at risk for high quality of life impairment in patients with vitiligo. Br J Dermatol. 2008;159(2):351–9.
7. Whitton ME, Pinart M, Batchelor J, Leonardi-Bee J, González U, Jiyad Z, et al. Interventions for vitiligo. Cochrane Database Syst Rev. 2015;(2):CD003263. doi:10.1002/14651858.CD003263.pub5.
8. Teovska-Mitrevska N, Eleftheriadou V, Guarneri F. Quality of life in vitiligo patients. Dermatol Ther. 2012;25(S1):S28–31.
9. Finlay AY, Khan GK. Dermatology Life Quality Index (DLQI) – a simple practical measure for routine clinical use. Clin Exp Dermatol. 1994;19(3):210–6.
10. Lewis-Jones MS, Finlay AY. The Children's Dermatology Life Quality Index (CDLQI): initial validation and practical use. Br J Dermatol. 1995;132(6):942–9.
11. Holme SA, Man I, Sharpe JL, Dykes PJ, Lewis-Jones MS, Finlay AY. The children's dermatology life quality index: validation of the cartoon version. Br J Dermatol. 2003;148(2):285–90.
12. Chren MM, Lasek RJ, Quinn LM, Mostow EN, Zyzanski SJ. Skindex, a quality-of-life measure for patients with skin disease: reliability, validity, and responsiveness. J Invest Dermatol. 1996;107(5):707–13.
13. Chren MM, Lasek RJ, Flocke SA, Zyzanski SJ. Improved discriminative and evaluative capability of a refined version of Skindex, a quality-of-life instrument for patients with skin diseases. Arch Dermatol. 1997;133(11):1433–40.
14. Chren MM, Lasek RJ, Sahay AP, Sands LP. Measurement properties of Skindex-16: a brief quality-of-life measure for patients with skin diseases. J Cutan Med Surg. 2001;5(2):105–10.
15. Lilly E, Lu PD, Borovicka JH, et al. Development and validation of a vitiligo-specific quality-of-life instrument (VitiQoL). J Am Acad Dermatol. 2013;69(1):e11–8.
16. Senol A, Yücelten AD, Ay P. Development of a quality of life scale for vitiligo. Dermatol. 2013;226(2):185–90.
17. Krishna GS, Ramam M, Mehta M, Sreenivas V, Sharma VK, Khandpur S. Vitiligo impact scale: an instrument to assess the psychosocial burden of vitiligo. Ind J Dermatol Venereol Leprol. 2013;79:205–10.

18. Gupta V, Sreenivas V, Mehta M, Khaitan BK, Ramam M. Measurement properties of the vitiligo impact scale-22 (VIS-22), a vitiligo-specific quality-of-life instrument. Br J Dermatol. 2014;171(5):1084–90.
19. Silverberg JI, Silverberg NB. Association between vitiligo extent and distribution and quality-of-life impairment. JAMA Dermatol. 2013;149(2):159–64.
20. Chan MF, Chua TL. The effectiveness of therapeutic interventions on quality of life for vitiligo patients: a systematic review. In J Nurs Pract. 2012;18(4):396–405.
21. Ongenae K, Dierckxsens L, Brochez L, van Geel N, Naeyaert JM. Quality of life and stigmatization profile in a cohort of vitiligo patients and effect of the use of camouflage. Dermatol. 2005;210(4):279–85.
22. Krüger C, Smythe JW, Spencer JD, Hasse S, Panske A, Chiuchiarelli G, et al. Significant immediate and long-term improvement in quality of life and disease coping in patients with vitiligo after group climatotherapy at the dead sea. Acta Derm Venereol. 2011;91(2):152–9.
23. Silverberg JI, Silverberg NB. Quality of life impairment in children and adolescents with vitiligo. Pediatr Dermatol. 2014;31(3):309–18.
24. Krüger C, Panske A, Schallreuter KU. Disease-related behavioral patterns and experiences affect quality of life in children and adolescents with vitiligo. Int J Dermatol. 2014;53(1):43–50.
25. Linthorst-Homan MW, de-Korte J, Grootenhuis MA, et al. Impact of childhood vitiligo on adult life. Br J Dermatol. 2008;159(4):915–20.
26. Linthorst-Homan MW, Spuls PI, de-Korte J, et al. The burden of vitiligo: patient characteristics associated with quality of life. J Am Acad Dermatol. 2009;61(3):411–20.
27. Karelson M, Silm H, Kingo K. Quality of life and emotional state in vitiligo in an Estonian sample: comparison with psoriasis and healthy controls. Acta Derm Venereol. 2013;93(4):446–50.
28. Kiprono S, Chaula B, Makwaya C, Naafs B, Masenga J, et al. Quality of life of patients with vitiligo attending the regional Dermatology Training Center in Northern Tanzania. Int J Dermatol. 2013;52(2):191–4.

Part IV
Other Management Options for Melasma and Vitiligo

Chapter 31
Photoprotection in Brown Skin

Vermén M. Verallo-Rowell

31.1 Introduction

Melasma is a hyperpigmentation that worsens with sun exposure; even with the use of high sun protection factor (SPF) broad-spectrum sunscreens alongside available therapies, it recurs repeatedly [1]. Most people with brown skin prefer a lighter skin color [2], use skin lightening products [3], and practice sun avoidance [4], yet melasma remains common among them [5]. In search for answers, the author embarked in 1999 on several studies working on the hypothesis that melasma may be a *subclinical* photosensitivity from *low-dose* photosensitizers (PS) reacting to *low-energy* indoor lights.

The first set of photopatch tests (PPT) to lamps of mixed spectral outputs but with dominant VL, UV, or NIR showed UVA, VL, and NIR *phototoxic* contact dermatitis (PTCD) with persistent pigmentation at UVA and VL – not with NIR – irradiated test sites. It was concluded that photoprotection must not only center against UVA and UVB but also against VL and IR. To this effect, the author published the first book incorporating all these relevant studies and results with the ultimate goal of making the populace, specifically the brown race, aware of these findings. A review on the publication was later published by Dr. H Lim [6].

Since PTCD is a nonspecific reaction, the author, in 2013, carried out LED – pure VL-PPTs. These elicited relevant crescendo and often delayed appearing reactions, leaving hyperpigmented irradiated test sites several months after the PPT; hence, a diagnosis of photoallergic contact dermatitis (PACD) was derived [7].

V.M. Verallo-Rowell
Department of Dermatology, Skin & Cancer Foundation, Inc,
Unit 1611 Medical Plaza Ortigas, San Miguel Avenue, Pasig City, Philippines
e-mail: vmvrmd@gmail.com

E.B. Handog, M.J. Enriquez-Macarayo (eds.), *Melasma and Vitiligo in Brown Skin*,
DOI 10.1007/978-81-322-3664-1_31

31.2 Melasma in Brown Skin: Photoprotection as Part of Therapy

Recent studies show that the most affected biological processes in melasma are lipid metabolism genes, such as peroxisome proliferator-activated receptor alpha (PPAR), arachidonate 15-lipoxygenase, PPAR gamma coactivator 1 alpha, and the Wnt inhibitory factor-1 which are downregulated [8]. These findings are supported by an impaired barrier function and solar elastosis in melasma lesional skin [9]. Downregulation occurs when a cell is overstimulated for a prolonged period of time, so expression of the receptor protein is decreased in order to protect the cell. In this process, a cell decreases the quantity of a cell component such as RNA or protein, in response to an external variable.

Our series of PPTs suggest that in individuals with melasma, the possible external variables are the subclinical photosensitivity, the low-dose PS from the environment and in personal products, and the low-energy indoor radiation that elicits the reaction. Also suggested is the need to perform photopatch tests to specifically identify both the PS and the eliciting radiation [7].

31.2.1 Photopatch Testing (PPT)

Unlike regular patch testing for straight contact allergy, PPT remains inaccessible and infrequently utilized. A survey in 2001 lists only 49 European centers performing a mean of 16 PPTs yearly. Cognizant of significant differences in methodology, the European Society for Photodermatology and the Society of Contact Dermatitis formed the Taskforce for Photopatch Testing which drew up the European consensus methodology [10]. PPT has mostly been done in Europe on individuals with skin phototypes I to III [11, 12]. Fewer PPT studies have been done on individuals with Phototypes II/III–V in the United States [13] and in similar groups in Latin America [14, 15]. Much fewer PPT studies originate from the brown-skinned populations across Asia, especially from tropical countries [16–18] where natural sunlight is strong all year long.

In 1999, the author started PPT in the Philippines, utilizing first the US guidelines then later, the European consensus. PPT (+) readings are interpreted as follows [19]:

Phototoxic is an immediate erythematous macule with well-defined borders that fades within 24–48 h postirradiation (decrescendo) that within a week becomes replaced by hyperpigmentation.

Photoallergic is when the erythematous macule increases in diameter and thickness, even itches, over a week or more (crescendo) and is replaced by hyperpigmentation as the papule subsides.

Thermal reaction to near infrared radiation (NIR) is immediate with slight to marked stinging and redness, and no pigmentation is seen up to 2 weeks of observation.

31.2.1.1 PPT Study 1 (2001) [20]

Verallo et al. used 67 photosensitizers from Chemotechnique, Sweden (24 fragrances, 13 plants, 22 North Americans) and eight cosmetic ingredients from Skin Sciences Laboratory, Inc. (SSLI), Pasig, Philippines in a cross-sectional study among 40 Filipino females who prefer to have lighter complexions, take measures to lessen sun exposure, and are of mixed heritage (mostly Malay, some Chinese) with skin phototypes IV and V, 20 subjects with melasma and a control group of 20 without melasma. Three test lamps were used, each one with a dominant spectrum: (a) VL400–760 nm, (b) UVA320–400 nm, and (c) NIR760–1500 and with a mix of much lower spectral outputs from other radiation types (Fig. 31.1).

Results were as follows: VL had the most number of (+) reactions that were reviewed and reported separately in 2008 [21]. All (+) reactions were of the phototoxic type and relevant, to make the diagnosis of VL-Phototoxic Contact Dermatitis, with persistent pigment at all (+) PPT sites. In the melasma group, 55 % ($N=11/20$) had 29 (+) PPT reactions to 11 fragrances, 11 North American, and seven plant photoallergens (PAs); no reactions were noted in the non-melasma group. This association was highly significant ($P=0.00$, two-tailed Fischer's exact test) such that compared to a (−) PPT, a (+) reaction predicted 12.67 times increased likelihood of having melasma ($P=0.05$; 1.402–114).

UVA irradiation had 10 (+) phototoxic type reactions with persistent pigment at (+) PPT sites. IR had 12 (+) phototoxic type reactions but showed no persistent pigmentation.

31.2.1.2 PPT Study 2 (2010) [22]

This consisted of a case series of 20 Filipinos with melasma and irregular melasma-like pigmentation, without dermatitis on their extensor arms and V-area of the neck. The same photosensitizers as in Study 1 were used, with a Birtcher lamp for PPT (Fig. 31.2).

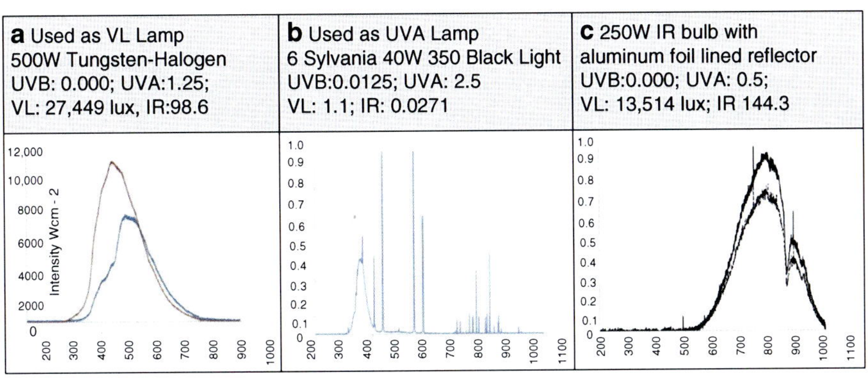

Fig. 31.1 Spectral signature and irradiance in mW/cm2 of three test lamps with mixed outputs used in PPT study 1 (**a**) VL lamp, (**b**) UVA tubes, and (**c**) IR bulb

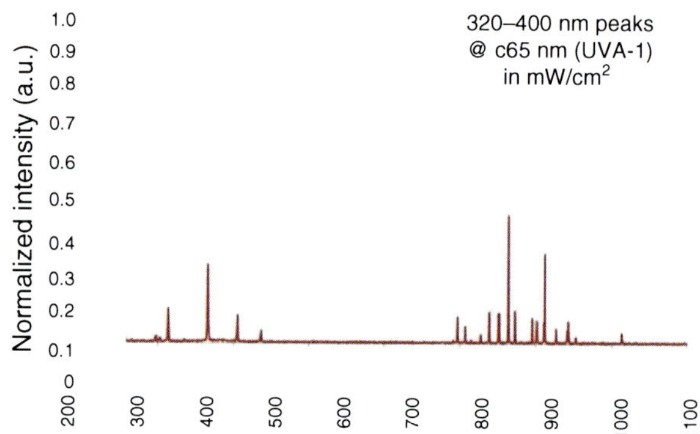

Fig. 31.2 Birtcher lamp: a 20 W mercury arc lamp with a barium silicate–nickel oxide filter

PPT using low-energy Birtcher or Wood's lamp has shown photoallergy [23] to musk ambrette [24] and to other men's perfumes [25].

In the case series (Fig. 31.2), many (+) decrescendo reactions to perfume (6/20, 30 %), plant (16/20, 80 %), Scandinavian series (11/20, 55 %), and SSLI sunscreen series (8/20, 40 %) were seen, all in concordance with persistent pigmentation at (+) test sites.

Diagnosis was UVA 1 – phototoxic contact dermatitis with pigment persistence at (+) PPT reaction sites.

For the first time, these PPTs showed (+) responses to VL and IR, not just to UV, the accepted action spectrum of most PS. These appeared to be phototoxic reactions (macular, non-spreading, and not pruritic). The persistent post-exposure hyperpigmentation clinically mimics post-inflammatory hyperpigmentation seen after most photosensitivity reactions in brown skin. Of relevance is that presently, it is now accepted that compact fluorescent lamps emit a mixed spectra of UV, VL, and IR [26, 27]. Despite the low radiation dosage emitted by these indoor lights, landmark papers have established the principle of "cumulative damage" referring to the repeated sub-erythemal radiation exposures that eventually result in erythema and lower the MED [28–30]. The next step was to find out if like UVA, the standard PPT test energy pure VL can also elicit PACD.

31.2.1.3 PPT Study 3 (2013–2015) [7]

This study used an LED lamp emitting pure VL (Fig. 31.3) for testing four patients with recalcitrant melasma and photosensitive hyperpigmentation even when using broad-spectrum sunscreens. Pure VL-PPT in four patients resulted in only a few (+) reactions of the crescendo type, with spreading borders, and pruritus lasting up to 2 weeks. These were interpreted as *photoallergic reactions*. The resulting pigmentation persisted for weeks to many months.

Figure 31.4a–f shows typical VL-PPT (+) reactions to p-Phenylenediamine in one of the patients. He had both allergic contact dermatitis and VL photoallergic contact dermatitis. Photoaggravated CD was ruled out because the (+) reactions lasted for at least 2 weeks and more.

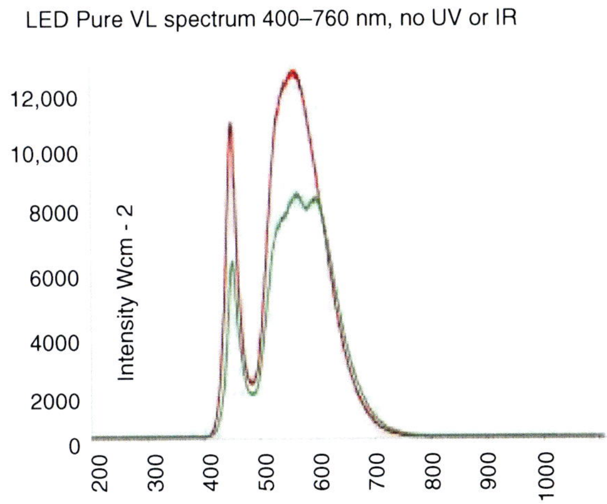

Fig. 31.3 LED pure VL spectrum 400–760 nm, no UV or IR, used in Study 3 VL-PPT

LED-VLirradiationVL–PPT					
Photo Aller-gen	Unirradiated				
	48 (1+)	72 (1+)	96 (1+)	Relevance, Dx	
Un-Irradiated			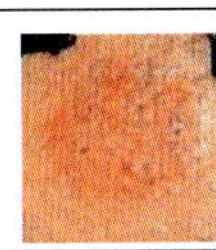	Palpable Ery-thema Novesicles	√Relevant Allergic Contact Dermatitis (ACD)
	Irradiated				
	24 (1+)	48 (2+)	72 (2+)	Relevance, Dx	
Irradiated				More Erythema More Palpable with tiny vesicles forming	√Relevant Photoallergic Contact dermatitis PACD or Photo Agg ravated ACD

Fig. 31.4 LED-VL-PPT to p-Phenylenediamine

A PPT done in 2007 used the UVA tubes (shown in Fig. 31.1b) and the PSs in PPT Studies 1 and 2. *Unirradiated* sites (Fig. 31.4a–c) had many (+) reactions: 10 of 13 plants, 8 of 21 Scandinavians, and 6 of 24 fragrance PSs. These results were interpreted as *angry back* or *excited skin* at *unirradiated* sites. UVA-*Irradiated* PSs were all (−) except for one fragrance PS (Fig. 31.4d–f). The minimal reaction at the *irradiated* sites was signed out as *photoinhibition*.

Persistence of a photo-distributed eruption led us to perform a follow-up PPT (2013) using a pure VL LED lamp and 64 PS: 55 from the American Contact Dermatitis Society (ACDS) 80-allergen series and nine sunscreen ingredients from SSLI. The same 64 PS served as unirradiated controls. While PPT to mixed energy lamps elicited *PTCD*, PPT using pure VL elicited *PACD* followed by clearance of the pigmentations on avoiding the PS, the eliciting lights, and with the use of daily sunscreens with protection factors to VL and IR (Fig. 31.5).

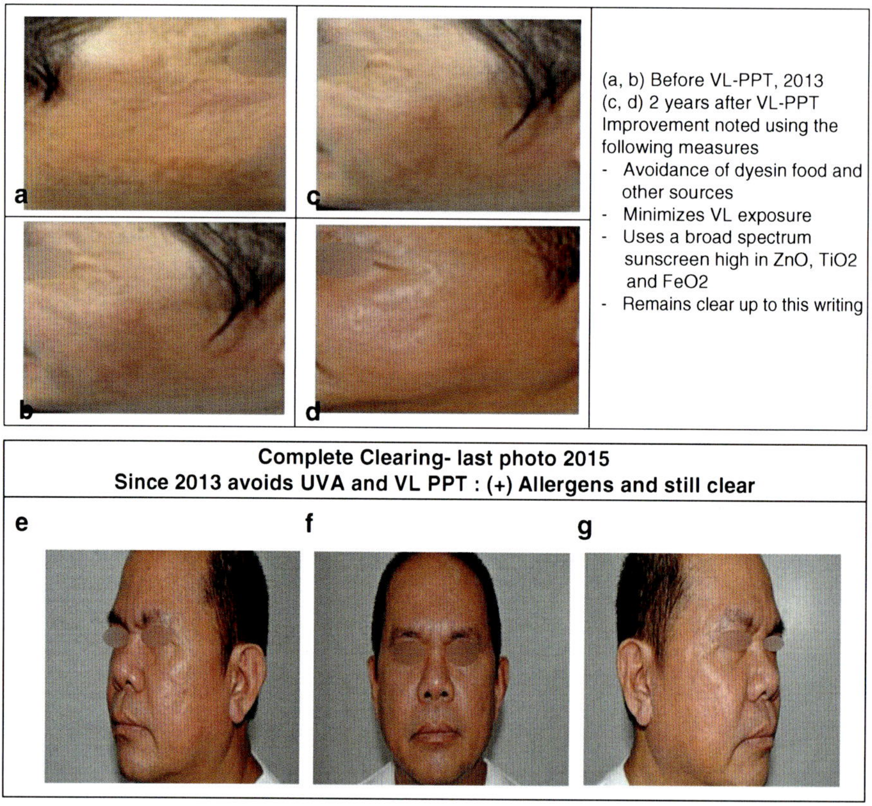

Fig. 31.5 Filipino male, 57 y/o, with recurrent melasma since the 1990s. VL-PPT done in 2013. 2013 Before VL-PPT (**a**) *right side* of the face, (**b**) *left side* of the face 2015 Same patient, after the 2013 VL-PPT and use of appropriate measures to control melasma (**c**, **g**) *right side* of the face, (**d**, **e**) *left side* of the face, (**f**) full front face

31.2.2 Pigmentation Induced by Radiation: In Normal Skin

Reaction to UVB starts with erythema followed by a protective tan from an increase in the number of melanocytes, new melanin production, and redistribution to keratinocytes. UVA-induced pigmentation is caused by neomelanogenesis and is brought about by immediate photooxidation of existing melanin/precursors/metabolites. The molecular and biologic changes of these UV-induced pigmentations are well studied, and current broad-spectrum sunscreens are protective [31, 32].

31.2.3 Beyond UV, VL, and IR Studies [33]

In electron spin resonance, activation of endogenous photosensitizers was shown in ex vivo skin explants exposed to filtered natural midday sunlight [34]. The reactive oxygen species (ROS) generated is calculated at 4% from UVB, 46% from

UVA, and 50 % from VL. In an in vitro study, exposure to VL resulted in increased ROS production, increased expression of MMP-1 and TNF-α mRNA in epidermal keratinocytes [35]. Aside from photooxidation, ex vivo hormonal/molecular and clinical studies showed that even in Caucasians, but more so in brown skin, VL also activates melanogenesis after multiple (preconditioning) VL exposures and even at lower doses of VL [36, 37]. These findings align well with the VL-induced skin pigmentation demonstrated in skin tests and in histopathology of Caucasian versus brown skin exposed to 400–800 nm artificial light at 80–480 mW/cm^2 [38–40].

Consistent with these findings is the persistent pigment at (+) PPT reaction sites of PS exposed to pure VL or to mixed spectrum indoor light sources. In the author's studies on normal subjects to determine the MED to VL for sunscreen protection factor, pigment likewise persisted for several weeks before fading away gradually [7].

Although indoor radiation fluences are low and minimized further by movements away from the light source, cumulative damage to chronic low-dose sub-erythemal radiation has long been shown in normal and in photosensitive skin [41, 42].

Studies of IR effects on photoaging which shows dyspigmentation are even more significant [43]. *Thus, in brown skin patients with melasma, whether known to be photosensitive or not, photoprotect against UV, VL, and IR* [44].

31.3 Vitiligo in Brown Skin: Photoprotection as Part of Therapy

Although normal skin of Fitzpatrick phototypes I to II and the vitiligo macule look similar to the naked eye, they differ at the molecular level. Normal phototypes I and II skin has melanin-producing melanosomes within melanocytes possessing dendritic connections to about 40 keratinocytes. Vitiliginous skin has few, if any, functioning melanocytes, melanosomes, or melanin; thus, cannot respond to sun exposure by increased production of sun-protective melanin [45].

Global studies have shown that chronic sun exposure and a history of sunburns contribute to the increasing incidence of melanomas and non-melanoma skin cancers (NMSC) in people with types I and II [46] skin and a similar, though smaller, increase in brown skin types III–V [47]. Clinicians are concerned about contradictory reports on the incidence of melanoma and NMSC in vitiligo patients prompting a recent paper on the subject [48]. Of the 1024 retrieved articles on melanoma and NMSC in vitiligo in this review, five were selected to assess best evidence.

A case-control questionnaire survey by Teulings, et al., (the Netherlands, mostly skin types II and III) on 1307 patients with vitiligo and their normal partners, found a threefold decreased probability of melanoma (odds ratio OR 0.32, 95 % CI 0.12–0.88) and NMSC (OR 0.28, 95 % CI 0.16–0.50) after adjusting for risk factors (>100 nevi and sunburn in childhood). Seven melanomas occurred in those with normal pigmented skin and two basal cell carcinomas (BCC) within vitiligo lesions. The questionnaires were answered by patients at their homes without the assistance of a trained physician; hence, accuracy of patient recall may be questionable [49].

The next four were cohort studies. In Paradisi et al.'s study, from a large reference center in Rome (no skin types given), 11 melanomas occurred in 10,040 vitiligo patients and 118 in the control group of 25,956 non-dermatological patients seen for vascular surgery (RR 0.24 95% CI 0.13–0.45). There were 37 NMSC in vitiligo patients, 509 in the control (RR 0.19 95% CI 0.14–0.17). This study had a large number of subjects and good internal validity, but there was an age distribution difference in the two groups [50].

Another relatively large prevalence study of Lindelof et al. from two Swedish hospitals (no skin type given) consisting of 1052 vitiligo patients found only one with melanoma and no SCC. The review authors calculated an absolute risk of developing melanoma at 0.001 (95% CI 0.0002–0.0054). This study did not elaborate on factors that could have influenced the outcome [51].

Schallreuter et al. reported on 136 Caucasians with vitiligo who were screened for NMSC. No melanomas, BCC, or SCC were seen. Despite a significant number of early childhood sunburns, there was no histologic evidence for sun-related damage and no increased risk for common photodermatoses [52].

Hexsel et al. screened 477 vitiligo patients for the occurrence of NMSC which resulted in a calculated absolute risk of 0.013 (95% CI 0.0058–0.0272). There was one basal cell carcinoma (BCC) and one squamous cell carcinoma (SCC) on vitiliginous skin, three BCCs and one SCC on normally pigmented skin [53].

While the above studies showed a decreased incidence of vitiligo skin cancers, in the largest cohort of 10,040 patients, Paradisi found that those who underwent phototherapy when compared with those who did not had a higher and statistically significant risk for skin cancers. The phototherapy group risk for melanoma was 7.54 (95% CI 1.99–28.56); for NMSC, it remained high at 4.7(95% CI 2.0–10.8). Anecdotal cases of SCC on exposed and non-exposed skin of vitiligo in brown skin, with or without phototherapy, also continue to be reported [54–59].

The authors of the Hammoud review [48] warn that since none of the studies described the extent of vitiligo nor included patients who died from melanoma or NMSC, risk underestimation is a possibility.

Racially, Hexsel's cohort of vitiligo patients were 42% Caucasian, 41% Brown (29% African-American, 6% Asian-Pacific Islander, 2% Hispanic, 2% Middle Eastern, 2% Native American) and 17% with unavailable racial designations. The small sample of 477 vitiligo patients was deemed not large enough to detect skin cancer in brown skin as only Caucasians had the six NMSC (four in vitiligo, two in normal pigmented skin). This was the only study on incidence rates comparing the vitiligo cohort with two general US populations. Their results suggest that there may be an increased or equal risk of NMSC in vitiligo patients, a finding that may run counter to the long-standing belief of decreased skin cancer risk in Caucasians with vitiligo. The authors caution that health care providers should not underestimate the risk of this common cancer in vitiligo patients [52]. Possible reasons for the negative association between melanoma and NMSC in individuals with vitiligo may be (1) patients with vitiligo probably have been told to protect their skin against the sun and (2) an over expression of the p53 tumor suppressor gene which can kill cells via a dual transcription-dependent and -independent function in the nucleus and at the mitochondria has been proposed to explain this low BCC and SCC risk.

In normal unstressed cells, p53 is a very unstable protein with a half-life from 5 to 30 min, present at very low cellular levels due to continuous degradation mediated by murine double minute 2 gene (MDM2) [60]. A study on phototypes III and IV brown-skinned Egyptians with vitiligo (all with outdoor occupations) demonstrated significantly strong expression of p53 and MDM2 proteins versus controls in normally pigmented and depigmented lesions at the epidermis, skin adnexa, and blood vessels and higher in those with generalized than with localized vitiligo. The rapid induction of high p53 protein levels may prevent inappropriate propagation of cells carrying potentially mutagenic damaged DNA such as after sun exposure [61].

Since skin cancer risk is still in flux, it is best to recommend sun avoidance and daily use of broad-spectrum sunscreen as recommended in the Vitiligo Treatment Guidelines for brown [62] or white [63] skin.

31.4 Sunscreens: Testing, Labeling, Efficacy, Safety

The US FDA 2011 Final Rule [64] is mostly aligned with the European cosmetic, toiletry and perfumery industry's COLIPA. These, the ISO, and regulatory bodies in the UK, Australia, New Zealand, Japan, and the ASEAN's harmonized rule differ in accepted ingredients, concentrations, and classification as over-the-counter (OTC), therapeutic drugs, or cosmetic. However, all agree that the ideal profile is uniform protection across the entire UVB/UVA range (290–400 nm) similar to that provided by sun avoidance [65].

Sun protection factor (SPF) protects in the UVB 290–320 nm range and is obtained through an in vivo methodology on at least ten subjects using a xenon arc solar simulator with specific guidelines on test light specifications, usage, and testing methodology. Labeling should include uses, warnings, directions, non- or water resistance, and the listing first of active and then inactive ingredients in alphabetical order.

UVA protection factor (UVA-PF) testing utilizes the more ethical in vitro method that is well on its way to being harmonized among the various regulatory bodies. The US FDA mandates determination of the critical wavelength (CW) at which 90 % of the UVB and UVA is absorbed, by a pre-irradiated test sunscreen film applied at 0.75 mg/cm^2 on a polymethyl methacrylate (PMMA) plate. CW greater than 370 nm is the simple pass/fail criterion for UVA-PF, which if 1/3 the SPF of 50+, the sunscreen can be claimed to be broad spectrum.

For the author, it is but proper that all sunscreen products must undergo aforementioned tests to prove the veracity of their claims of "broad spectrum" and protection factor number; efficacy cannot be based on ingredients alone. These details on how sunscreens are evaluated for efficacy and safety are mentioned here because in some countries, there are products that claim "broad-spectrum sunscreen" and protection factor numbers based just on ingredients in the formulation and unsupported by the above testings. An informal survey by the residents of the Skin and Cancer Foundation, Inc. (Philippines) showed several such "sunscreens" sold as cheaper products to the public and even to dermatologists who dispense them with labels as claimed by the sellers who often are compounding pharmacists or chemists without a photo laboratory to support their label claims.

VL and IR protection factors: There are as yet no standard guidelines on determination of protection factor (PF) determinations for VL and IR but some companies are already responding to this need [66, 67]. At our center, these VL and IR-PPT studies were initiated and the need to photoprotect against VL and IR was substantiated. We have adapted the methodology of UVA for in vivo PF testing but used the LED-VL for VL and un-/cooled IR for IR. These studies achieved up to 6 VL-PF and 6 IR-PF.

31.5 Conclusion

Guide to photoprotection in vitiligo and melasma of brown skin:

Photoprotect exposed skin from sun and indoor lights by avoidance practices
Always seek the shade and cover up with clothing
Use umbrellas and other shading devices
Minimize overhead lights and the use of wide-screen monitors
Use indirect or shaded lamps with double envelope CFLs and LED bulbs
Avoid heat while cooking or using hair dryer, in the sauna, and other heat-emitting surfaces

Apply daily a reputable broad-spectrum sunscreen
With a 50+ SPF, protection factors for UVA and as regulatory bodies and/or manufacturers respond to our needs
Watch out for and use sunscreens with VL and IR protection factors [68]
With high amounts of low but not nano-sized inorganic particles (zinc oxide and titanium dioxide) [69]
Also with high (more than 3.2 %) iron oxide content in colored foundations or moisturizers [70]

Add potent oral/dietary antioxidants such as
Niacinamide, turmeric, and green tea and always remember the polyphenols in fruits, vegetables, wine, tea, and caffeine [71]
The more anti-inflammatory medium-chain saturated coconut oil [72]
Omega-3 polyunsaturated fatty acids that are especially high in fish oils and nonsteroidal anti-inflammatory chemicals in food substances [73]

Photopatch test
If despite using the above sunscreens, melasma persists or continually recurs, and especially if it is darkened by lasers and IR or other heat devices
Photopatch not just to UVA but also VL or cooled IR
Based on the patient's energy exposures at work, play, or home and
Choose PS based on a thorough history of lifestyle, occupation, habits, and environment
With the results of the PPT, *Avoid* the Test *radiation* and the Relevant (+) *PS* that elicit the (+) reactions

Acknowledgment Maria Turner, MD and Percival Almoro, PhD for their invaluable scientific and technical help from conceptualizing to data gathering and interpretation and to manuscript writing and to all the residents of the Skin and Cancer Foundation, Inc. who from 1999 to 2015 rotated through and helped in doing and documenting the photo patch testing of these patients with the staff of the VSRC Photodermatology Laboratory.

References

1. Sardesai VR, Kolte JN, Srinivas BN. A clinical study of melasma and a comparison of the therapeutic effect of certain currently available topical modalities for its treatment. Indian J Dermatol. 2013;58(3):239.
2. Jablonski NG. Aspiring to lightness in living color: the biological and social meaning of skin color. Berkley and Los Angeles: University of California Press; 2012. p. 169–81.
3. Anekwe O. The global phenomenon of skin bleaching: a crisis in public health. Part I. Practice sun avoidance Jan 29, 2014. Voices in Bioethics. Online J Columb Univ. http://voicesinbioethics.org. Accessed 15 Sep 2015.
4. David EJR. Neocolonialism and contemporary oppression. In: Brown skin, white minds: Filipino-/American postcolonial psychology. North Carolina, USA: Information Age Publishing, Inc. 2013:37–49.
5. Sarkar R, Arora P, Garg VK, et al. Melasma update. Indian Dermatol Online J. 2014;5:426–35.
6. Lim H. Book review of Verallo-Rowell skin in the tropics: sunscreens and hyperpigmentations 2001 Anvil Publishing. J Am Acad Dermatol. 2004;50(2):329–30.
7. Verallo-Rowell VM, Turner MC, Almoro P. Review article: UVA, visible light, infrared photopatch testing of recalcitrant melasma: Philippines, 1999 to 2015. Manuscript under editorial review.
8. Kang HY, Suzuki I, Lee DJ, Ha J, Reiniche P, Aubert J, et al. Transcriptional profiling shows altered expression of want pathway-and lipid metabolism-related genes as well as melanogenesis related genes in melasma. J Invest Dermatol. 2011;131(8):1692–700.
9. Lee A-Y. An updated review of melasma pathogenesis. Dermatol Sin. 2014;32(4):233–9.
10. Bruynzeel DP, Ferguson J, Andersen K, Gonçalo M, English J, Goossens A, et al.; European Taskforce for Photopatch Testing. Photopatch testing: a consensus methodology for Europe. J Eur Acad Dermatol Venereol. 2004;18(6):679–82.
11. Sarkany RPE. Photopatch testing comes of age. Br J Dermatol. 2012;166(5):912–3.
12. The European Multicentre Photopatch Test Study (EMCPPTS) Task Force. A European multicentre photopatch test study. Br J Dermatol. 2012;166(5):1002–9.
13. Scalf LA, Davis MDP, Rohlinger AL, Connolly SM. Photopatch testing of 182 patients: a 6-year experience at the Mayo Clinic. Dermatitis. 2009;20(1):44–52.
14. Suzuki HS, Hammerschmidt M, Kakizaki P, Mukai MM. Phototype comparison between original Caucasian and Asian skin types. Cosmet Dermatol. 2011;3(3):193–6.
15. Valbuena Mesa MC, Hoyos Jiménez EV. Photopatch testing in Bogota (Colombia) 2011-2013. Contact Dermatitis. 2015;74(1):11–7.
16. Chuah SY, Leow YH, Goon AT, Theng CT, Chong WS. Photopatch testing in Asians: a 5- year experience in Singapore. Photodermatol Photoimmunol Photomed. 2013;29(3):116–20.
17. Sindhvananda J, Chunhasewee C, Panichluechachai N. The significance of photopatch testing and photoallergic contact dermatitis: 10-years experience. J Health Sci. 2014;23(4):753–61.
18. Tzu-Lin H, Chia-Yu C. Chronic actinic dermatitis: a clinical study of 15 cases in northern Taiwan. Dermatol Sin. 2014;32(2):82.
19. Goncalo M. Phototoxic and photoallergic reactions. In: Johansen JD, Frosch PJ, Lepoittevin JP, editors. Contact dermatitis. Springer: Berlin Heidelberg. 2011. (IV). p. 361–76.
20. Verallo-Rowell VM, Villacarlos-Bautista D, Oropeza NS, Gepaya-Resurreccion B, Mendoza SA. Indoor lights used in the photopatch testing of a case-controlled group of melasma and

non-melasma patients. In: Verallo-Rowell VM, ed. Skin in the Tropics Sunscreens and Hyperpigmentations. Anvil Publishing Inc. Philippines. 2001:102–31.
21. Verallo-Rowell VM, Pua JM, Bautista D. Visible light photopatch testing of common photocontactants in female Filipino adults with and without melasma; a cross-sectional study. J Drugs Dermatol. 2008;7(2):149–56.
22. Verallo-Rowell VM. Photopatch testing of melasma with hyperpigmentation at classic photosensitivity sites: a sequential case report series on twenty patients from the Philippines. Dermatitis. 2010;21(6):350–1.
23. Jillson OF. Wood's light an incredibly important diagnostic tool. Cutis. 1981;28:620–6.
24. Cronin E. Photosensitivity to musk ambrette. Contact Dermatitis. 1984;11:88–92.
25. Raugi GJ, Storrs FJ, Larsen WG. Photoallergic contact dermatitis to men's perfumes. Contact Dermatitis. 1979;5:251–60.
26. Mironova T, Hadjiargyrou M, Simon M, Rafailovich MH. The effects of UV emission from compact fluorescent light exposure on human dermal fibroblasts and keratinocytes in vitro. Photochem Photobiol. 2012;88(6):1497–506.
27. Fenton L, Ferguson J, Ibbotoson S, Moseley H. Energy saving lamps and their impact on photosensitive and normal individuals. Br J Dermatol. 2013;169(4):910–5.
28. Kaidbey KH, Kligman AM. Cumulative effects from repeated exposures to ultraviolet radiation. J Invest Dermatol. 1981;76:352–5.
29. Parrish JA, Zaynoun S, Anderson RR. Cumulative effects of repeated sub threshold doses of ultraviolet radiation. J Invest Dermatol. 1981;76:356–8.
30. Lavker RM, Gerberick GF, Veres D, Kaidbey KH. Cumulative effects from repeated exposures to suberythemal doses of UVB and UVA in human skin. J Am Acad Dermatol. 1995;32:53–62.
31. Handel AC, Miot LDB, Miot HA. Melasma: a clinical and epidemiological review. An Bras Dermatol. 2014;89(5):771–82.
32. Nouveau S, Agarwal D, Kohli M, Bernerd F, Misra N, Nayak CS. Skin hyperpigmentation in Indian population: insights and best practice. Ind J Dermatol. 2016:61(5):487–95.
33. Dupont E, Gomez J, Bilodeau D. Beyond UV radiation; a skin under challenge. Int J Cosmet Sci. 2013;35:1–9.
34. Zastrow L, Groth N, Klein F, Kockott D, Lademann J, Ferrero L. The missing link–light-induced (280–1600 nm) free radical formation in human skin. Skin Pharmacol Physiol. 2009;22:31–44.
35. Zastrow L, Groth N, Klein F, Knockout D, Lademann J, Ferrero L. UV, visible and infrared light: which wavelengths produce oxidative stress in human skin? Hautarzt. 2009;60:310–7.
36. Liebel F, Kaur S, Ruvolo E, Kollias N, Southall MD. Irradation of skin with visible light induces reactive oxygen species and matrix-degrading enzymes. J Invest Dermatol. 2012;32:1901–7.
37. Rhandawa M, Seo I, Liebel F, Southall MD, Kolas N, Ruyolo E. Visible light induces melanogenesis in human skin through a photo adaptive response. PLoS One. 2015;10(6): e0130949.
38. Duteil L, Cardot-Leccia N, Quille-Roussel C, Maubert Y, Harmelin Y, Boukari F, et al. Differences in visible light induced pigmentation according to wavelengths: a clinical and histological study in comparison with UVB exposure. Pigment Cell Melanoma Res. 2014;27:822–6.
39. Mahmoud BH, Hexsel CL, Hamzavi IH, Lim W. Review. Effects of visible light on the skin. Photochem Photobiol. 2008;84(2):450–62.
40. Sklar LR, Almutawa F, Lim HW, Hamzavi I. Effects of ultraviolet radiation, visible light, and infrared radiation on erythema and pigmentation: a review. Photochem Photobiol Sci. 2013;12(1):54–64.
41. Fenton L, Moseley H. Review article. UV emissions from low energy artificial light sources. Photodermatol Photoimmunol Photomed. 2014;30:153–9.
42. Korgavkar K, Xiong M, Weinstock MA. Compact fluorescent lamps and risk of skin cancer. J Cutan Med Surg. 2013;17(50):308–12.

43. Soyun C, Lee MJ, Chung JH. Infrared plus visible light and heat from natural sunlight participate in the expression of MMP and type I procollagen as well as infiltration of inflammatory cell in human skin in vivo. J Dermatol Sci. 2008;50(2):123–33.
44. Grether-Beck S, Marini A, Jaenicke T, Krutmann J. Review article: photoprotection of human skin beyond ultraviolet radiation. Photodermatol Photoimmunol Photomed. 2014;30:167–74.
45. Kumar S, Singh A, Prasad RR. Role of histopathology in vitiligo. J Indian Med Assoc. 2011;109(9):657–65.
46. Young AR, Wikonal NM. The chronic effects of ultraviolet radiation on the skin photocarcinogenesis. In: Lim HW, Honigsmann H, Hawk JLM, editors. Photodermatology. NewYork: Informa Healthcare USA; 2007. p. 107–17.
47. Gloster Jr HM, Neal K. Skin cancer in skin of color. J Am Acad Dermatol. 2006;55:741–64.
48. Hammoud SM, Kruis RWJ, Sigurdsson V. Prediction of the occurrence of melanoma and non-melanoma skin cancer in patients with vitiligo. Acta Derm Venereol. 2016;96:106–7.
49. Teulings HE, Overkamp M, Ceylan E, Nieuweboer-Krobotova L, Bos JD, Nijsten T, et al. Decreased risk of melanoma and nonmelanoma skin cancer in patients with vitiligo: a survey among 1307 patients and their partners. Br J Dermatol. 2013;168:162–71.
50. Paradisi A, Taboli S, Didona B, Sobrino L, Russo N, Abeni D. Markedly reduced incidence of melanoma and non-melanoma skin cancer in a nonconcurrent cohort of 10,040 patients with vitiligo. J Am Acad Dermatol. 2014;71:1110–6.
51. Lindelöf B, Hedblad MA, Sigurgeirsson B. On the association between vitiligo and malignant melanoma. Acta Derm Venereol. 1998;78:483–4.
52. Schallreuter KU, Tobin DJ, Panske A. Decreased photodamage and low incidence of non-melanoma skin cancer in 136 sun-exposed Caucasian patients with vitiligo. Dermatology. 2002;204:194–201.
53. Hexsel CL, Eide MJ, Johnson CC, Krajenta R, Jacobsen G, Hamzavi I, Lim HW. Incidence of nonmelanoma skin cancer in a cohort of patients with vitiligo. J Am Acad Dermatol. 2009;60:929–33.
54. Gangopadhyay A, Das JK, Agarwal AK. Squamous cell carcinoma in a patient with vitiligo of photo-covered skin. Indian J Dermatol. 2014;59(2):193–4.
55. Dhawan AK, Verma P, Singal A, Sharma S. Squamous cell carcinoma complicating vitiligo in an Indian man. J Cutan Aesthet Surg. 2012;5(1):36–7.
56. Park HS, Lee YS, Chun DK. Squamous cell carcinoma in vitiligo lesion after long-term PUVA therapy. J Eur Acad Dermatol Venereol. 2003;17:578–80.
57. Seo SL, Kim IH. Squamous cell carcinoma in a patient with generalized vitiligo. J Am Acad Dermatol. 2001;45(S):S227–9.
58. Akimoto S, Suzuki Y, Ishikawa O. Multiple actinic keratoses and squamous cell carcinomas on the sun-exposed areas of widespread vitiligo. Br J Dermatol. 2000;142:824–5.
59. Takeda H, Mitsuhashi Y, Kondo S. Multiple squamous cell carcinomas in situ in vitiligo lesions after long-term PUVA therapy. J Am Acad Dermatol. 1998;38:268–70.
60. Moll UM, Petrenko O. The MDM2-p53 interaction. Mol Cancer Res. 2003;1(14):1001–8.
61. Bakry OA, Hammam MA, Abdel Wahed MM. Immnohistochemical detection of P53 and Mdm2 in vitiligo. Indian Dermatol Online J. 2012;3(3):171–6.
62. Antoniou C, Katsambas A. Guidelines for the treatment of vitiligo. Drugs. 1992; 43(4):490–8.
63. Gawkrodger DJ, Ormerod AD, Shaw L, Mauri-Sole I, Whiten ME, Watts MJ, et al. Guidelines for the diagnosis and management of vitiligo. Br J Dermatol. 2008;159(5):1051–76.
64. Wang SQ, Lim HW. Current status of the sunscreen regulation in the United States: 2011 Food and Drug Administration's final rule on labelling and effectiveness testing. J Am Acad Dermatol. 2011;65:863–9.
65. Osterwalder U, Sohn M, Herzog B. Global state of sunscreens review article. Photodermatol Photoimmunol Photomed. 2014;30:62–80.
66. Bissonnette R, Nigen S, Bolduc C, Mery S, Nocera T. Protection afforded by sunscreens containing inorganic sunscreening agents against blue light sensitivity induced by aminolevulinic acid. Dermatol Surg. 2008;34(11):1469–76.

67. Schalka S, Addor FASA, Agelune CM, Pereira VMC. Sunscreen protection against visible light: a new proposal for evaluation. Surg Cosmet Dermatol. 2012;3(4):45–52.
68. Castanedo-Cazares JP, Hernandez-Blanco D, Carlos-Ortega B, Fuentes-Ahumada C, Torres-Alvarez B. Near-visible light and UV photoprotection in the treatment of melasma: a double blind randomized trial. Photodermatol Photoimmunol Photomed. 2014;39(1):35–42.
69. Boukari F, Jourdan E, Fontas E, Montaudie H, Castela E, Lacour JP, Passerine T. Prevention of melasma relapses with sunscreen combining protection against UV and short wavelengths of visible light: a prospective randomised comparative trial. J Am Acad Dermatol. 2015;72(1):189–90.
70. Bissonnette R. Update on sunscreens. Skin Therapy Lett. 2008;13(6):5–7.
71. Chen AC, Damian DL, Halliday GM. Review article. Oral and systemic photoprotection. Photodermatol Photoimmunol Photomed. 2014;30:102–11.
72. Verallo-Rowell VM. The skinny on saturated fat … it can be good for you. Rx: Coconuts! The Perfect Health Nut. Anvil, Philippines. 2005:39–52.
73. Pilkington SM, Gibbs NK, Friedmann PS, Rhodes LE. Nutritional abrogation of photoimmunosuppression: in vivo investigations. Photodermatol Photoimmunol Photomed. 2014;30:112–27.

Chapter 32
Camouflage for Brown Skin with Melasma or Vitiligo

Rashmi Sarkar, Sumit Sethi, and Narendra Gokhale

32.1 Introduction

External appearance plays an important role in personality development and influencing social interactions. Imperfections on the face can lead to poor body image and decrease in self-confidence. Camouflage techniques can be useful to conceal congenital or acquired lesions in patients who have failed to achieve satisfactory results with skin treatments. Camouflage makeup can normalize the appearance of the skin and improve the quality of life [1, 2].

32.2 Indications for Camouflage Makeup

There are various therapeutic indications for camouflage makeup. Though the best results are seen with pigmentary alterations, raised lesions and even scars can also be camouflaged. Pigmentary disorders requiring camouflaging include vitiligo,

R. Sarkar (✉)
Department of Dermatology and Venereology, Maulana Azad Medical College and Associated Hospitals, New Delhi 110 002, India
e-mail: rashmisarkar@gmail.com

S. Sethi, MBBS, MD, DNB
Genesis Centre of Dermatology, Janakpuri, New Delhi 110 002, India
e-mail: sethi1587@gmail.com

N. Gokhale
Dr. Narendra Gokhale's Skin Clinic,
101, Morya Arcade, 1/2 – Old Palasia, Near Palasia Thana, Indore, Madhya Pradesh 452001, India
e-mail: docngokhale@gmail.com

E.B. Handog, M.J. Enriquez-Macarayo (eds.), *Melasma and Vitiligo in Brown Skin*,
DOI 10.1007/978-81-322-3664-1_32

chloasma, solar lentigo, nevi, lentigines, post-inflammatory hypopigmentation or hyperpigmentation, café au lait spots, dark circles of the eyes, and tattoos [1–3].

32.3 Camouflaging of Pigmentary Disorders

Pigmentary disorders are camouflaged by applying an opaque cosmetic that hides the underlying skin hues or by applying shades of complementary colors. Patches with decreased or increased pigmented compared to the surrounding skin can be hidden by camouflaging with foundations with an appropriate amount of tint [1, 2].

32.4 Camouflage in Vitiligo

Patients with vitiligo feel stigmatized as they face discrimination from society. They suffer from poor body image and low self-respect, which leads to profound social and psychological effects. Most of the treatment options for vitiligo need a long time to produce good desirable results, and camouflage therapy becomes indispensable for those patients, especially when the neck, face, and hands are affected [4, 5].

32.5 Classification of Camouflage in Vitiligo

Temporary and permanent options are available for camouflaging in vitiligo. Foundation-based cosmetic camouflages, liquid dyes, and self-tanning products are included in temporary camouflage. Micropigmentation/medical tattooing helps in achieving permanent camouflage in vitiligo [4, 5].

32.5.1 Permanent Camouflage/Tattoo

Permanent camouflage in vitiligo is achieved with a cosmetic tattoo. The pigments used in the inks of tattoos and permanent makeup are made up of inert materials and classified as color additives and cosmetics. They are insoluble in most organic solvents and water. The practice of tattooing is not controlled by the Food and Drug Administration (FDA); however, the pigments used for tattooing are subject to FDA regulation. None of the pigments are approved for implantation or injection and most are not even approved for skin contact.

Permanent makeup is waterproof, time saving, hassle-free, and always fresh and permanent. People with physical difficulty in applying regular, temporary makeup or with allergies to conventional cosmetics choose this procedure. The color cannot be washed off, as specialized techniques are used to implant the pigment into the dermal layer. When only small areas of the face are involved such as the perioral area and the dorsal hands, very pleasing results are obtained. It is easy to treat the dark phenotypes than lighter ones. Perfect matching of the color of the tattoo with the surrounding skin for a good cosmetic result is highly dependent on the doctor's/technician's skill. Performance of the procedure in sensitive areas such as the lips and eyelids is best done under local anesthesia. Periodic maintenance every 2–5 years is usually required since the color of the tattoo naturally fades over time. To prevent the risk of transmitting infectious diseases, tattooing should be performed using sterile technique under universal precautions. Tattooing has been reported to cause allergic, photoallergic, foreign body, and granulomatous reactions [4–6]. Misapplication, migration, and fanning of pigment are the most frequent complications, leading to patient dissatisfaction.

32.5.2 *Temporary Camouflage*

32.5.2.1 Liquid Dyes

Indigo carmine, potassium permanganate, and henna pastes were commonly used to camouflage vitiligo. An amber-like, natural shade is afforded by these dyes. A single layer provides a lighter shade and an additional layer gives a darker color. A disadvantage however is the difficulty to find a suitable color match for patients. Also, in areas associated with friction on movement such as the neckline and cuffs, there is a tendency for the temporary camouflage to be rubbed off [4, 5].

32.5.2.2 Foundation-Based Cosmetic Camouflage

The visual impact of vitiligo can be reduced by the uniform application of selected opaque cosmetics with light-reflecting ingredients. Camouflage products provide an excellent coverage and natural appearance by forming an opaque cover over the white patches in vitiligo [1, 2, 4, 5].

32.5.2.3 Self-Tanning Products

Dihydroxyacetone (DHA) is used as a self-tanning product. It is a sugar that binds with the amino acids tryptophan and histidine present in the stratum corneum layer, forming brown chromophores known as melanoidins. These melanoidins change color from yellow to brown, giving the skin a tanned effect. DHA (3–5 %) is neither greasy nor dirty and easy to apply. The pigmentation appears a few hours later (Fig. 32.1a, b), and repeated application is done until the desired effect is obtained.

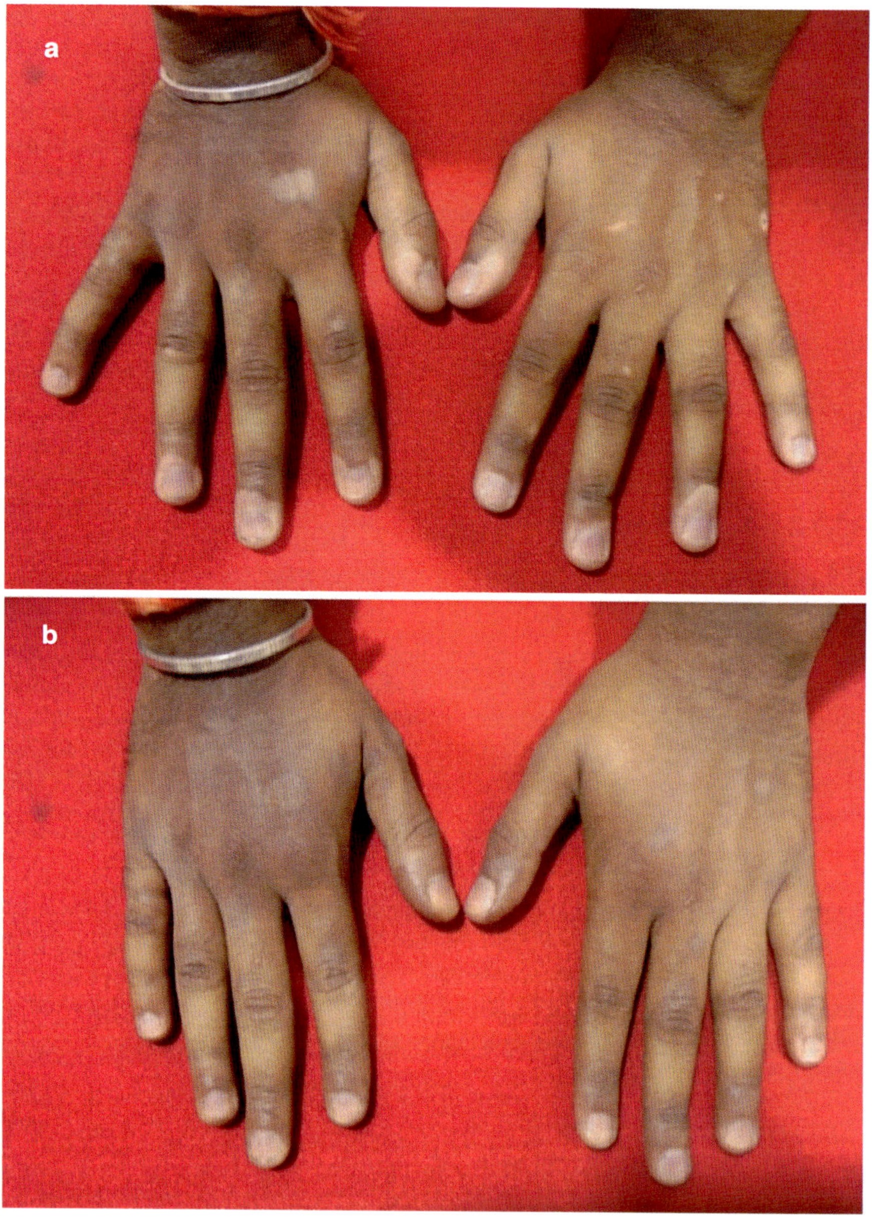

Fig. 32.1 Vitiligo on the hands (**a**), camouflaged with application of dihydroxyacetone (**b**)

Frequent applications of DHA are required to maintain desired effect as the normal epidermal turnover exfoliates the epidermis. The staining usually lasts up to 3–5 days. DHA binds only with the stratum corneum layer, and thus the intensity of the tan correlates with the compactness and thickness of the horny layer. Old, mottled hyperkeratotic, or rougher skin takes up an uneven finish. Lighter skin requires a lower concentration of DHA cream than subjects with dark skin. The advantage of DHA is its high substantivity and water resistance, avoiding discoloration of cloth on staining. Its innate sun protection properties however have little practical application due to its low SPF which decreases after application with each passing day. Obtaining a proper color match is difficult as blending with the surrounding skin is tricky [4, 5].

After the formulation becomes 6–9 months old, it starts to impart a greenish color to the skin; thus, product storage requires special care.

DHA is an economical, effective, and safe therapeutic option for patients with recalcitrant vitiligo. It is advantageous over camouflage cream involving the hands and feet as the cover creams are just waterproof and not rub proof [4, 5, 7].

DHA is applied every alternate night on perfectly dry skin. The lesions are cleaned with water and scales are gently removed with a towel, prior to application. Using a cotton bud, a finger, or a paintbrush, a thin layer of the cream is applied with circular movements to obtain a homogeneous result. Application on the mucosa and areas near the forehead hairline and eyebrows should be avoided. The areas which take to self-tanners quite well such as the face and neck should have sparing application. In case the hairs are short, the application of the product should be behind the ears. Nails and hair may take color, whereas mucous membranes do not. In order to avoid staining, the fingers should be cleaned immediately after application. Contact with textiles is avoided for the first 30 min, and no water contact is allowed over the next 2 h. Bathing, swimming, or any activity that will lead to sweating must be avoided for 1 h; no belts, brassieres, and shoes should be worn for 1 h, if the products have been used on the body. During periods with high UV exposure, sun protection is recommended with potent sunscreens of a high UVA and UVB protection factor [7, 8].

32.6 Camouflage in Melasma

Dyspigmentation of the face caused by melasma is a cosmetic challenge, and camouflage cosmetics are an important part of treating the melasma patient. Not only do they provide additional photoprotection, but they also restore the patient's self-confidence while dermatologic treatment is under way. The difficulty lies in blending the various brown tones associated with the condition. Topical prescription medications intended to lighten the darkened skin usually take a minimum of 3 months to produce clinically acceptable results, necessitating the need for camouflage techniques in the interim. It is very difficult to completely eliminate the uneven pigmentation, especially in hypermelanotic disorders accompanied by melanophages in the dermis such as dermal and mixed melasma. In such patients camouflaging uneven pigmentation can be achieved with corrective cosmetics such as Dermablend®, Covermark®, or Dermacolor®. These cosmetics provide broad-spectrum sunscreen activity along with good coverage. They are especially useful in hyperpigmented conditions in which sunlight plays an aggravating and perpetuating role [9].

Most sunscreen products are colorless and get absorbed directly into the skin, leaving no trace. Tinted sunscreen combines the benefits of sun protection with camouflage. Self-tanning lotions that have sunscreen properties and so-called "invisible color" lotions for children are sometimes also described as tinted. Tinted sunscreen products are manufactured by including ultraviolet A (UVA) and ultraviolet B (UVB) protection in makeup foundations.

32.7 Principles of Camouflaging Pigmentation Defects

There are three basic techniques for camouflaging skin defects.

Concealing is hiding discoloration by completely covering them with makeup. Concealers are creamy products, different from regular foundation in being more thick and opaque, and are available in a variety of colors to match the natural shade of the skin.

Color correcting is neutralizing red, blue, or yellow tones to more natural tones of complementary color. Skin color is contributed by underlying tones including hemoglobin producing red, keratin/degenerated elastin producing yellow, and melanin producing brown tone. Application of a complementary green foundation can help to camouflage a red pigmentation defect, yielding a brown tone, easily covered with a conventional facial foundation. Brown tones also result when yellow skin tones are blended with complementary purple-colored foundations. Thicker skin possesses more yellow tones, while thinner skin appears red. For these reasons, only one shade is insufficient to mimic the natural skin tone.

Contouring is creating the illusion of highlights and shadows to disguise the irregular facial surface. It creates dimension by using shadow and light (darker areas recede, while lighter areas appear to come forward). A contour shadow is required which is about two shades darker than the concealer, and a highlighter which is about two shades lighter.

To meet different needs of each defect to be concealed, many formulations of camouflage cosmetics are designed. Makeup bases, facial foundations, lining colors, and rouges are the basic products required to create the desired skin color. Camouflage products contain fillers endowed with optical properties and are different from makeup products as they contain up to 25–50 % more pigment. They impart a normal, natural appearance by concealing skin discoloration. Camouflage cosmetics are designed to mask and cover a problem but must be mixed to match the patient's skin tone. A good cover cosmetic should be opaque, natural looking, greaseless, easy to apply, waterproof, 100 % fragrance-free, long lasting, applicable to all skin types, non-sensitizing, nonirritating, non-photosensitizing, and noncomedogenic. Sun protection can be an additional benefit. Depending on the requirement of the patient, different types of camouflage cosmetics are available which may provide partial and full concealment or just pigment blending.

Hue, intensity, and value are the three color coordinates to be kept in mind while selecting a suitable camouflage cosmetic. These will determine which form of makeup (e.g., paste, liquid, or mineral) is most suitable as well as proper application technique. The name of the pure color is denoted by hue, intensity determines the brightness (saturation) of the color, and value refers to the darkness or lightness of the color. Brown and pink are the common hues required in vitiligo patients of darker skin types [1–3, 9].

32.8 Types of Camouflage Cosmetics

Skin areas that are lighter than the natural skin color can be camouflaged with a darker brown cosmetic, while darker areas can be minimized by applying facial foundations of a lighter hue. Makeup bases and facial foundations are the primary cosmetics designed to camouflage underlying dyspigmentation. Facial foundations are available as soft or hard grease paints, pancake makeup, and liquid makeup.

32.8.1 Camouflage Procedure

The camouflage procedure includes application of a base cream followed by covering with a foundation suitable for each patient and finally drying up with a finishing powder. The best camouflage facial foundations to cover dyspigmentation are the creamy soft grease paints which can be applied to the back of the hand for warming and blending. They are the easiest to use since they exhibit a long playtime (i.e., time before the cosmetic dries), minimal application skill, excellent coverage, good blending characteristics, and adequate wear ability for most people.

32.8.1.1 Technique of Application

Match the correct camouflage color using normal skin closest (preferably adjacent) to the area to be camouflaged. The makeup color that "disappears" into the adjacent normal skin is the correct selection. Small amount of the makeup can be applied to the back of the hand for blending and then held up to the face to evaluate the color match. Blending makeup on the back of the hand also warms the product, allowing for easier mixing and application. Finally, the foundation color mix is dabbed from the central face outward to approximately 0.25 in. into the hairline and is blended beneath the chin and over the ears. To obtain a more natural appearance, feathering of cosmetic at the margins of application is necessary. Unpigmented, finely ground, talc-based powder is used to set the cosmetic once the makeup has dried. It helps to improve wearability, makes it waterproof, prevents smudging, and imparts a matte finish.

32.8.1.2 Color Matching

It is very difficult to match a color from different manufacturers because of the number of tints and shades that can be produced by combination of various colors and varying the amount of white in them. Ten to twelve shades are required to match black skin, but for white skin only 7–8 shades are required. If more than two shades are selected for color blending, the camouflage process becomes time-consuming and costly for the patient. Also, the final color is muddy.

In patients having pigmentation problem, the underlying dyspigmentation of the skin counts as one color. It is recommended to avoid mixing more than two cream foundation colors in a patient of melasma to achieve an attractive final color match. In vitiligo patients, the underlying color is red in dark skin and yellow in sallow skin. In case the color contrast is too prominent, an opaque surgical foundation with a high coverage to cover all underlying skin tones may be a better camouflage selection. After selecting the closest foundation match for the patient, blend in red for ruddy complexion and yellow for a sallow complexion. If the patient has mild melasma and does not require an opaque cosmetic, a traditional facial foundation can be used and applied in three consecutive layers, allowing 5 min of drying time after each application. If an acceptable color match is desired, the final blend should represent all facial tones. The patient must realize that after camouflage therapy, it will be obvious that he/she is wearing a cosmetic [1–3, 8].

A camouflage product requires thorough matching with the surrounding skin because unlike regular foundation, it is applied to only a part of the face. The cosmetic outcome should be documented with pictures before and after the application of cosmetic product. Camouflage products should be worn on as a needed basis and should be removed before sleeping. Oily cleansers are provided by most companies for removal, and subsequent cleansing with water and soap is also recommended [1–3, 8].

A high concentration of oils is present in camouflage cosmetics, which may, though rarely, cause comedone formation in predisposed individuals. The foundation should be use-tested by the patient to rule out comedogenicity. They are easy to apply, lightweight, and free from contact allergens. With fragrances and preservatives present in some brands, allergic reactions and dermatitis may rarely occur [9].

32.9 Camouflage Therapy and Quality of Life

Health-related quality of life (QOL) is a method used to measure social, physical, and psychological well-being, thereby evaluating the burden of disease on daily living. Psychological well-being is based on multiple factors, one of which is satisfaction with physical appearance. Significant psychological morbidity may result from the presence of visible skin lesions. Corrective cosmetics rapidly enhance QOL by improving skin appearance. They are reported to have high satisfaction rates and are well tolerated by patients with continued use [3].

Camouflage helps those patients who need adjustment to an altered self-image and also helps them to cope with altered appearance. The immediate visual effect of camouflage therapy helps patients to regain confidence and self-esteem. Without making any permanent alteration to the structure or function of the skin, it helps them return to normal social and economic activities, thus improving their quality of life [10].

32.10 Conclusion

Dyspigmentary cutaneous conditions can be psychologically devastating to men, women, and children, irrespective of skin group classification, race, or religion. People seeking skin camouflage have a great desire for their skin to appear normal. Camouflage therapy provides an immense benefit to these patients by helping them to cope with the psychological implications of facial disfigurement or blemishes.

Camouflage products provide a natural appearance with excellent coverage of the defect and thus are an ideal adjunct to other therapies for successful treatment of such skin conditions. They help to minimize stigmatization by helping to cover the visible signs of the disease, and the results are extremely gratifying for both patients and physicians. They are readily available, safe, and inexpensive.

References

1. Bouloc A. Camouflage techniques. In: Draelos ZD, editor. Cosmetic dermatology: products and procedures. 1st ed. Oxford: Wiley-Blackwell; 2010. p. 176–83.
2. Draelos ZD. Facial scarring and camouflaging. In: Draelos ZD, editor. Cosmetics and dermatological problems and solutions: a problem based approach. Thirdth ed. New York: Informa Healthcare; 2011. p. 47–51.
3. Antoniou C, Stefanaki C. Cosmetic camouflage. J Cosmet Dermatol. 2006;5:297–301.
4. Kaliyadan F, Kumar A. Camouflage for patients with vitiligo. Indian J Dermatol Venereol Leprol. 2012;78(1):8–15.
5. Sarveswari KN. Cosmetic camouflage in vitiligo. Indian J Dermatol. 2010;55(3):211–4.
6. De Cuyper C. Permanent makeup: indications and complications. Clin Dermatol. 2008;26(1):30–4.
7. Fesq H, Brockow K, Strom K, Mempel M, Ring J, Abeck D. Dihydroxyacetone in a new formulation–a powerful therapeutic option in vitiligo. Dermatology. 2001;203(3):241–3.
8. Jouary T, Pase DA. Camouflage. In: Picardo M, Taieb A, editors. Vitiligo. Berlin Heidelberg: SpringerVerlag; 2010. p. 423–9.
9. Draelos ZD. Camouflaging melasma dyspigmentation. Cosmet Dermatol. 2007;20:281–2.
10. Holme SA, Beattie PE, Fleming CJ. Cosmetic camouflage advice improves quality of life. Br J Dermatol. 2002;147(5):946–9.

Chapter 33
What's in the Pipeline for Melasma and Vitiligo

Nada Elbuluk and Pearl E. Grimes

33.1 Melasma

33.1.1 Overview

Melasma is a common acquired disorder of hyperpigmentation characterized by irregular light brown to dark brown patches of hyperpigmentation commonly affecting the face. The trunk and arms are also occasionally involved. Multiple studies have documented the negative impact of melasma on quality of life [1]. Moreover, new research has led to an increased understanding of the complex pathogenesis of this disorder [2]. Key etiologic factors include a genetic predisposition, solar damage, barrier abnormalities, and unique sensitivities to hormonal changes including pregnancy, oral contraceptives, and hormone replacement therapy. New technological and pharmacological advances have facilitated expansion of approaches for the prevention, diagnosis, and long-term management of this difficult and challenging chronic pigmentary disorder.

N. Elbuluk, MD, MSc
Dermatology, NYU School of Medicine, New York, NY, USA

P.E. Grimes, M.D. (✉)
Vitiligo & Pigmentation Institute of Southern California, Division of Dermatology, David Geffen School of Medicine, University of California,
5670 Wilshire Blvd. #650, Los Angeles, CA 90036, USA
e-mail: pegrimesmd@aol.com

E.B. Handog, M.J. Enriquez-Macarayo (eds.), *Melasma and Vitiligo in Brown Skin*,
DOI 10.1007/978-81-322-3664-1_33

33.1.2 Melasma Assessment

Polarized light photography, colorimeters, mexameters, and spectrophotometers are all helpful tools used to assess melasma [3]. New tools, such as in vivo reflectance confocal microscopy, have further enhanced the ability to evaluate melasma. This tool provides a noninvasive method to diagnose melasma and monitor treatment response as well as therapeutic side effects [4]. In several studies, it has been found to be more accurate than prior techniques for diagnosing and monitoring melasma by providing real-time high-resolution imaging of the skin with more precise information about the location and extent of pigment as well as other epidermal and dermal cellular components. It may also help predict the efficacy of melasma treatments through baseline and follow-up evaluations [5–7]. Dermoscopy has also recently been used to better characterize the features of melasma [8]. Future studies with the use of these technologies will provide greater insight into understanding features of melasma and its response to various treatment options.

33.1.3 Melasma and Photoprotection

Given the ability of wavelengths outside of the ultraviolet range to also induce pigmentary changes in the skin, recent studies are evaluating the appropriate photoprotection needed in patients with melasma. A study examining the effects of UVA1 and visible light found that both led to pigmentation in skin types IV–VI, with visible light inducing dark and sustained pigmentation [9]. A prospective randomized comparative trial examined the use of tinted and untinted ultraviolet (UV) sunscreen with iron oxide and found that melasma relapses in both groups were prevented through protecting against UV and short wavelengths of visible light [10]. Another study compared the use of UV broad-spectrum sunscreen to UV broad-spectrum sunscreen with iron oxide as a visible light-absorbing pigment, and the latter group also showed greater improvement of their melasma [11]. Continued understanding of the wavelengths of light which can trigger melasma may lead to future sunscreens with broader and improved photoprotection.

33.1.4 Therapeutic Interventions

33.1.4.1 Tranexamic Acid (TA)

Triple-combination creams (TCC), retinoids, and hydroquinone (HQ) remain a mainstay in the therapeutic armamentarium of melasma [12]. However, recent studies have shed light on newer therapies for melasma, which have been studied as monotherapies and in combination with older traditional treatments, to yield improved clinical efficacy (Table 33.1). Tranexamic acid, a plasmin inhibitor, known

Table 33.1 Melasma therapeutic interventions

Topicals	Chemical peels	Lasers and lights	Transdermal drug delivery modes
Retinoids	Glycolic acid	ND:Yag (QS and long pulsed)	Skin needling
Hydroquinone	Salicylic acid	QS ruby	Microneedling
Corticosteroids	Jessner's	QS alexandrite	Iontophoresis
Triple-combination cream	Mandelic acid	Non-ablative lasers[a]	Monopolar radiofrequency
Novel skin-lightening agents: Botanicals Vitamins Alternative	Trichloroacetic acid	Intense pulse light: Fractionated Pulse-in-pulse mode	
Tranexamic acid[b]	Retinol	Ablative lasers[a]	
Kojic acid		Variable pulsed light	
Azelaic acid		Pulsed dye laser	

[a]Includes fractional and non-fractional

[b]Also used in oral and injectable form

as an antifibrinolytic medication, is a newer melasma treatment which has been studied in an oral, topical, and injectable form [13]. TA specifically inhibits plasminogen activator from converting plasminogen, which resides in epidermal basal cells and keratinocytes, to plasmin [14]. UV exposure can induce the keratinocyte-plasminogen activator system resulting in melanogenesis. TA's inhibitory effects on melanogenesis include decreasing tyrosinase, TRP-1, and TRP-2 [15].

Studies have shown varied clinical benefits of TA. A double-blind, randomized, controlled, split-face clinical trial investigated topical TA 5 % compared to vehicle and found no significant difference in Melasma Area and Severity Index (MASI) score reduction on both sides, with TA also causing erythema [16]. Another study compared TA 3 % to HQ 3 % with dexamethasone 0.01 % in a double-blind, split-face trial and found that both decreased MASI scores, but there was no significant difference between the improvements in the two groups [17]. Topical liposomal tranexamic acid 5 % has been studied in comparison to HQ 4 % in a split-face trial in which both topicals were applied twice daily and both resulted in significantly reduced MASI scores [13].

Oral TA given as two pills, twice a day for 6 months in a Chinese study of 74 patients, resulted in nearly 64 % of the patients having a good to excellent response with no significant complications [18]. A larger study of oral TA, given as 250 mg twice daily for 3 months, found that patients who took the medication had a significant reduction in MASI [19]. Oral TA has also been studied in combination with topical TA. In one study, patients took oral TA (two tablets, three times daily) and used topical tranexamic acid twice daily for 8 weeks, and the subjects had decreased epidermal pigmentation and erythema, as well as a decrease in dermal melasma changes including vessel number and mast cell count [20].

TA has also been studied in a microinjection form and with microneedling. In a randomized, open-label study comparing these two treatment modalities, both were found to improve MASI scores with greater improvement in the microneedling group, which may have been due to deeper and more uniform delivery of the TA through the microchannels created by microneedling [21].

Side effects of TA can include nausea, diarrhea, orthostatic reactions, hypomenorrhea, and, rarely, skin reactions, acute renal cortical necrosis, and color vision disturbances [14, 18].

In the future, as further studies are done on TA, it may become a more commonly used treatment for those with melasma.

33.1.4.2 New Drug Delivery Vehicles

New vehicles for topical drug delivery are being investigated. Ethosomes® and Transferomes® have been studied in vitro for topical drug delivery of compounds such as linoleic acid which are used to treat disorders of hyperpigmentation [22]. By using these drug delivery carriers for topical medications, there may be increased skin penetration past the stratum corneum, which may lead to improved local and systemic delivery, as well as higher clinical efficacy.

New conjugates of traditional melasma medications may also be on the horizon. Treatments that typically cause skin irritability, such as salicylic acid (SA) and HQ, have been combined into new formulations which have higher lipophilicity, less aqueous solubility, and lower crystallinity than each medication separately [23]. These new conjugates may improve skin absorption and skin tolerance.

33.1.4.3 Novel Skin-Lightening Agents

Novel skin-lightening agents are also being developed, many of which have shown promising results. The number of studies done on these newer agents however is very limited, and therefore larger studies will be needed to truly determine their safety and efficacy. One of these agents, undecylenoyl phenylalanine, an antagonist to alpha-melanocyte-stimulating hormone and beta-adrenergic receptors, has been found to significantly lighten melasma with minimal side effects [24]. Given that hormones are thought to play a role in the pathogenesis of melasma, topical flutamide 1 %, an antiandrogenic agent previously used for hair loss, has been studied in an RCT and was found to be as effective as topical HQ 4 % in improving melasma by mexameter assessment and was superior to HQ when comparing MASI scores [25]. Cysteamine, an intrinsic antioxidant that protects against ionizing radiation and that can inhibit melanin synthesis, was used topically in melasma patients and in comparison to placebo was found to significantly reduce MASI scores at 2 and 4 months [26].

33.1.4.4 Alternative Topical Therapies

Natural ingredients have been gaining popularity in the treatment of pigmentary disorders including melasma. Topical lignin peroxidase, a purified active enzyme derived from the fermented fungus *Phanerochaete chrysosporium,* has been studied in a 9-week single-center, open-label, prospective study in 31 Chinese women and was found to improve melasma through decrease in skin pigmentation and improvement in skin luminance [27]. *Rumex occidentalis*, an Asian herb that inhibits tyrosinase activity and blocks melanin formation, was studied in a randomized double-blind placebo-controlled trial in which 45 subjects either received 3 % *R. occidentalis* cream or 4 % HQ cream, and both were found to be comparable in efficacy and safety [28]. Plant extracts containing catechins/polyphenols, which have inhibitory effects on tyrosinase, have resulted in a significant decrease in melanin levels when compared to placebo [29]. Another plant-derived ingredient, silymarin, derived from the milk thistle plant, contains silybin, a potent antioxidant with photoprotective properties and the ability to inhibit L-dopa oxidation activity of tyrosinase. When studied in 96 melasma patients, a significant improvement was seen in a dose-dependent manner along with prevention of UV-induced skin damage and no significant side effects [30]. Mulberry extract, which has flavonoids and antioxidant properties as well as tyrosinase inhibiting properties, was evaluated in a randomized, single-blind, placebo-controlled trial and was found to significantly improve MASI and quality of life scores [31]. Topical niacinamide (4 %), which has anti-inflammatory properties and can decrease melanosome transfer, has been studied against HQ 4 % in an 8-week, 27-subject study and was found to similarly improve pigmentation in melasma as HQ, but also had the added benefit of reducing mast cell infiltrate and solar elastosis [32].

Various skin-brightening ingredients are also being marketed into commercial products that are hydroquinone free. A topical cream with disodium glycerophosphate, L-leucine, phenylethyl resorcinol, and undecylenoyl phenylalanine was used to treat mild to moderate melasma twice daily for 12 weeks in 20 female patients and resulted in a significant reduction in melasma severity and appearance with high tolerability [33]. Methimazole, an antithyroid medication, was formulated into a 5 % topical cream and used once daily in two patients with HQ-resistant melasma and after 8 weeks led to significant melasma improvement with high tolerability and no significant side effects [34].

33.1.4.5 Chemical Peels, Lasers, and Lights

Various chemical peels, lasers, and lights continue to be studied as treatment modalities for improving melasma [35]. Chemical peels recently studied include glycolic acid (GA), salicylic acid (SA), Jessner's, mandelic acid (MA), and trichloroacetic acid (TCA) [36, 37]. Chemical peels have also been used in combination with topical creams.

Lasers and lights recently studied include Q-switched (QS), ablative, and non-ablative lasers that are fractional and non-fractional, long pulsed ND:Yag, intense pulsed light (IPL), copper bromide, and pulse dye lasers (PDL) [38–42]. Q-switched lasers, including ND:Yag, ruby, and alexandrite lasers, are continuing to be studied at various settings in different skin types with varied success rates [43, 44]. Although some laser and light treatments have caused improvement in melasma, other studies have found worsening rebound melasma, postinflammatory hyperpigmentation (PIH), and/or hypopigmentation.

Ablative and non-ablative lasers including CO_2 and Erbium Yag in fractional and non-fractional forms have also shown promise in melasma treatment particularly in targeting dermal melasma [45, 46]. The use of ablative lasers, however, has been more limited due to the increased risk of PIH and difficulty in maintaining long-term results [47].

A new type of IPL, called fractionated IPL, has recently been studied as a weekly treatment for melasma in Asian women and, when compared to biweekly conventional IPL, was found to result in decreased MASI scores with no melasma rebound [48]. Another new type of IPL uses a pulse-in-pulse mode, which releases multiple fractionated subpulses in one pulse width [49]. When compared to traditional IPL, both significantly decreased MASI scores, with the former being preferred by patients due to decreased discomfort during and after treatments. Another light treatment similar to IPL called variable pulsed light is also being investigated. Unlike IPL, it disperses energy as a few small, rapid microflashes instead of one flash of light. It offers the advantage of decreased pain and better absorption into select layers of the skin with decreased amounts of heat entering neighboring tissues [50].

Lasers targeting the vascular component of melasma are also garnering interest. Two recent studies examining the use of copper bromide laser which has wavelengths of 578 nm and 511 nm targeting vascular lesions and pigmentation, respectively, have found the laser to not be efficacious in treating melasma and when compared to Kligman's combination cream formula , the latter was found to be more effective [51, 52]. In contrast, another report of a woman treated with PDL and Kligman's formula found that the PDL treatment prevented recurrence of melasma in treated areas [2].

33.1.4.6 Laser Combination Treatments

Combination treatments for melasma continue to show promise in further improving melasma and helping those with refractory melasma. Traditional topical treatments are being studied in combination with other topical and procedural treatments and have been found to have various degrees of therapeutic efficacy.

QS ND:Yag 1064 nm laser has been studied in combination with several other treatments. When used with IPL, it has been found to be more effective, particularly for refractory melasma and then when each is used as a monotherapy [39, 53, 54]. When QS ND:Yag laser toning has been combined with vitamin C ultrasonic application, it has led to higher physician and patient assessments [55]. QS ND:Yag laser done after microdermabrasion and maintained with a topical regimen of tretinoin or vitamin C along with sunscreen has been shown to be efficacious in inducing melasma remission for up to 6 months with minimal risk and recovery time [56].

IPL and fractional erbium glass laser, each combined with TCC, have shown greater efficacy together than when each treatment is used alone [57, 58]. Another recent study found that patients treated with oral TA, IPL, and QS ND:Yag laser treatments compared to those who had the laser and light treatments without TA found that the patients in the former group had improved clinical efficacy without significant side effects [59]. This result was supported by another Korean study, which examined the use of oral TA in patients receiving low fluence (LF) 1064-nm QS ND:Yag and found that those in the combination group had overall greater clinical improvement than those who had the laser treatment alone [60].

33.1.4.7 Transdermal Drug Delivery: Needling, Iontophoresis, and Energy Devices

Additional treatments being investigated for melasma include modes of transdermal drug delivery including skin needling, microneedling, iontophoresis, and radiofrequency. Skin needling has been found to enhance the penetration of topical products, and in a study combining skin needling with a depigmenting serum (containing rucinol and sophora-alpha), the combination resulted in significant improvement of the melasma in comparison to the use of the serum alone [61]. Iontophoresis can increase drug penetration of a compound into the skin in a controlled fashion by applying current through the tissue [62]. Vitamin C iontophoresis has been used successfully in the treatment of melasma and when used in a nanosome formulation has even been found to have better clinical results than 70 % GA [63]. It has also shown efficacy in melasma treatment when followed by a home maintenance regimen consisting of MA [39].

Platelet-rich plasma (PRP) has recently been studied in a single patient who underwent three treatments and had regression of her melasma with greater than 80 % reduction in epidermal pigmentation [64]. The mechanism of action is not fully understood but may involve the effects of TGF-β1 on inhibition of melanin synthesis along with an increase in skin volume.

Energy devices, such as monopolar radiofrequency, have also been combined with transdermal drug delivery of a product containing kojic acid 1 % and were found to decrease MASI scores, average melanin, and erythema with no significant side effects [65].

33.2 Vitiligo

33.2.1 Overview

Vitiligo is a relatively common acquired, idiopathic pigmentary disorder characterized by one or more depigmented patches of the skin. The disorder can be cosmetically disfiguring and severely impacts quality of life. Patients with vitiligo often experience low self-esteem, depression, stigmatization, and isolation [66, 67]. The mechanisms involved in the destruction of melanocytes in vitiligo are complex and include genetic influences, self-destruction, oxidative stress, neural defects, and autoimmunity. Current research places autoimmune and oxidative stress at the forefront of mechanisms mediating the destruction of melanocytes in vitiligo.

33.2.2 Treatment Strategies

New approaches for vitiligo address stabilization of the disease as well as repigmentation. While no consensus is available on the concept of stabilization in vitiligo, the vitiligo disease activity (VIDA) score has been utilized in several publications. It is a 6-point scale in which the activity of the disease is evaluated based on the appearance of new vitiligo patches, or the enlargement of preexisting patches assessed during a period ranging from less than 6 weeks to 1 year [68]. New therapies for stabilization of the disease include minocycline, methotrexate, and narrowband UV phototherapy (NB-UVB) (Table 33.2). Emerging therapies for repigmentation include prostaglandin analogues, rituximab, afamelanotide, and JAK inhibitors.

33.2.2.1 Therapies for Stabilization

Minocycline

Minocycline is a broad-spectrum bacteriostatic antibiotic commonly prescribed for acne vulgaris. Studies document that it also has anti-inflammatory and immunomodulatory properties [69]. It inhibits cytokine production, free radical formation,

Table 33.2 Pipeline therapies for vitiligo

Stabilization	Repigmentation
Oral corticosteroids	Afamelanotide
NB-UVB phototherapy	Prostaglandin F2α analogues
Minocycline	Rituximab
Methotrexate	Alternative phototherapy
	JAK inhibitors
	Simvastatin

and apoptosis. Recently, minocycline was compared to oral minipulse dexamethasone therapy for stabilization of active vitiligo [70]. Twenty-five patients were treated with minocycline 100 mg daily for 6 months, and 25 patients received dexamethasone 2.5 mg on 2 consecutive days weekly. Both drugs were significantly effective for stabilization of vitiligo. Side effects were minimal in each group. This study expands our therapeutic options for stabilization of vitiligo.

Methotrexate

Methotrexate is an antimetabolite and competitively inhibits dihydrofolate reductase. It inhibits DNA, RNA, thymidylates, and protein synthesis. In addition, it inhibits T-cell activation and intracellular adhesion molecule expression by T cells. Methotrexate also downregulates B cells [71]. In a recent study of 42 patients, methotrexate was compared to oral minipulse corticosteroid therapy for stabilization of vitiligo. Half were treated with methotrexate 10 mg weekly and half with dexamethasone OMP 2.5 mg on two consecutive days weekly for 6 months. Both were equally effective in controlling vitiligo disease activity [72].

Narrowband UVB Phototherapy

Recent studies document the beneficial effects of NB-UVB phototherapy for stabilization of vitiligo. Forty-two patients were evaluated in a prospective comparative 3-month trial. Half were treated with NB-UVB twice weekly and the remainder with minocyclinc 100 mg daily. Stabilization occurred in 76 % of the NB-UVB group compared to 33 % of patients treated with minocycline. These findings suggest that NB-UVB phototherapy is indeed effective in stabilizing active vitiligo [73]. In addition, NB-UVB has been shown to be effective in reversing oxidative stress in patients with vitiligo. This may be essential for stabilization of the disease [74]. This investigation is one of the very first to document the stabilizing effects of NB-UVB in a comparative trial.

33.2.2.2 Therapies for Stabilization

Afamelanotide

Afamelanotide is a potent synthetic analogue of alpha-melanocyte-stimulating hormone. It stimulates melanogenesis and melanocyte proliferation. When compared to α-MSH, afamelanotide exerts prolonged physiologic effects with stronger binding affinity to the melanocortin receptor (MC1R). Several studies have demonstrated defects in the melanocortin system in vitiligo patients [75, 76]. These defects include low physiologic plasma α-melanocyte-stimulating hormone, decreased α-MSH in lesional skin areas, and decreased expression of prohormone convertase.

Clinically, afamelanotide combined with NB-UVB was found to be significantly superior to NB-UVB monotherapy in a randomized multicenter study involving 55 patients with non-segmental vitiligo [76, 77]. Patients were treated for 6 months and observed 6 months thereafter. Twenty-eight patients were treated with afamelanotide and 27 with NB-UVB alone. The time to onset of repigmentation with combination group was significantly lessened, especially on the face and upper extremities, and more evident in skin types IV–VI. Moreover, there was significantly greater repigmentation in the combination group versus NB-UVB monotherapy. Notable side effects from combination treatment versus monotherapy were nausea, fatigue, and hyperpigmentation. Overall, the drug was well tolerated. However, the optimum dosage, administration frequency, and further side effects need to be determined.

Prostaglandin Analogues

Prostaglandin E2 (PGE2) is a novel and potentially beneficial treatment for localized stable vitiligo. PGE2 controls the proliferation of melanocytes through stimulant and immunomodulatory effects. In a consecutive series, repigmentation occurred in 40 of 56 patients with stable vitiligo treated with translucent PGE2 0.25 mg [78]. The patients applied the PGE2 gel twice daily for 6 months. The mean onset of repigmentation was 2 months. The response was excellent in 22 of 40 patients, with complete repigmentation observed in eight patients. The patients with disease duration of 6 months showed the most significant response. Repigmentation occurred the earliest on the face and scalp.

Bimatoprost, a synthetic prostamide (prostaglandin-ethanolamine) F2α analogue, is associated with hyperpigmentation of periocular skin caused by increased melanogenesis [79]. In a study by Narang et al. with ten patients, three had 100 % repigmentation, three had 75–99 %, and one had 50–75 %. The best responses were observed on the face [80]. A recent study documented efficacy of bimatoprost in 18 patients with non-facial vitiligo [81].

Latanoprost, also a prostaglandin F2α analogue, has also been evaluated for repigmentation of vitiligo in 22 patients. It was superior to placebo and has comparable efficacy of NB-UVB in achieving repigmentation of vitiliginous lesions [82].

Alternative Phototherapy

Natural sunlight emits a spectrum of accessible UV radiation, including sufficient amounts of NB-UVB beneficial for vitiligo. However, it also emits nontherapeutic wavelengths increasing the erythrogenic response. A topical cream was subsequently developed which filtered nontherapeutic radiation for solar exposure with a bias for 311 nm, allowing NB-UVB to pass through for treatment [83].

In a double-blind placebo-controlled study, 15 vitiligo patients exposed themselves to natural sunlight thrice weekly following the use of the selectively permeable topical cream allowing exposure to NB-UVB [84]. This was compared against a placebo sunscreen with SPF4. Only acrofacial vitiligo was treated. UV exposure was determined by an MED chart and measurement of solar ultraviolet light using a UV radiometer. Mean repigmentation at 12 weeks was 49 % for the topical cream and 3 % for the placebo group. Additional studies are warranted.

Rituximab

Rituximab is a chimeric monoclonal antibody against the protein CD20, primarily expressed on the surface of B cells. B cells are responsible for antibody formation. Rituximab destroys B cells and is used to treat diseases characterized by increased numbers of B cells or B-cell dysfunction. Anti-melanocyte antibodies have been shown to mediate the destruction of melanocytes in vitiligo [67, 85]. A 6-month pilot study was conducted in five vitiligo patients with active disease. They received intravenous rituximab 1 g in a single dose and were followed for 6 months. After 6 months, three of five patients showed marked repigmentation. One had slight improvement and the remaining patients showed no change. This repigmentation was correlated with biopsy findings of an increased number of melanocytes, decreased lymphoid infiltration, and decreased melanocyte apoptotic markers (Bcl-2, Apaf-1, caspase-9). As expected, circulating CD20 lymphocytes were decreased; however, melanocyte-specific antibodies and immunoglobulin levels showed no difference [86].

JAK Inhibitors

Tofacitinib is a JAK 1/3 inhibitor approved to treat severe rheumatoid arthritis. Tofacitinib inhibits the production of IL-17 and proliferation of CD4 cells. In addition, it inhibits γ-interferon signal transduction [87]. Current studies suggest that interferon γ-induced expression of the chemokine CXCL 10 mediates depigmentation in vitiligo [88, 89].

Recently a vitiligo patient was treated with oral tofacitinib citrate at a dose of 5 mg every other day. After 3 weeks, the dose was increased to 5 mg daily. At 2 months, partial repigmentation of the face and upper extremities was evident, and after 5 months, there was significant repigmentation of the forehead and hands. The patient experienced no adverse events related to the drug [90]. This case elicited much interest given its mechanism of action and the recent advances in our understanding of the pathogenesis of vitiligo. Proof of concept and clinical trials are indeed warranted to further assess the impact of JAK inhibitors in patients with vitiligo.

Simvastatin

Simvastatin, a HMG-CoA reductase inhibitor, is a widely used cholesterol-lowering medication which has also been documented to have significant anti-inflammatory properties. Such effects include scavenging free radical formation and increasing the production of TL10 and TGF-beta. Simvastatin also decreases TNF alpha, IL-6 and IL-2 production. It is an inhibitor of interferon-γ-induced STAT 1 activation [91, 92].

Recent studies have reported that the interferon-γ-induced chemokine CXCL 10 is critical for the progression and maintenance of depigmentation in vitiligo [93]. In a recent study of a mouse model of vitiligo, simvastatin prevented and reversed depigmentation [94]. It reduced the number of infiltrating autoreactive CD8+T cells in vitiligo. Treatment of melanocyte-specific CD8+T cells in vitro with simvastatin decreased proliferation and IFN-γ production. These findings strongly suggest simvastatin should be tested in clinical trials for vitiligo.

33.3 Summary

Melasma and vitiligo are indeed therapeutically challenging diseases. Recent advances in our knowledge of the pathomechanisms of both disorders will significantly impact the flow of new drugs and new approaches for the treatment of these psychologically devastating disorders of pigmentation.

References

1. Yalamanchili R, Shastry V, Betkerur J. Clinico-epidemiological study and quality of life assessment in melasma. Indian J Dermatol. 2015;60:519.
2. Passeron T. Melasma pathogenesis and influencing factors – an overview of the latest research. J Eur Acad Dermatol Venereol. 2013;27(S1):5–6.
3. Molinar VE, Taylor SC, Pandya AG. What's new in objective assessment and treatment of facial hyperpigmentation? Dermatol Clin. 2014;32:123–35.
4. Ardigo M, Cameli N, Berardesca E, Gonzalez S. Characterization and evaluation of pigment distribution and response to therapy in melasma using in vivo reflectance confocal microscopy: a preliminary study. J Eur Acad Dermatol Venereol. 2010;24:1296–303.
5. Kang HY, Bahadoran P. Application of in vivo reflectance confocal microscopy in melasma classification. J Am Acad Dermatol. 2012;67:157–8.
6. Costa MC, Eljaiek HV, Abraham LS, Azulay-Abulafia L, Ardigo M. In vivo reflectance confocal microscopy in a typical case of melasma. An Bras Dermatol. 2012;87:782–4.
7. Funasaka Y, Mayumi N, Asayama S, Takayama R, Kosaka M, Kato T, Kawana S. In vivo reflectance confocal microscopy for skin imaging in melasma. J Nippon Med Sch. 2013;80:172–3.
8. Li Y, Liu J, Sun QN. Characteristic dermoscopic features of melasma. Zhongguo Yi Xue Ke Xue Yuan Xue Bao. 2015;37:226–9.
9. Mahmoud BH, Ruvolo E, Hexsel CL, Liu Y, Owen MR, Kollias N, et al. Impact of long-wavelength UVA and visible light on melanocompetent skin. J Invest Dermatol. 2010;130:2092–7.
10. Boukari F, Jourdan E, Fontas E, Montaudie H, Castela E, Lacour JP, Passeron T. Prevention of melasma relapses with sunscreen combining protection against UV and short wavelengths of visible light: a prospective randomized comparative trial. J Am Acad Dermatol. 2015;72:189–90e1.

11. Castanedo-Cazares JP, Hernandez-Blanco D, Carlos-Ortega B, Fuentes-Ahumada C, Torres-Alvarez B. Near-visible light and UV photoprotection in the treatment of melasma: a double-blind randomized trial. Photodermatol Photoimmunol Photomed. 2014;30:35–42.
12. Gong Z, Lai W, Zhao G, Wang X, Zheng M, Li L, et al. Efficacy and safety of fluocinolone acetonide, hydroquinone, and tretinoin cream in Chinese patients with melasma: a randomized, double-blind, placebo-controlled, multicenter, parallel-group study. Clin Drug Investig. 2015;35:385–95.
13. Banihashemi M, Zabolinejad N, Jaafari MR, Salehi M, Jabari A. Comparison of therapeutic effects of liposomal Tranexamic Acid and conventional Hydroquinone on melasma. J Cosmet Dermatol. 2015;14:174–7.
14. Bagherani N. The efficacy of tranexamic acid in the treatment of melasma. Dermatol Ther. 2015;28:265.
15. Kim MS, Bang SH, Kim JH, Shin HJ, Choi JH, Chang SE. Tranexamic acid diminishes laser-induced melanogenesis. Ann Dermatol. 2015;27:250–6.
16. Kanechorn N, Ayuthaya P, Niumphradit N, Manosroi A, Nakakes A. Topical 5% tranexamic acid for the treatment of melasma in Asians: a double-blind randomized controlled clinical trial. J Cosmet Laser Ther. 2012;14:150–4.
17. Ebrahimi B, Naeini FF. Topical tranexamic acid as a promising treatment for melasma. J Res Med Sci. 2014;19:753–7.
18. Wu S, Shi H, Wu H, Yan S, Guo J, Sun Y, Pan L. Treatment of melasma with oral administration of tranexamic acid. Aesthetic Plast Surg. 2012;36:964–70.
19. Monheit GD, Dreher F. Comparison of a skin-lightening cream targeting melanogenesis on multiple levels to triple combination cream for melasma. J Drugs Dermatol. 2013;12:270–4.
20. Na JI, Choi SY, Yang SH, Choi HR, Kang HY, Park KC. Effect of tranexamic acid on melasma: a clinical trial with histological evaluation. J Eur Acad Dermatol Venereol. 2013;27:1035–9.
21. Budamakuntla L, Loganathan E, Suresh DH, Shanmugam S, Suryanarayan S, Dongare A, et al. A randomized, open-label, comparative study of tranexamic acid microinjections and tranexamic acid with microneedling in patients with melasma. J Cutan Aesthet Surg. 2013;6:139–43.
22. Celia C, Cilurzo F, Trapasso E, Cosco D, Fresta M, Paolino D. Ethosomes(R) and transfersomes(R) containing linoleic acid: physicochemical and technological features of topical drug delivery carriers for the potential treatment of melasma disorders. Biomed Microdevices. 2012;14:119–30.
23. Hsieh PW, Aljuffali IA, Fang CL, Chang SH, Fang JY. Hydroquinone-salicylic acid conjugates as novel anti-melasma actives show superior skin targeting compared to the parent drugs. J Dermatol Sci. 2014;76:120–31.
24. Katoulis A, Alevizou A, Soura E, Mantas N, Bozi E, Gregoriou S, et al. A double-blind vehicle-controlled study of a preparation containing undecylenoyl phenylalanine 2% in the treatment of melasma in females. J Cosmet Dermatol. 2014;13(2):86–90.
25. Adalatkhah H, Sadeghi-Bazargani H. The first clinical experience on efficacy of topical flutamide on melasma compared with topical hydroquinone: a randomized clinical trial. Drug Des Devel Ther. 2015;9:4219–25.
26. Mansouri P, Farshi S, Hashemi Z, Kasraee B. Evaluation of the efficacy of cysteamine 5% cream in the treatment of epidermal melasma: a randomized double-blind placebo-controlled trial. Br J Dermatol. 2015;173:209–17.
27. Zhong SM, Sun N, Liu HX, Niu YQ, Wu Y. Reduction of facial pigmentation of melasma by topical lignin peroxidase: a novel fast-acting skin-lightening agent. Exp Ther Med. 2015;9:341–4.
28. Mendoza CG, Singzon IA, Handog EB. A randomized, double-blind, placebo-controlled clinical trial on the efficacy and safety of 3% Rumex occidentalis cream versus 4% hydroquinone cream in the treatment of melasma among Filipinos. Int J Dermatol. 2014;53:1412–6.
29. Khan BA, Akhtar N, Hussain I, Abbas KA, Rasul A. Whitening efficacy of plant extracts including Hippophae rhamnoides and Cassia fistula extracts on the skin of Asian patients with melasma. Postepy Dermatol Alergol. 2013;30:226–32.

30. Altaei T. The treatment of melasma by silymarin cream. BMC Dermatol. 2012;12:18.
31. Alvin G, Catambay N, Vergara A, Jamora MJ. A comparative study of the safety and efficacy of 75% mulberry (Morus alba) extract oil versus placebo as a topical treatment for melasma: a randomized, single-blind, placebo-controlled trial. J Drugs Dermatol. 2011;10:1025–31.
32. Navarrete-Solis J, Castanedo-Cazares JP, Torres-Alvarez B, Oros-Ovalle C, Fuentes-Ahumada C, Gonzalez FJ, et al. A double-blind, randomized clinical trial of niacinamide 4% versus hydroquinone 4% in the treatment of melasma. Dermatol Res Pract. 2011;2011:379173. doi:10.1155/2011/379173.33.
33. Gold MH, Biron J. Efficacy of a novel hydroquinone-free skin-brightening cream in patients with melasma. J Cosmet Dermatol. 2011;10:189–96.
34. Malek J, Chedraoui A, Nikolic D, Barouti N, Ghosn S, Abbas O. Successful treatment of hydroquinone-resistant melasma using topical methimazole. Dermatol Ther. 2013;26:69–72.
35. Bae MI, Park JM, Jeong KH, Lee MH, Shin MK. Effectiveness of low-fluence and short-pulse intense pulsed light in the treatment of melasma: a randomized study. J Cosmet Laser Ther. 2015;17:292–5.
36. Lee DB, Suh HS, Choi YS. A comparative study of low-fluence 1064-nm Q-switched Nd:YAG laser with or without chemical peeling using Jessner's solution in melasma patients. J Dermatolog Treat. 2014;25:523–8.
37. Puri N. Comparative study of 15% TCA peel versus 35% glycolic acid peel for the treatment of melasma. Indian Dermatol Online J. 2012;3:109–13.
38. Attwa E, Khater M, Assaf M, Haleem MA. Melasma treatment using an erbium:YAG laser: a clinical, immunohistochemical, and ultrastructural study. Int J Dermatol. 2015;54:235–44.
39. Cunha PR, Pinto CA, Mattos CB, Cabrini DP, Tolosa JL. New insight in the treatment of refractory melasma: Laser Q-switched Nd: YAG non-ablative fractionated followed by intense pulsed light. Dermatol Ther. 2015;28:296–9.
40. Kroon MW, Wind BS, Beek JF, Van Der Veen JP, Nieuweboer-Krobotova L, Bos JD, Wolkerstorfer A. Nonablative 1550-nm fractional laser therapy versus triple topical therapy for the treatment of melasma: a randomized controlled pilot study. J Am Acad Dermatol. 2011;64:516–23.
41. Choi CP, Yim SM, Seo SH, Ahn HH, Kye YC, Choi JE. Retrospective analysis of melasma treatment using a dual mode of low-fluence Q-switched and long-pulse Nd:YAG laser vs. low-fluence Q-switched Nd:YAG laser monotherapy. J Cosmet Laser Ther. 2015;17:2–8.
42. Ho SG, Yeung CK, Chan NP, Shek SY, Chan HH. A retrospective study of the management of Chinese melasma patients using a 1927 nm fractional thulium fiber laser. J Cosmet Laser Ther. 2013;15:200–6.
43. Fabi SG, Friedmann DP, Niwa Massaki AB, Goldman MP. A randomized, split-face clinical trial of low-fluence Q-switched neodymium-doped yttrium aluminum garnet (1,064 nm) laser versus low-fluence Q-switched alexandrite laser (755 nm) for the treatment of facial melasma. Lasers Surg Med. 2014;46:531–7.
44. Jang WS, Lee CK, Kim BJ, Kim MN. Efficacy of 694-nm Q-switched ruby fractional laser treatment of melasma in female Korean patients. Dermatol Surg. 2011;37:1133–40.
45. Jalaly NY, Valizadeh N, Barikbin B, Yousefi M. Low-power fractional CO_2 laser versus low-fluence Q-switch 1,064 nm Nd:YAG laser for treatment of melasma: a randomized, controlled, split-face study. Am J Clin Dermatol. 2014;15:357–63.
46. Neeley MR, Pearce FB, Collawn SS. Successful treatment of malar dermal melasma with a fractional ablative CO_2 laser in a patient with type V skin. J Cosmet Laser Ther. 2010;12:258–60.
47. Morais OO, Lemos EF, Sousa MC, Gomes CM, Costa IM, Paula CD. The use of ablative lasers in the treatment of facial melasma. An Bras Dermatol. 2013;88:238–42.
48. Yun WJ, Lee SM, Han JS, Lee SH, Chang SY, Haw S, et al. A prospective, split-face, randomized study of the efficacy and safety of a novel fractionated intense pulsed light treatment for melasma in Asians. J Cosmet Laser Ther. 2015;17:259–66.
49. Chung JY, Choi M, Lee JH, Cho S, Lee JH. Pulse in pulse intense pulsed light for melasma treatment: a pilot study. Dermatol Surg. 2014;40:162–8.

50. Augustyniak A, Erkiert-Polguj A, Rotsztejn H. Variable pulsed light treatment of melasma and post-inflammatory hyperpigmentation - a pilot study. J Cosmet Laser Ther. 2015;17:15–9.
51. Hammami Ghorbel H, Boukari F, Fontas E, Montaudie H, Bahadoran P, Lacour JP, Passeron T. Copper bromide laser vs triple-combination cream for the treatment of melasma: a randomized clinical trial. JAMA Dermatol. 2015;151:791–2.
52. Eimpunth S, Wanitphakdeedecha R, Triwongwaranat D, Varothai S, Manuskiatti W. Therapeutic outcome of melasma treatment by dual-wavelength (511 and 578 nm) laser in patients with skin phototypes III-V. Clin Exp Dermatol. 2014;39:292–7.
53. Vachiramon V, Sirithanabadeekul P, Sahawatwong S. Low-fluence Q-switched Nd: YAG 1064-nm laser and intense pulsed light for the treatment of melasma. J Eur Acad Dermatol Venereol. 2015;29:1339–46.
54. Yun WJ, Moon HR, Lee MW, Choi JH, Chang SE. Combination treatment of low-fluence 1,064-nm Q-switched Nd: YAG laser with novel intense pulse light in Korean melasma patients: a prospective, randomized, controlled trial. Dermatol Surg. 2014;40:842–50.
55. Lee MC, Chang CS, Huang YL, Chang SL, Chang CH, Lin YF, Hu S. Treatment of melasma with mixed parameters of 1,064-nm Q-switched Nd:YAG laser toning and an enhanced effect of ultrasonic application of vitamin C: a split-face study. Lasers Med Sci. 2015;30:159–63.
56. Kauvar AN. Successful treatment of melasma using a combination of microdermabrasion and Q-switched Nd:YAG lasers. Lasers Surg Med. 2012;44:117–24.
57. Tourlaki A, Galimberti MG, Pellacani G, Bencini PL. Combination of fractional erbium-glass laser and topical therapy in melasma resistant to triple-combination cream. J Dermatolog Treat. 2014;25:218–22.
58. Goldman MP, Gold MH, Palm MD, Colon LE, Preston N, Johnson LA, Gottschalk RW. Sequential treatment with triple combination cream and intense pulsed light is more efficacious than sequential treatment with an inactive (control) cream and intense pulsed light in patients with moderate to severe melasma. Dermatol Surg. 2011;37:224–33.
59. Cho HH, Choi M, Cho S, Lee JH. Role of oral tranexamic acid in melasma patients treated with IPL and low fluence QS Nd:YAG laser. J Dermatolog Treat. 2013;24:292–6.
60. Shin JU, Park J, Oh SH, Lee JH. Oral tranexamic acid enhances the efficacy of low-fluence 1064-nm quality-switched neodymium-doped yttrium aluminum garnet laser treatment for melasma in Koreans: a randomized, prospective trial. Dermatol Surg. 2013;39:435–42.
61. Fabbrocini G, De Vita V, Fardella N, Pastore F, Annunziata MC, Mauriello MC, et al. Skin needling to enhance depigmenting serum penetration in the treatment of melasma. Plast Surg Int. 2011;2011:158241. doi:10.1155/2011/158241.
62. Huh CH, Seo KI, Park JY, Lim JG, Eun HC, Park KC. A randomized, double-blind, placebo-controlled trial of vitamin C iontophoresis in melasma. Dermatology. 2003;206:316–20.
63. Sobhi RM, Sobhi AM. A single-blinded comparative study between the use of glycolic acid 70% peel and the use of topical nanosome vitamin C iontophoresis in the treatment of melasma. J Cosmet Dermatol. 2012;11:65–71.
64. Cayirli M, Caliskan E, Acikgoz G, Erbil AH, Erturk G. Regression of melasma with platelet-rich plasma treatment. Ann Dermatol. 2014;26:401–2.
65. Cameli N, Abril E, Mariano M, Berardesca E. Combined use of monopolar radiofrequency and transdermal drug delivery in the treatment of melasma. Dermatol Surg. 2014;40:748–55.
66. Grimes PE. Pathogenesis and treatment of vitiligo. In: Post TW, editor. Waltham: UpToDate. In Press.
67. Ezzedine K, Eleftheriadou V, Whitton M, Van Geel N. Vitiligo. Lancet. 2015;386:74–84.
68. Njoo MD, Das JD, Bos JD, Westerhof W. Association of the Koebner phenomenon with disease activity and therapeutic responsiveness in vitiligo vulgaris. Arch Dermatol. 1999;4:407–13.
69. Song X, Xu A, Pan W, Wallin B, Kivlin R, Lu S, et al. Minocycline protects melanocytes against H2O2-inducedcell death via JNK and p38 MAPK pathways. Int J Mol Med. 2008;22(1):9–16.

70. Singh A, Kanwar AJ, Parsad D, Mahajan R. Randomized controlled study to evaluate the effectiveness of dexamethasone oral minipulse therapy versus oral minocycline in patients with active vitiligo vulgaris. Indian J Dermatol Venereol Leprol. 2014;80:29–35.
71. Benedek TG. Methotrexate: from its introduction to non-oncologic therapeutics to anti-TNF. Clin Exp Rheumatol. 2010;28:53–8.
72. Singh H, Kumarin MS, Bains A, Parsad D. A randomized comparative study of oral corticosteroid minipulse and low-dose oral methotrexate in the treatment of unstable vitiligo. Dermatology. 2015;231:286–90.
73. Siadet AJ, Zeinali N, Iraji F, Naeini B, Nilforoushzadeh MA, Jamshidi K, et al. Narrowband ultraviolet B versus minocycline for unstable vitiligo. A prospective comparative trial. Dermatol Res Pract. 2014;2014:856–900.
74. Karsli N, Akcal C. Narrowband UVB for stabilization of vitiligo. J Int Med Res. 2014;42:799–805.
75. Graham A, Westerhof W, Thody AJ. The expression of α-MSH by melanocytes is reduced in vitiligo. Ann N Y Acad Sci. 1999;885(1):470–3.
76. Grimes PE, Hamzavi I, Lebwohl M, Ortonne JP, Lim HW. The efficacy of afamelanotide and narrowband UV-B phototherapy for repigmentation of vitiligo. JAMA Dermatol. 2013;149:68–73.
77. Lim HW, Grimes PE, Agbai O, Hamzavi I, Henderson M, Haddican M, et al. Afamelanotide and narrowband UVB phototherapy for the treatment of vitiligo: a randomized multicenter trial. JAMA Dermatol. 2015;151(1):42–50.
78. Kapoor R, Phiske MM, Jerajani HR. Evaluation of safety and efficacy of topical prostaglandin E2 in treatment of vitiligo. Br J Dermatol. 2009;160(4):861–3.
79. Kapur R, Osmanovic S, Toyran S, Edward DP. Bimatoprost-induced periocular skin hyperpigmentation: histopathological study. Arch Ophthalmol. 2005;123:1541–6.
80. Narang T. Topical bimatoprost may hold promise as a treatment for vitiligo. World Congr Dermatol Poster. 2011 May 24–29; Seoul.
81. Grimes PE. Efficacy and safety of bimatoprost for repigmentation of vitiligo. J Clin Dermatol. 2016. Submitted.
82. Anbar TS, El-Ammawi T, Abdel-Rahman AT, Hanna R. The effects of latanoprost on vitiligo: a preliminary comparative study. Int J Dermatol. 2014;29:1–7.
83. Mccoy J, Goren A, Lotti T. In vitro evaluation of a novel topical cream for vitiligo and psoriasis that selectively delivers NB-UVB therapy when exposed to sunlight. Dermatol Ther. 2014;27:117–20.
84. Goren A, Salafia A, Mccoy J, Keene S, Lotti T. Novel topical cream delivers safe and effective sunlight therapy for vitiligo by selectively filtering damaging ultraviolet radiation. Dermatol Ther. 2014;27(4):195–7.
85. Gilhar A, Zelickson B, Ulman Y, Etzioni A. In vivo destruction of melanocytes by the IgG fraction of serum from patients with vitiligo. J Invest Dermatol. 1995;105:683–6.
86. Ruiz-Arguelles A, Garcia-Carrasco M, Jimenez-Brito G, Sanchez-Sosa S, Perez-Romano B, Garces-Eisele J, et al. Treatment of vitiligo with a chimeric monoclonal antibody to CD20: a pilot study. Clin Exp Immunol. 2013;174:229–36.
87. Gooderham M. Small molecules. Skin Therapy Lett. 2013;18:7–14.
88. Harris JE, Harris TH, Weninger W, Wherry EJ, Hunter CA, Turka LA. A mouse model of vitiligo with focused epidermal depigmentation requires IFN –gamma for autoreactive CD8 (+) Tall accumulation in the skin. J Invest Dermatol. 2012;132:1869–76.
89. Richmond JM, Harris JE. Immunology and skin in health and disease. Cold Spring Harb Perspect Med. 2014;4(12):a015339.
90. Craiglow B, King BA. Tofacitinib citrate for the treatment of vitiligo. A pathogenesis-directed therapy. JAMA Dermatol. 2015;151:110–2.
91. Krysiak K, Gdula – Dymek A, Scieszka J, Okopie B. Anti-inflammatory and monocyte-suppressing effects of simvastatin in patients with impaired fasting glucose. Basic Clin Pharmacol Toxicol. 2011;108:131–7.

92. Feily A, Baktash A, Mohebbipour A. Potential advantages of simvastatin as a novel anti-vitiligo arsenal. Eur Rev Med Pharmacol Sci. 2013;17:1982–3.
93. Rashighi M, Agarwal P, Richmond JM, Harris TH, Dresser K, Su MW, et al. CXCL10 is critical for the progression and maintenance of depigmentation in a mouse model of vitiligo. Sci Transl Med. 2014;6(223):223ra23.
94. Agarwal P, Rashighi M, Essien KI, Richmond JM, Randall L, Pazoki-Toroudi H, Hunter CA, Harris JE. Simvastatin prevents and reverses depigmentation in a mouse model of vitiligo. J Invest Dermatol. 2015;135(4):1080–8.